What People Are Saying

"In this fascinating, instructive book, dancer-turned-training guru Tammy Wise guides the reader into the heart of the emotional body, and the healing power that lies within. Combining Taoist philosophy, energy medicine, physiology, and self-inquiry -- along with extensive experience helping clients attune mind and body -- Wise introduces BodyLogos, her powerful, original method for healing physical and emotional pain. "A gift is required of each of us," she teaches, in the process of becoming fully human beings. This is a clear road map to changing our stories by healing our pain, becoming conscious of how we move through space, where we're resistant and where we are free. If you truly care about claiming your gifts and moving through the world with more power and grace, this is the book you've been waiting for".

~ MARK MATOUSEK
AUTHOR of WHEN YOU'RE FALLING, DIVE: LESSONS IN THE ART OF LIVING

"An extraordinary book that combines physical conditioning with Taoist meditation methods for the ultimate body/mind workout. Ms.Wise's knowledge of proper strength training techniques is extensive, but it is her insights regarding the connection between muscle and mind that sets her apart. I heartily endorse this book to anyone interested in stepping beyond mere body sculpting to a more complete approach to healthy, self-improvement".

~ JULIO BELBER
CENTER CARE PRESIDENT & CEO

"As an editor at Martha Stewart, Tammy was a go-to fitness pro, and I could always count on her to deliver a fresh, insightful, mind-body takes on run-of-the-mill strength and fitness training. She never ceased to wow me, and the stories we worked on together were among the most popular pieces we ran".

~ TERRI TRESPICIO
FORMER SENIOR EDITOR of WHOLE LIVING MAGAZINE

"BodyLogos® teacher training has been one of the most treasured gifts of my life. Tammy's work empowers and heals the practitioner. I now not only sculpt the body during my workouts, but also use it as a sacred time. I see myself and other people with more clarity by exploring how consciousness is being mapped on the body. BodyLogos is the work of a master, a work of art".

~ HIIE SAUMAA PhD
INSTITUTE for IDEAS and IMAGINATION, COLUMBIA UNIVERSITY

"BodyLogos® philosophy and systems are fundamentally sound, healthy, helpful, and beneficial to the wellbeing of all types of people regardless to background. Tammy Wise is an extraordinary person, physically fit, mentally balanced, realistic, and spiritually uplifting. She is BodyLogos".

~ RAUL LUGO M.D.
F.A.C.S. SURGICAL ONCOLOGY CAROLINA SURGICAL ONCOLOGY P.C.

"Let's be honest about this. I am an 84-year-old woman in great health but I am winding down. What Tammy has done is nothing short of miraculous. I feel strong. I feel confident. I feel good. Quite simply, Tammy has changed my life".

~ PATRICIA BOSWORTH
CONTRIBUTING EDITOR of VANITY FAIR

"Strength is more than just a measurement of power; it is about resilience and injury avoidance. BodyLogos® goes beyond strength training; it trains the mind and the body, ensuring that you build muscle while quieting the mind".

~ DAVID D. ROTHSCHILD
MEDICAL TECHNOLOGY INVESTOR

"This work is not for the faint-hearted. BodyLogos® is as much a mental and emotional workout as it is a physical one. Wise has written that in creating BodyLogos she uncovered "a map to find my way back to me." This map is her gift to all of us".

~ DONIA ALLEN
BODYLOGOS® INSTRUCTOR

From Master to Minister

"I am overwhelmingly impressed and appreciate your wonderful creation.

From your book, I can see that BodyLogos® has become your way of teaching Taoism using a movement/physical fitness approach. It utilizes the principles of yin and yang and of the cyclical nature of energy, while emphasizing the inseparable union of body and mind.
As a dancer, you have automatically incorporated the principles of Taoism into movement. Hence the name BodyLogos, with "Logos" to express Taoism's essential reverence for the Laws of the Universe. BodyLogos is based upon not only your appreciation for the body but the influence the body can have on one's personal growth. Though the specific technique was born out of your personal experience, it is inseparably connected to our philosophy."

~ DR. STEPHEN T. CHANG
AUTHOR of THE GREAT TAO

Mary,
Just take one step at a time —

The Art of Strength

Sculpt the Body—Train the Mind

In love & light,

[signature]

Tammy Wise

BALBOA
PRESS
A DIVISION OF HAY HOUSE

Copyright © 2018 Tammy Wise.

Cover credits:
Author photo: Steve Friedman
3D stills: Dmitriy Starkov
Graphic artist: Teri Elefante

Interior credits:
Graphic artist: Teri Elefante
Exercise photos: Jeff Sanders
Head shot photos: Steve Friedman

All rights reserved. No part of this book may be used or reproduced by any means, graphic, electronic, or mechanical, including photocopying, recording, taping or by any information storage retrieval system without the written permission of the author except in the case of brief quotations embodied in critical articles and reviews.

Balboa Press books may be ordered through booksellers or by contacting:

Balboa Press
A Division of Hay House
1663 Liberty Drive
Bloomington, IN 47403
www.balboapress.com
1 (877) 407-4847

Because of the dynamic nature of the Internet, any web addresses or links contained in this book may have changed since publication and may no longer be valid. The views expressed in this work are solely those of the author and do not necessarily reflect the views of the publisher, and the publisher hereby disclaims any responsibility for them.

The author of this book does not dispense medical advice or prescribe the use of any technique as a form of treatment for physical, emotional, or medical problems without the advice of a physician, either directly or indirectly. The intent of the author is only to offer information of a general nature to help you in your quest for emotional and spiritual well-being. In the event you use any of the information in this book for yourself, which is your constitutional right, the author and the publisher assume no responsibility for your actions.

Any people depicted in stock imagery provided by Getty Images are models,
and such images are being used for illustrative purposes only.
Certain stock imagery © Getty Images.

ISBN: 978-1-9822-0946-9 (sc)
ISBN: 978-1-9822-0947-6 (e)

Library of Congress Control Number: 2018910397

Print information available on the last page.

Balboa Press rev. date: 10/27/2018

Contents

Acknowledgments xiii
The BodyLogos Story xv
    It's Time for BodyLogos xviii
How to Read This Book xxi
Basic Principles of BodyLogos xxiii
    Energy Principles of Relaxed Strength xxiii
    Theory of Yin and Yang xxiii
    The Five-Element Theory xxvi
    Principles of Spirit xxviii

Part 1: A Life Practice: From the Inside Out

Overview 1

Mind Chapter 4
    Lesson: 1 The Art of Meditation 5
        Meditation as a Phenomenon 5
            Tao Eagle Active Meditation 6
        Active Meditation 7
        BodyLogos Psyche-Muscular Components 11
        Five Forms of Expression 12
        Connect to Your Breath 13
            Breathing Exercise 14
        Trauma Takes Your Breath Away 15
        Active Stillness 17
        Neutral Attention Offers Awareness 18
            Neutral Witness Exercise 19
        The Self within the self 21

Emotion Chapter 24
    Lesson: 2 The Practice of Meditation 25
        Meditation Breakdown 27
        Fear: Feel Your Body 27
        Anger: Experience Your Truth 29
        Joy: Allow What Is 30
        Reflection: Align Mind and Body 31
        Sorrow: Surrender Judgment 32

Body Chapter 34
    Lesson: 3   The Art of Strength 35
        Strength's Beauty 35
        Alignment Flow 36
        Neutral Alignment Reference Points 39
            Experience Neutral Alignment 39
        Adjusting Alignment 40
        Alignment Stabilizer Reference Points 42
            Experience Alignment Stabilizers 44
        Bones Don't Move—They're Moved 45
            Experience the Bone 46
        Vertical Relaxation 47
        Gathering Universal Energy 48
            Experience Essential Alignment 49

Movement Chapter 52
    Lesson: 4   The Practice of Strength 53
        Movement Breakdown 56
        Drilling: Wrists, Shoulder Blades, Ankles, and Thumbs 56
        Crushing: Elbows, Knees, and Digits 57
        Pounding: Shoulders and Hips 58
        Crossing: Head and Spine 59
        Splitting: Sternum and Discs 61

Connection Chapter 64
    Lesson: 5   The Art of Alignment 65
        Connect to Your Unique Purpose 65
        Balance versus Alignment 66
        Mindfulness Delivers Equipoise 67
            Experience Equipoise Exercise 67
        Replenish Your Energy 69
            Centripetal of Centrifugal Force Exercise 71
        Learning to Listen 73
        BodyLogos Orientations 73
        Energy versus Physical Movement 74
        Skeleton 74
        Muscles 75
        Feeling versus Thinking 75

Direction Chapter 78
    Lesson: 6   The Practice of Alignment 79
        Workout Breakdown 81
        Winter: Getting Started 81

Spring: Warm-Up 82

Summer: Strength Training 83

Indian Summer: Endurance Training 83

Autumn: Cool Down 85

Part 2: Our Life Practice: From the Outside In

Overview 89

Practice Chapter 92

Lesson: 7   The Art of Practice 93

A Current of Life Runs through You 93

Isolated Connection 95

Unified Connection 96

Five Energy Patterns 97

Meeting Resistance 97

Connection Point Exercise 99

Your Energy Body Is the Container for Your Meditation 101

BodyLogos Exercise Structure 104

Creating Change Chapters 106

Lesson: 8   Coming Home Energy Pattern: Abdominals, Biceps, Shoulders 107

Coming Home—Seated Lap Lay and Active Meditation 108

Practice Change 109

Coming Home Energy Pattern as It Relates to the Abdominal Muscles 110

How to Isolate the Abdominal Muscles 113

Lower Abdominal Exercises 115

Upper Abdominal Exercises 125

Oblique Abdominal Exercises 137

BodyLogos Psyche-Muscular Observations for Abdominal Muscles 144

Meet the Models 147

Coming Home Energy Pattern as It Relates to the Biceps Muscles 148

How to Isolate the Biceps Muscles 151

Biceps Exercises 153

BodyLogos Psyche-Muscular Observations for Biceps Muscles 162

Meet the Models 165

Coming Home Energy Pattern as It Relates to the Shoulder Muscles 166

How to Isolate the Shoulder Muscles 169

Shoulder Exercises 171

BodyLogos Psyche-Muscular Observations for Shoulder Muscles 182

Meet the Models 185

Lesson: 9   Determined Power Energy Pattern: Back, Triceps 187

Determined Power—Standing Ponder and Active Meditation 188

Practice Change 189
Determined Power Energy Pattern as It Relates to the Back Muscles 190
How to Isolate the Back Muscles 193
Back Exercises 195
BodyLogos Psyche-Muscular Observations for Back Muscles 204
Meet the Models 207
Determined Power Energy Pattern as It Relates to the Triceps Muscles 208
How to Isolate the Triceps Muscles 211
Triceps Exercises 213
BodyLogos Psyche-Muscular Observations for Triceps Muscles 222
Meet the Models 225

Lesson: 10   Creating Forward Energy Pattern: Chest, Quadriceps 227
        Creating Forward—T-Shirt Strip and Active Meditation 228
Practice Change 229
Creating Forward Energy Pattern as It Relates to the Chest Muscles 230
How to Isolate the Chest Muscles 233
Chest Exercises 235
BodyLogos Psyche-Muscular Observations for Chest Muscles 244
Meet the Models 247
Creating Forward Energy Pattern as It Relates to the Quadriceps Muscles 248
How to Isolate the Quadriceps Muscles 251
Quadriceps Exercises 253
BodyLogos Psyche-Muscular Observations for Quadriceps Muscles 262
Meet the Models 265

Lesson: 11   Suspending Judgment Energy Pattern: Hamstrings 267
        Suspending Judgment—Standing Prayer and Active Meditation 268
Practice Change 269
Suspending Judgment Energy Pattern as It Relates to the Hamstring Muscles 270
How to Isolate the Hamstring Muscles 273
Hamstring Exercises 275
BodyLogos Psyche-Muscular Observations for Hamstring Muscles 284
Meet the Models 287

Lesson: 12   Universal Connection Energy Pattern: Buttocks, Inner Thighs, Calves 289
        Universal Connection—Standing Corkscrew and Active Meditation 290
Practice Change 291
Universal Connection Energy Pattern as It Relates to the Buttock Muscles 292
How to Isolate the Buttock Muscles 295
How to Find the Iliopsoas Muscles 296
Buttock Exercises 299

BodyLogos Psyche-Muscular Observations for Buttock Muscles 308
Meet the Models 311
Universal Connection Energy Pattern as It Relates to the Inner-Thigh Muscles 312
How to Isolate the Inner-Thigh Muscles 315
Inner-Thigh Exercises 317
BodyLogos Psyche-Muscular Observations for Inner-Thigh Muscles 324
Meet the Models 327
Universal Connection Energy Pattern as It Relates to the Calf Muscles 328
How to Isolate the Calf Muscles 331
Calf Exercises 333
BodyLogos Psyche-Muscular Observations for Calf Muscles 342

Part 3: Life Is Outside Resistance
Overview 345

Physical Transformation Chapter 346
   Lesson: 13   Sculpt the Body 347
      Attend to the Moment 347
      Holistic Self-Appraisal 349
      Discerning Your Condition 350
      Create Your Own Workout 351
      Correcting Physical Complaints 352
      Cultivating Physical Strength Workouts 355
      Meeting a Challenge 366

Emotional Transmutation Chapter 368
   Lesson: 14   Train the Mind 369
      The Purpose of Spirit 369
      Becoming Conscious 370
      Correcting Psychological Complaints 372
      Cultivating Psychological Strength Workouts 375
      Evolve Your Intention 386

Living Change Chapter 388
   Lesson: 15   Aligned Living 389
      When You Align with Spirit, Spirit Aligns with You 389
      Surviving to Thriving 390
      Time Is of the Essence 391
      Relieving Crisis and Conflict 393
      The Will to Align 404
      Venture Forth 404

Index 407

Acknowledgments

My mother, father and sister set the stage for me to learn who I could be. My extended family of friends has extended my capacity to love. And my teachers have influenced me to carve my own path. I am grateful to have had the influence of these people to learn about myself. They helped to set me on my call to action, which I hope I've captured here, at long last, in this book *The Art of Strength*.

John Mederos stands out as the dance teacher and choreographer who prepared me for Broadway and gave me opportunity to teach dance in a professional setting. He aligned with my uncrafted belief that expression was communicated by releasing tension, not holding fast to an ideal. A cornerstone to the technique I developed called BodyLogos®, which I teach in this book.

John Lindseth, the founder of The School of Classical Tao, inspired me to delve deeply into my studies and encouraged me to choose Tao as a Ministry. He gave me the atmosphere to explore my body as a Divine structure and the language to share BodyLogos principles.

This book wouldn't exist without the many students who were willing to commit to the process and explore the theories in real life and in real time. I treasure my students in group fitness and private practice who allowed me to utter the first concepts of BodyLogos as my beliefs. Those were terrifying moments for me, but students responded with genuine interest that inspired me to continue on the path and organize the method for others.

Hiie Saumaa and Donia Allen are two students who motivated me to create the BodyLogos teacher-training program so they could learn more about the philosophy and gain greater agency in developing themselves and others in the work. As it turns out, they inspired me to include videos in this book and informed me which concepts needed that added support.

Sharon Lerner, Karen McAuley, Jane Mushabac and Angela Marvin, Lise Liepmann, Hiie Saumaa, Donia Allen, Sarah Montana, and the Balboa editorial team together transformed my thesis of BodyLogos into a practical method that flows for reading and doing. Without these highly sensitive writers my expertise would be hidden under the dogma of theories and principles.

We brought these theories to life through story. And I especially want to thank my clients who were willing to share theirs with me, and with you in the pages of this book.

Another major effort for this beast of a book was to create the images to support and explain the theories. *(You will notice I started this book with long red hair and completed it with short grey hair! Don't even ask how many years!!)*

Steve Friedman and Jeff Sanderson created the original photo library for the book. Both of them playful and skilled made all the talent relaxed, joy-filled and beautiful. And of course, my gratitude goes out to the models. They all generously offered their image to the work making every shoot heartfelt and fun!

To that end, I want to thank Teri Elefante, who worked tirelessly on the graphics from start to finish with such an invested interest in the journey. She spoke of our work together as a calming force that nurtured her in her whole life, a sentiment that touches my heart deeply. I will treasure our friendship forever.

The last piece, and what makes this book so special, is the 3D videos. Dmitriy Starkova, a 3D animator living in the Ukraine managed to decipher my needs through Skype chat and my elementary storyboards. A relationship based on only writings and pictures, we never spoke. He made the world I was about to publish in feel a little smaller and less scary.

This video effort also required an Indiegogo Fundraiser to manage. The donors made this element of the project possible and I am happy to report worth every penny. Thank you all for your generosity, interest and trust. Thank you to those donors: Cynthia McDowell, Ken & Debra Sofer, Laura Dwight, Marie Weilman, Marion Kokot, Judy Tobey, Susan Rosi, John Califano, Alfred Hemlock, Susan Dalsimer, Cynthia Vance, Sherri Kendricks, Ronny Meyer, Venisa Hoeflinger, Barbara Ehlers, Angela Marvin, Lise Liepman, Terri Landi, Keith Brandwen, Natalie Reuss, Suzy Grant, Nanette Walsh, Bob Weeck, Silvia Oseguera, Jane Mushabac, Sarah Papier, Julia Robbins, Patricia Bosworth, David Rothchild, Marty Plevel, Denise Shalev, JOE, Elisa Colas, Lise Liepmann, Elizabeth McGuy, Sandra & Guy Moszkowski, Barbara Ricigliano, Hiie Saumaa, Kirsten Maxwell, Carolee Goodgold, gdw12, Etric Slayton, Kari McCabe, Jennifer Snowdon, Roberta Espie, Gail & John Horton, Irving Allen, Donia Allen, Peter Kavuma, Joyce Nawy, Jacqulyne Arrington, Toby Miroff & Stephen Lino, and Barbara Burge. You are one of 56 donors who supported a vision into a living dream.

Aminta de Lara coached me on speaking, Jennifer Snowdon made me look beautiful with her high-definition make-up artistry, and David Margolin Lawson made me sound clearer than I sometimes felt and composed music that gently carried my words. These artists believed in my vision as I did, giving the gift of comradery.

Chris Shelby, my producer-director-videographer-editor was my rock. From start to finish, he was always calm, always had a solution, and always had my back. Without him these videos could not have evolved with the grace they behold. I treasure his involvement, integrity and friendship.

When a project takes years you need both a release valve and a spear raiser to keep things moving. Monica Velez released my fears with her sensitive touch and innovative massage style that transported me from the sedentary writing demands back to dance; Margarite Westley raised my bar as a body technician challenging me in a ballet technique class that transforms unconscious habits into conscious expression. They are the yin and yang of my physical world. Thank you for keeping me whole.

Nature is my guide. My four-legged, finned and winged ones are my connection point.

The BodyLogos Story

Each of us is called to honor nature's golden rule: to leave the world a better place than we found it. Some of us bring tiny, perfectly imperfect humans into the world. Some of us create soul-shaking art. Some of us make paradigm-shifting discoveries. But a gift is required of each of us.

BodyLogos is my life's gift. But like any treasure worth having, this gift was formed under intense pressure, excavated in sweat using every tool at my disposal, and forged in fire to become an indestructible and beautiful practice. It has been a long process of learning how to prove what I've learned through experience. Our bodies are continually telling us what our story is through our pain. We can either continue living the same story or set out on a new path. BodyLogos is the road map to changing our story.

BodyLogos was birthed at a time rife with endings. I had just completed my seminary course work to become a Taoist minister, and I was deeply entrenched in developing my thesis on how to bring Tao into the modern world. My marriage of ten years was crumbling, and I'd finally summoned the courage to end it. I was completely disheartened, frustrated, and not at all like my strongest self. I felt vulnerable and exposed like a crab with no shell.

And yet here I was, at the gym and obsessed with back exercises—chin-ups. Chin-ups, of all things, were particularly difficult at a time when I was feeling my weakest. "Chin up" is the flippant advice we give people when they need to be strong. Suddenly, I felt a download of wisdom. Of course, I was doing chin-ups. I wanted to strengthen my back, which offers protection. I wanted to exercise my triceps, the muscles designed to push things away. I had spent most of my life basing my decisions on guilt, other people's expectations, and a desire to please. I desperately needed space to figure out what I wanted. My body's choice of muscle groups carried convictions that strengthened my mind's changing beliefs. My body's wisdom was greater than my own life's experience.

The whole psyche-muscular blueprint became clear to me. I practically sprinted home and drew up a psychological map of the muscular body, drawing on the philosophy of five elements and the natural and physical function of each muscle group. I researched, explored, and finally summoned the courage to put my theories to the test with my group fitness class.

"Okay now, your biceps are the muscles that pull desirables toward you," I said. "So while you're doing this exercise, visualize something you'd like to pull closer to you. Whether it's part of your outer world or your inner world, what would you like to create in your life?"

"This tension collapses our chests and compresses our hearts. Our backs are then overprotective, and our hearts hide in them like a cave. We can encourage our hearts to move forward by using the muscles in our chests."

It was hands down one of the scariest moments of my life. I was sure I was going to be laughed out of the studio. Instead, tears flowed. Students found release—experienced as relief—in their strength training. That old, outdated fitness-industry tenet that strength training has to be "no pain, no gain" came crashing down on me. I realized the fitness industry at large wasn't teaching strength. It was blindly building the body's greatest irritant, tension. It became abundantly clear through this work that we cannot build strength through tension because strength is the flow of force, while tension is the stagnation of force. As my clients and I learned to integrate our emotional and spiritual selves into our exercise to deliberately release tension, I noticed that a real and lasting strength was generated. There, in this merger, it was possible to become totally aligned, to create a body and spirit strong enough to contain the universe inside us all.

That flicker of curiosity that started with chin-ups birthed an epiphany: I must bring Tao into the world through movement. This was my thesis. No, the real truth was simpler. I'd been bringing Tao into the world through unconscious movement my whole life, and now it was time to own it, name it, and teach others how to do the same.

The roots of BodyLogos started in childhood. When I was growing up, my body's wisdom saved my soul. Though I was a promising athlete, I threw myself—body, mind, and spirit—into dance partially because, as I once said in an interview, "I don't have to speak in dance." I'd become known to my high school peers as "Smiley" because I preferred smiling over speaking. Through dance, I could throw all that expression into my body, into movement, into a sense of agency and self-mastery, into regaining a sense of control. Though my ballet teachers barked to "squeeze my butt cheeks together until I couldn't sit down," I was always searching for a way to fill each moment with release, which I desperately needed due to a tumultuous household.

My father's sickness was the elephant in the room, and we all tiptoed around it. Unspoken anger, resentment, and fear permeated the household. My mother's anger toward my father simmered, boiled, and burned. My father drank. And drank more. My sister reacted, exploded, and ran to her room, slamming the door. I sat stoically at the dining room table, trying to hold the world together, frozen in place to keep from making waves.

My father started coming into my room at night when I was ten or eleven years old. My body would curl itself into the fetal position with the innate, primal urge to protect myself without confronting him. As he slipped into my bed, I would disassociate completely. It was as if some hand from the heavens came, plucked me out of my body, and cocooned me in alignment between earth and sky, safe and tucked away. I would stay there, occasionally jerked back into my body, back into the trauma and terror of not knowing what was happening, but somehow recognizing deeply that someone I thought loved me was causing me the darkest pain I could imagine. But then, when it was all too much, I would disassociate again, transported back to where I felt held by the expanse of the entire universe—safe in the power of something bigger than even the worst, darkest forces on earth. I was safe, held, aligned—there was no way I could believe there wasn't a greater power. It was here, in the depths, that I first discovered my body's divine wisdom and resilience.

Eventually, my parents divorced. I talked less and danced more. And more. And more. Until finally, I booked the first bus and truck tour of *A Chorus Line* right out of high school. As dancers cycled through the brilliant but brutally taxing show in short bursts, I quickly found after a year that I was the youngest member of the bus and truck company but the most senior member. It's clear to me in hindsight that my dedication to finding an equal release to every element of tension allowed me to listen to my body's wisdom and give it what it needed to stay strong, flexible, and happy.

That happiness poured into my career and life. I observed with shock the misery of one of my older cast members. I thought, *How can you not be happy? You're starring in a production of the best show on Broadway! The only thing better than this is Broadway, and they will inevitably cast Broadway from this tour.* (And they did within twelve months.) What was the problem? In fairness, I was nineteen, doing what I loved, and didn't have a home to miss. I was totally out of line to judge her—and, at the same time, still totally right. (See, yin and yang at work, even then.) But I promised myself in that moment that if my spirit ever looked that lost, it was time to leave show business.

And after a long, fulfilling, and prolific dance career, that day arrived. I found myself less interested in using my body and more curious about how my body used energy. How do we keep energy levels up in the body? I figured I should start with what we put into our bodies—and I signed up at Annmarie Colbin's nutritional cooking school, the Natural Gourmet Institute. It was there that I first encountered the Tao theory of five elements. Little did I know that it would propel me on a journey to explore not only how to keep energy levels up in the body but also how energy has the power to transform and heal our entire being. One course simultaneously opened a door to my future and unveiled an illuminating window into the disassociations of my childhood.

That class was in Chinese herbology with John Lindseth. I was so fascinated by what I learned that I immediately transferred to his school, the School of Classical Taoist Herbology. I was like a sponge, absorbing any and all information on how to most optimally work with energy. I became certified in nutrition, meditation, herbs, and acupressure. As I sat in lectures, a light bulb went off as they described Taoism's principles about energy.

I'd think to myself, *Oh yeah! That's how I land a double pirouette! That's how I do an arabesque without hurting my back!*

I finally had a language for all the theories I'd been putting into practice as a dancer over my entire life. I finally had words and methodologies to describe the meditative encounters that saved me in my darkest moments. The sun was rising on a new chapter for me, one in which I could not only survive but also organize this information into a truly healing, transformative practice that could be integrated into all aspects of life.

Long story short, after three and a half years, John pulled me aside and let me know I'd completed enough course work that I qualified to present myself to the Foundation of Tao for my ministry. I needed to create my thesis about how I would bring Taoism into the world. That thesis, which flickered into existence over a chin-up bar when I felt my absolute lowest, has completely changed the frequency of my life and countless clients. It is a practice that, after trauma crumpled me into a ball after years of repression, gave me the strength to release my pain and change my story.

BodyLogos is the gift of true, total alignment. It's not merely the alignment of spinal discs or sinewy muscle. By integrating this active meditation, BodyLogos aligns the empty voids in our bodies that hold energy. I have seen clients' lives change. People who feel like their lives are too crowded, their apartment too small, and their job too stifling use this work to go inward and discover they are actually too crowded inside. And alignment offers them expansion. Your inner world—physically and spiritually—is like the rowers on a crew team. If one person isn't in sync with the rest of the team, the boat either stops gliding or starts going in circles.

When you are in alignment, you learn to get out of your own way. You have the shock absorbent system and strength in place to handle whatever life throws at you. Once you have made contact with the empty space inside you, it is yours—your space, from which you can escape the chaos of the world and be a neutral witness to your life. It is the space from which you are reminded that no matter the situation—no matter how out of control you may feel—you always have a choice. You can move toward something, move away, or go inward. You can protect yourself. You can open yourself. You can stand in your power, because that's what your body does and teaches you to do every day.

This practice is gradual, granular work. It starts small and simply. Even transforming the feeling of deprivation by meditating on the idea that "I'm actively pushing away that chocolate cake" while you work triceps can imbue an element of elegance to self-care that affects your whole life. I've seen clients use it to start strong second acts as authors, entrepreneurs, and artists. My clients have unearthed the courage to buy their first home, purchase the boat they always wanted, and turn their passion projects into real businesses.

I used it myself to work up the nerve to purchase the motorcycle I'd always wanted. This glamorous, badass woman used to carry her motorcycle helmet into the gym every day. And every day I would muse about how awesome it would be to be her, if I only had the nerve—but I didn't. Then I put BodyLogos into practice. As I pulled in strength and pushed away apprehension, I began to meditate on what it might be like to have that motorcycle and become my own inspiration. One day, with mind and body aligned, I was ready.

I purchased a full-sized Harley-Davidson and said to the seller, "Listen, I've got great balance, and I ride a bicycle every day. But I don't know how to use a clutch. I will pay you in cash if you agree to teach me how to ride this thing." After a howl of laughter, he agreed. We quickly became riding buddies. I not only ride a motorcycle all over Manhattan, but I take it on a new adventure all over the country every summer. Thanks to BodyLogos, I don't muse about how glamorous or cool it would be to be anyone else—I am continually becoming the person I want to be. My gift to you—my deepest, sincerest wish for you—is the power to do the same.

You picked up this book because there's something you need from this work—to heal your pain, to change your life, or to build a stronger, healthier body. This practice will challenge you to consider what you need. Do you just need to improve your personal life, or are you ready to take responsibility for healing the collective of humanity and, by extension, yourself?

The exercises in this book will help you develop a practice that summons the warrior, healer, and creator in you. It will help you tap into the power you have as being one with the universe and as a microcosm of existence yourself. You have everything you need within you to become the person you imagine. May this practice give you the strength and alignment to become your highest self, as it has for me.

It's Time for BodyLogos

East Meets West

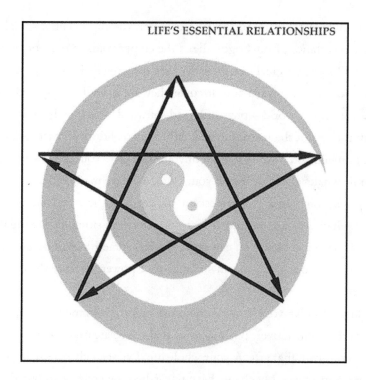

When the changing fads in fitness moved away from my sensibilities, I became curious about the industry's history. In a 1960 *Sports Illustrated* article, President John F. Kennedy named US citizens "The Soft American."[1] He said, "We are under-exercised as a nation; we look instead of play; we ride instead of walk." Since this proclamation, exercise has gained momentous popularity. Kennedy's words spurred a massive boost in health and fitness

---

[1] J. F. Kennedy, "The Soft American," 1969, *Sports Illustrated*, 13:15–17.

education—and the fitness industry made it fun. As we cycled out of the twentieth century, the United States started to explore Eastern fitness modalities as well, embracing the connection between the mind and body through yoga, meditation, and other holistic practices.

But in the twenty-first century, rivalry for superiority crept into the fitness hype, turning personal pride into private humiliation. A tension-producing environment has now emerged. Class titles have evolved from "Whole Fitness" to "Burn Out!" This competitive atmosphere poses no distinction between strength and tension. As the fitness industry booms to 34,460 clubs and 54.1 million club members in 2015 in the United States alone, up from 26,830 clubs and 41.3 million club members in 2005, [2]it now brings with it an onslaught of exercise injuries. IDEA Health and Fitness Ass. reported at this time that three to five million Americans were injured by recreational exercise and sports-related activities each year. And while the primary causes of these injuries are physical, they continued, psychological issues are a growing cause for this rising factor, and fitness professionals need to pay attention to it. The fitness culture's tone, however, evolved from encouraging people to take responsibility for their health to goading them to prove they are healthy. The message is that the harder you work out, the healthier you are. Instead of focusing on fitness to support wholeness, the current craze—"Burn Out," "Power Yoga," "HIIT"—encourages us to assault ourselves in the pursuit of becoming fit. Even those who aren't typically drawn into a competitive or self-loathing frame of mind can become prey to the ringing chorus of "You're not enough" that permeates the fitness industry.

On the other hand, many who follow Eastern philosophies have understood for centuries that personal suffering occurs when the conscious mind and the unconscious body are in conflict. To alleviate suffering, we must align the mind and body.

Eastern philosophy elaborates further that our life's work is to actively maintain a pure, inward alliance and enjoy the spiritual belonging we inherited at birth. To me, this means that by recognizing where I hold tension in my body and using my mind to deliberately surrender it, my personal story will challenge me back to the pureness of spirit I was born with.

Our bodies are our guide home—our therapists, so to speak. Even with the best of intentions to align, our spirit selves can remain obscured by unintended and unconscious blocks in mind and body. These times of confusion or agitation can exhaust us into lethargy or rouse us into hyperactivity. Shedding light on the spirit self—and seeing behind our personal barricades—requires a willingness to believe there is something precious beneath our surface, something worth unearthing. We are more than we are aware of. By believing that our greatest value is found in what we don't know yet, our wills are inspired to light the way, and our workouts become a place to witness the subtle, unconscious realities of our lives.

This active meditation practice is right for those who believe they are an extension of creation—and consequently they are creators themselves. This fundamental belief is independent of religious faith or upbringing. It is a scientific and philosophical concept. By definition, we as human beings are creators of life, and we birth more than our children. We create every aspect of our lives daily; each day is a new canvas on which we create. Do we, however, recognize ourselves as creators? Our relationships with the outside world—be they interpersonal, material, intellectual, presentational, or a combination thereof—reflect what we have created. Do we celebrate, honor, and acknowledge these creations as our own? Aligning the spirit self with mind and body is the counterpart to aligning the spirit self with the universal spirit. This holistic alignment, supported by BodyLogos practice, is an act of cooperation, both within and without, that can transform conflict into serenity.

---

[2] U.S. Bureau of Labor Statistics, https://blog.gyminsight.com/859-most-current-fitness-industry-ststistics.

This book explains my journey toward strength and my way of balancing alignment as a three-dimensional being—mind, body, and spirit. It also illustrates how the founding principles of this journey lie in Tao's theory of yin and yang and Tao's five-element theory. Tao recognizes all manifestations in mind and body, positive or negative, as the result of these two theories; and all life oscillates between and revolves around these theories.

The powerlessness that challenged my youth no longer describes my general emotional state, but I can still be triggered into feeling powerless. By applying the basic principles of Taoism—the theory of yin and yang and the five-element theory—and using the BodyLogos psyche-muscular blueprint to understand the basis of my misalignment, I experience immediate energy, stability, and relaxed strength.

My contribution to the fitness industry is to neutralize the implication that suffering is required to look and feel good. My offering to you is relaxed strength and a profound connection with, and respect for, your body's knowledge. BodyLogos practice brings you home to an inner alignment that improves your strength rather than proving your toughness. It frees you from the burden of being defined by your pain. It's the confidence to make choices and craft a life simply because it contributes to a soundness of body, mind, and spirit—and not because it adheres to an external pressure to do or be anything else. It's the will to align mind, body, and spirit to create the life you want and deserve.

> When the Tao is taught,
> People know where to go and what to learn,
> Because they know that they will not be harmed,
> But will receive great peace.
>
> The teacher of Tao is like one who gives real food
> To fish just to see them lead a happy life;
> He does not feed them colorful bait
> With the intention of catching them.
>
> Tao is something flavorless,
> With nothing much to offer the mouth,
> Neither does it offer much
> To be enjoyed by the eyes or entertain the ears,
> Yet its usefulness is inexhaustible.

—Lao Tzu, *Tao Te Ching*

How to Read This Book

In meditation practice, stimulus comes to you and passes through you. You remain open for stimuli to come through you again and again.

Practice meditation as you read this book. Let each word come to you and pass through you rather than leaning into the words to understand and conquer their meaning.

This is active meditation.

This is the art of feeling and the craft of creating positive change.

Book Structure

This book will present a unique breakdown of traditional strength-training exercises, introduce a psyche-muscular understanding of your posture, and acquaint you with active meditation. You will learn the emotional root of your physical tension. The book is aided by fifteen video guides at the following:

mindthebody.bodylogos.com/resources

A 3-D avatar and live video model demonstrate internal and external movement. You will see how energy optimally flows through the body, how tension obscures that flow, and how you can dissolve or resolve that tension. For best results, experience the videos as you read each chapter. From this synthesis, you will have the tools to unlock your body's tension and build relaxed strength.

In the BodyLogos practice, muscle groups fall under one of five energy patterns. Each of these five patterns cycles energy slightly differently, and each generates a unique outcome or quality of strength. Because different muscle groups challenge different psyche-muscular expressions, active meditations are offered that focus not on the end result of an exercise but more significantly on the integrity, balance, and grace of each moment of movement.

> Focus on an end result and you will get the end result;
> focus on the way to the end result and you will be fulfilled when you get there.
>
> —Lao Tzu, *Tao Te Ching*

In the exercise breakdowns, you will be guided to experience the action (yang) and counter-action (yin) as individual yet coexisting aspects of each movement. You will then be guided to cycle these forces (five-element theory) to release unwanted static energy (tension) and recover wanted creative energy (strength). This step aligns you with gravity and gives you a balanced, centered, and safe relationship with resistance.

Learning this technique will unite your experience of living in a body with your experience of living with the outside world. This all-inclusive view of your self and this alliance with nature's way keep you on the journey of growing with, from, and for your environment—a journey viewed, in Tao thought, as a responsibility to the continued existence of the universe. *Practice active meditation to cultivate meditative action.*

The virtue of the universe is wholeness.
It regards all things as equal.
The virtue of the sage is wholeness.
She too regards all things as equal.

The universe may be compared to a bellows.
It is empty, yet it never fails to generate.
The more it moves, the more it brings forth.
Many words lead one nowhere.
Many pursuits in different directions only bring about exhaustion.
Rather, embrace the profound emptiness and silence within.

—Lao Tzu, *Tao Te Ching*

Value emptiness, and you will experience wholeness.

Experience the silent stillness that lives in the center of movement.
It will clarify and fortify a connection to all things.

—Tammy Wise, BodyLogos

Basic Principles of BodyLogos

Energy Principles of Relaxed Strength

What I have witnessed and come to understand through Taoism is that the mind and body, though independent of each other, operate as one. Any change in mind or body—positive or negative—shifts their internal relationship. If you make changes only to one, the other will be triggered into maintaining the status quo. Of course, it does. Biologically, maintaining the status quo is tantamount to survival. Creating change—stepping into your strength—is a committed, multidimensional balancing act between a relaxed mind and a strong body. And for all our good intentions, the hypercompetitive mentality of the West may value a strong body, but it makes a relaxed mind almost impossible.

Tao is a way of being. Its thought recognizes balance as a life-sustaining necessity for all life forms. There is no supremacy outside you that is responsible for your own, or our world's, state of being. BodyLogos practice shifts your state of being from a competitive Western fitness mentality to one of *relaxed strength*.

Being relaxed is a calmed-down, released state of being. Strength is a built-up possession of power. To possess relaxed strength, we are asked to stretch through the full gamut of movement and emotion so we become comfortable in any interval of our life experience. This stretch between opposites is described in the theory of yin and yang.

Theory of Yin and Yang

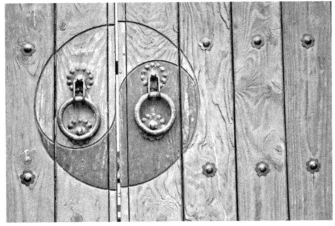

The theory of yin and yang is the belief that there is a natural duality in all things. Yin defines the resultant, passive, destructive principle: death. Yang is the causative, active, creative principle: life. Feminine and masculine, dark and light, cold and hot, and the moon and the sun are all considered external manifestations of yin and yang. Duality exists, however, in every dimension. Happy and sad, relaxed and anxious, accepted and rejected, lovable and detestable, and courageous and fearful are internal manifestations of yin and yang.

Known worldwide to represent balance, the Taijitu symbol, conceived by ancient Tao philosopher Zhou Dunyi in the Song dynasty (1017—1073 CE), encourages us to deliberately attend to manifesting personal balance to maintain well-being. The Taijitu illustrates that everything inherently has both yin and yang aspects, while each thing outwardly exhibits one more strongly than the other. The symbol characterizes this with a spot of yin in yang and a spot of yang in yin. And because the ratio of yin and yang aspects, both within and without, will inevitably ebb and flow in the wake of opposition, a curved line separates yin and yang aspects to characterize this movement.

Active meditation—alignment of mind, body, and spirit through movement—is the tool BodyLogos uses to create this balance within the self and in relationship with resistance amid this wake of yin and yang dynamics.

In dance, I exercised this opposition by dropping away from a lift and lifting away from a drop in equal proportions. Balancing yin and yang external forces made me an aligned dancer. But balancing yin and yang internal forces is what later made me a spirited dancer.

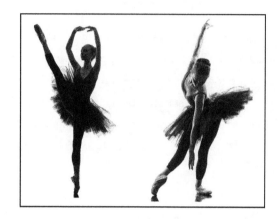

So how does this principle apply to your strength-training workout?

In the BodyLogos practice, opposing muscle groups are recognized as aspects of yin and yang. Like a pulley system, one muscle group contracts as its opposing muscle group expands. The contraction produces an action; the expansion produces a counter-action. The action creates movement, while the counter-action allows movement. The counter-action expands with as much force as the action contracts to maintain muscular balance. So when your body (or mind) meets with an outside resistance, BodyLogos practice first balances the opposing forces within the body and then adds the amount of force needed to allow both yin and yang aspects to move. Both the contracting and expanding forces are considered in all movements at all times.

When you are sensitive to your energy's force, you begin to feel your muscle's release and another muscle's contraction simultaneously, and that pattern teaches you to recognize imbalance and protect your joints when challenged. This opposition of energy is also exercised in basic posture without muscle movement to guide you. Energy balance protects the joints during challenges, produces a muscular release that gives stagnant energy a direction to move, allows you to slow down and be present, creates mental and emotional space, and conserves vital energy.

A client of mine started experiencing significant shoulder pain after a two-year period of extreme stress and one-hundred-hour workweeks. During this period, his attention became increasingly distracted. His workouts regrettably became a place to restlessly let off steam. Pain thankfully has its magical way of rescuing one's attention; it refocused him inwardly, breaking him free from his battle against outside resistance (life conflicts). He acknowledged his shoulder distress was rooted in a psychological holding pattern,[3] his need to defend his own life path and have his choices respected, which explained both his outward fixed attention and inward physical condition. Learning to release tension from his triceps before demanding action from his biceps or shoulders would balance and stabilize his shoulder joints. Along with physical therapy exercises to rehabilitate the injury, we directed his attention to channeling the stress-filled energy out through his triceps and balancing that degree of force inwardly through his biceps. Then he could neutralize the shoulder muscles' hyperactivity.

This channeling properly aligned the shoulder joints for safe use, created greater space in the shoulder joint for healing of the soft tissue, and gave his emotions a platform to be felt and deliberately let go. Balance was restored within four weeks, and the pain retreated in his shoulder. The outcome of this mind-body training brought about even more reward than being pain free; his newfound optimism generated innovative and exciting business ideas that brought in new partners and business opportunities. By balancing yin and yang forces, he learned to stop assaulting his body and his life simultaneously.

> I have been working with Tammy for more than a decade. Tammy's approach and the BodyLogos philosophy helped me navigate periods of extreme stress that manifested in injuries and pain that were serious enough to warrant trips to a physician and occupational therapist (OT). Not much changed with my months of OT. But work with Tammy helped heal the injury. BodyLogos is about balance and integration. Tammy could see from my body language and my expression not only how I was doing physically but how I was feeling. BodyLogos is training the mind and the body.
>
> —David

After Julio was rescued from a life-threatening condition with emergency surgery, his surgeon recommended training with me. Resistant to comply but recognizing the seriousness of his health condition, he rallied three of his top executives to be his training mates. I was asked to come into his corporate headquarters and discuss a training program for him and his posse. I was terrified. I had never been in corporate offices, and the thought of convening around a board table with four less-than-enthusiastic executives who would love to see me fail made me mute. What words could possibly convey the importance of aligning within themselves while they sat back in their cushy seats, smoking their cigars?

I prepared by imagining my boardroom conversation while running an upward rise of energy through my chest and a downward release of energy through my back until the tension in my lower back uncoiled its fear-based tension.

When the discussion ensued, I stood at the head of the table, running that same energy pattern, and spoke of alignment and balanced strength as a powerful foundation for a successful and active life without defenses and with complete conviction of my training method. There was no denying the result of mind-body alignment as they witnessed this young lady in my satin *Chorus Line* jacket standing with commanding grace, insisting that each of them align with me, not with each other, in the gym. And I required them to each have one private training session with me before I coached them as a group. They complied, and I worked with that CEO for well over a decade.

Focusing mind and body on a single aspect of existence in these cases and creating balanced yin and yang

---

[3] https://rhvillegas.wordpress.com/2013/05/16/what-is-a-chronic-holding-pattern.

forces describe the basic practice of active meditation. BodyLogos practice is a modern-day approach to the original Tao practices of active meditation—tai chi and chi gong—which were designed to symptomatically calibrate mind and body.

When you feel drained by living, chances are, you're not balanced and are resisting opposition. Recognizing and employing the opposing forces that exist in all aspects of living both inwardly and outwardly offer an ultimate stretch between polar opposites that allow for all that lies between. With awareness and deliberate management of your energy in each moment of movement, you can create balance and acceptance—rather than resistance—and stretch into alignment with your life and the ways of the universe.

Using the theory of yin and yang when training offers physical balance, mental understanding, and emotional harmony. By understanding opposition in alignment, you generate physical strength and mental clarity. The gift is a pure connection with your inner intelligence—spirit self—in your personal and interpersonal exchanges.

The Five-Element Theory

While the theory of yin and yang defines universal elements, the five-element theory explains the relationship between them. The ancient Taoists devised it as a systematic understanding of balance between complementary and antagonistic forces in the universe. Tao sages understood that the universe maintained balance through the cyclical interplay of five elements: fire, earth, metal, water, and wood. They believed our bodies were a microcosm of the universe, achieving physical and mental harmony in the same way.

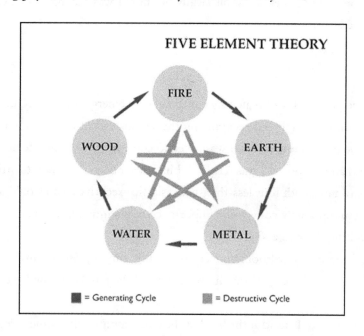

These elements are observed in nature through the changing expressions of seasons, colors, and textures. They are also observed in our human existence through the varying expressions of organs, senses, and emotions. For example, fire is connected to joy, the heart, the small intestines, and summer. Water is connected to fear, the kidneys, the bladder, and winter. The five-element theory offers us a cohesive system to balance all energy manifestations—physical, mental, or emotional. With it, mind and body can develop grace, a free-flowing interplay between us and our environment. And by using the BodyLogos practice, we strengthen that grace through movement.

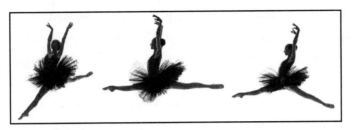

The five-element theory breaks down the elements of movement. In fact, working at the ballet barre is really hours of breaking down the elements of a single expression. A grand jeté, a leaping split in the air, can be divided into five elements. Mastering each element at the barre enabled me to coordinate them into a graceful and multidimensional (body, mind, and spirit) expression center floor. The essential elements of my barre work were to learn how to experience energy, like water seeping up through my body's softening (plié); feel alignment stabilize my body, like wooden trunks stabilize tree branches (tendu); stretch energetically beyond my body's physical limits, like the heat of fire stretching beyond its flames (dégagé); understand that grounding into the earth frees me to extend toward the sky (grand battement), and gain the explosive conviction to slice through the air, like metal slices through wood (jeté) so my expression (grand jeté) could be balanced. This progressive cycle encourages energy flow and is referred to as the generating cycle in the five-element theory.

Conversely, the five-element theory's destructive cycle shows what happens when an element is skipped. For example, if I experience energy seeping through my body as it softens (plié) but don't stabilize my alignment (tendu) when I stretch beyond my body's physical limits (dégagé), I descend into the floor as if swooning in slow motion. This is a technique used in skiing; when you're falling, you soften and are less likely to hurt yourself. This technique also adds drama to interpretive dance and storytelling. The destructive cycle skips a progressive element to reduce energy flow and produce a specialized outcome.

This systematic breakdown points out what is interfering with the cyclical nature of free-flowing energy. By following the five-element theory's generating cycle, whereby each element generates or produces the succeeding element, you can determine or adjust what is needed to progress. By recognizing the five-element theory's destructive cycle, whereby each element destroys or absorbs the succeeding element, you can determine or adjust what is needed to slow down.

By understanding opposition—theory of yin and yang—I mastered skeletal alignment; by understanding that a whole is made up of parts—five-element theory—I mastered muscular balance. Using these theories unconsciously as a youth made me able to freely express myself through my movements. Using these theories consciously as an adult makes me able to freely experience myself as part of a much greater whole and recognize the unique power and influence of my actions.

So how does this theory apply to your strength-training workout?

Let's recognize an isolated muscle group as an isolated element. Any isolated muscular release (yin) is balanced by an opposing muscular contraction (yang). For example, when your hamstrings release, their opposing muscle group, the quadriceps, contract. Visualize these two forces as an uninterrupted orbit of energy. This energy orbit cycles the releasing muscles' force into the contracting muscles' force, creating greater strength. When this muscular isolation extends its orbit of energy and includes the energy orbits of the whole body (five-element theory), it unifies the body to support that isolation.

A client of mine with meniscus knee problems grew anxious about walking. As a New Yorker, she walked predominantly on hard concrete, dodging potholes and avoiding the onslaught of people with their heads buried in their cell phones. This situation made her feel unsteady and rushed, which made her wonder whether her age was beginning to inhibit her lifestyle. Together, we strengthened all the isolated muscle groups that supported the structure of her knees—quadriceps, buttocks, and inner thighs. But not until she was able to establish a current of force that integrated these parts into a cohesive whole was she able to feel stable again. This cohesiveness cycled energy through these isolated muscle groups toward her center of gravity—her abdominal support. This balanced the direction of force throughout her muscular system to subtly and precisely align her bones with gravity. As balance improved, pain subsided. The body-wide tension holding her up relaxed, allowing her strength to step up with greater confidence.

Her knee pain receded, but more notably her newfound wholeness strengthened her trust in herself. She was at a common crossroad, where the challenge of living made her fear her mortality. Many of us have surrendered prematurely into compromised lifestyles because we believe we have no power in the aging process. Using the five-element theory as it related to her body, she reconnected herself to her center, stabilized her strength, and aligned her bones. By committing to her alignment, she freed herself from living a feeble life. She is a walking testimonial of the fountain of youth being a deliberate state of mind.

> Tammy has taught me to be aware of my posture, my muscles, my breathing. I stand up straight when I walk—and I walk a lot—always in comfortable shoes. It's all about practice. I am more confident now when I walk. I feel steady on my feet. I feel strong. I feel good. Quite simply, Tammy has changed my life.
>
> —Patricia

In the beginning of my BodyLogos journey, I experienced dance as orbits of force cycling from my body's center of gravity and balancing my muscular effort—the same center of gravity that aligns my bones between earth and sky. The more I "cycle energy," the more I realize that what I'm channeling goes far beyond my musculoskeletal system, beyond my body's ability and mind's cognition. Cycling energy supports the relationships that sculpt my entire life. I now experience strength as the ability to create deliberately. I believe that with the power invested in me, I can deliberately create change in my life, relationships, and world.

Principles of Spirit

It is a Tao belief that by connecting to the universe, we experience the intelligence—Logos—of spirit and are guided toward our own spirit selves. As a minister of Tao, I am convinced that this connection can be made through our relationship with nature's universal forces—gravity and centrifugal and centripetal forces. Our physical posture is the conduit that establishes the quality of this connection. To align with universal forces is to inadvertently align with our selves. The more aligned we are outwardly, the more aligned we are inwardly. Everything we need to know can be found within our alliance with nature.

After seminary, the same energy that had aligned my body in dance was now aligning my mind in life. When my alignment had deliberate intent, I could witness my own suffering and the suffering of others from an expanded viewpoint, whereby I could step beyond blame and shame. I was able to step outside the bubble of my mental and physical suffering on purpose rather than by accident. Before my Tao training, this viewpoint seemed intuitive rather than intentional—by chance, not by design. In seminary, however, I learned that there actually was something tangible informing my impressions.

I learned that the body is a victim of the mind's constant scrutiny. It's as if there is a war going on within the confines of our bodies, questioning and defending our value in the world at large, exhausting our strength. Expectations to be better than we are and accusations that blame others for our own feelings of inadequacy assault the body from the inside out. Tao thought expresses the danger of the mind's skirmish for importance.

> If you let yourself be blown to and fro,
> You lose touch with your root.
> If you let restlessness move you,
> You lose touch with who you are.
>
> —Lao Tzu, *Tao Te Ching*

Your body is the recipient of your inner restlessness. The emotional charge of your beliefs lives in your tissue. When your emotions are resolved, the tissues remain supple and healthy. But when your emotions are unresolved, holding patterns create blockages that lead to "dis-ease" in body, mind, and heart. And when that mind-body connection point is blocked, it causes "dis-association" around those unresolved feelings, causing your energy to drain.

Imagine your body is a screen window. When air (or energy) flows through it, the environment inside and out remains harmonious. But if the screen gets clogged with debris (judgments and beliefs stored as physical tension), the internal environment will become static due to a lack of air (or energy) flow. Low-grade tensions are felt only when triggered, while high-grade tensions are constant irritants. When energy can't flow through these areas, posture is compromised, and physical fatigue or pain ensues—in addition to mental "restlessness" and feeling "lost," as the Tao verse warns.

Like your fingerprint, your posture is the only one of its kind. In witnessing what your posture is doing, you become aware of the conscious and unconscious aspects of your body print. And by purposely creating balance in your alignment, you can deliberately sculpt balance in your life. This release of tension creates a flow of energy that not only influences your posture and vitality but also gets you in touch with *who you are*—physically, mentally, and spiritually—rather than being defined by *what you are doing*. By using the self-centering alignment techniques of BodyLogos, you strengthen mind and body, and connect to your spiritual self.

Sarah had an intense, unbreakable knot in her right shoulder for eight years. It seemed to coincidentally appear right after the murder of her mother and brother. She'd been to massage therapists, acupuncturists, and neurologists to receive injections, but eventually she was resolved to live with the pain. She couldn't shake the eerie timing of the knot, and though doctors concurred that it must be loosely stress related, she couldn't get any answers.

When she began editing the BodyLogos manuscript, she agreed to do the exercises in this book and follow the videos to understand the full scope of the work. As she worked with the neutral alignment and alignment stabilizer exercises in Lesson 3, she breathed relaxation into her shoulders, found her best alignment, and felt the knot start to relax. She burst into tears, feeling intense relief.

She asked me what, according to the psyche-muscular blueprint (more on that in Lesson 1), was happening in her body. I explained that the shoulders are connected to our hearts and hold our values—what we believe about the world. Because the right side of the body is more connected to the external world, grief often manifests itself physically in the right shoulder.

Sarah had spiritually, mentally, and emotionally grieved and processed her loss. But as the knot released itself, Sarah paid attention to an important meditative insight that arose. She may not be grieving anymore, but until the knot released, she continued to let her loss define and influence how she engaged with the world. She still clung to an outdated idea that the world was an inherently dangerous place long after the idea had stopped protecting her. As Sarah released this idea and let her chest come forward, she found herself more willing to receive joy and more eager to invest in the things that made her heart sing.

> I came to BodyLogos as an editor and am now a full-blown believer. Using this method to reconnect to my body, particularly after disassociating from my body to cope with trauma, has not only brought me back into my physical self—it's reconnected me to my spirit in ways I couldn't have anticipated.
>
> —Sarah

I am asking you to consider your body as a blueprint of your life story and a vessel of spiritual significance. Tao thought warns that the noisy fretting of mind-body mortality drowns the more subtle nature of spirit out. And the more deaf to spirit you become, the more tension accumulates mentally and physically. The separation disperses your energy, and you are left feeling powerless. When this happens, your body experiences the defensive tension of a victim, your mind experiences the assaultive judgment of a perpetrator, and the spirit becomes the unheard bystander of your internal ambivalence.

The universe, on the other hand, energizes creation from a free-flowing, everlasting source of energy. When aligned in mind and body, Tao says, you become a conduit for universal life force to flow through. You plug into the source of creation and become a body ROCKET.

Rest On Creation to Keep Energy True

It's my mission to keep you connected to *why* you are challenging yourself in the gym, because the significance of that *why* energizes your relationship with life. The journey of aligning with your personal *why* takes the courage to recognize personal weakness and allow interpersonal uncertainty. BodyLogos trains you to realize your truth and stand in your life wholly—holistically. Rather than being triggered into victimhood, be triggered toward self-discovery. This is relaxed strength.

Part 1
A Life Practice: From the Inside Out

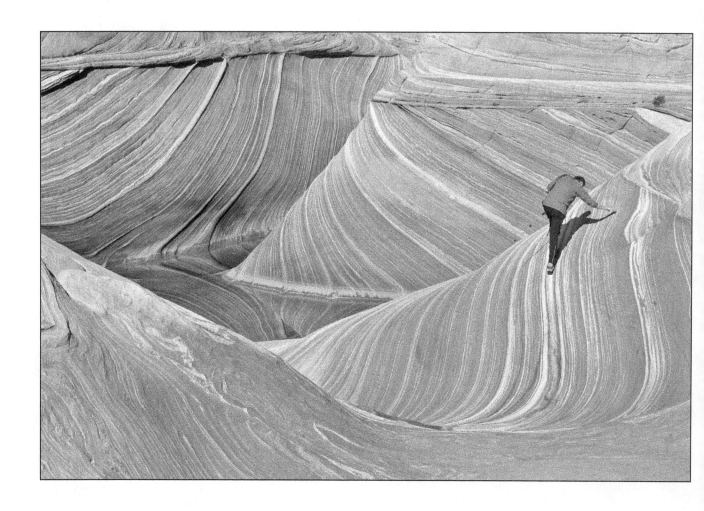

Overview

Lesson Chapters 1–6

Meditation is a way of connecting, not rest from movement.
Meditation is, in fact, the balance of movement.
The way of Tao is the way of the universe and the way of movement.

—Tammy Wise, BodyLogos

Through BodyLogos strength-training practice, you are bringing the inward connection of meditation into outward movement, recognizing your muscular body as a psychological blueprint, and learning a fitness discipline that brings clarity to life's obstacles through your connection to physical challenges.

The BodyLogos journey begins with valuing you. In Part 1, you will be introduced to and instructed in active meditation as a way to

- connect with and observe your energy movement;
- learn to "feel" versus "think" about the subtle happenings that block your strength and produce your tension; and
- discover how to unite energy movement, muscular coordination, and skeletal alignment for greater access to your supreme intelligence—your spirit self—so your workouts become self-centering and universally aligned.

When you learn to feel energy movement as rivers of force—separate from your actual physical movement—you realize you're not only an informed mind controlling the body's gestures but also a knowing body informing the mind's intellect.

Part 1 expands your understanding of how the Tao theory of yin and yang and the five-element theory apply to the human form and its movement. This is a breakdown of multidimensional movement—a practical understanding of the mind, body, and spirit as a united force that creates your posture, movement, and ultimately the quality of your life.

Part 1 uses three theoretical chapters (mind, body, and connection) and three practical chapters (emotions, seasons, and movements) to help you apply Tao theory to your workouts. This foundation positions your mind and body as co-creators of how you hold psychological beliefs in your physical body, how your tension interferes with your muscular balance, and how your skeleton's alignment diminishes your vitality. You learn to witness yourself objectively, observing muscular, skeletal, and emotional bodies as separate aspects of the whole. This witnessing allows you to observe an emotion without becoming the emotion and adjust single aspects of your musculoskeletal system to restore alignment and balance. This, in turn, increases your awareness of unresolved holding patterns before they interfere with the quality of your life as physical injury or emotional hardship.

Part 1 will convince you that balancing energy trains you to balance life and that strength training is a means to creating the life you want.

> True wisdom seems foolish …
> The Master allows things to happen.
> She shapes events as they come.
>
> —Lao Tzu, *Tao Te Ching*

Mind Chapter

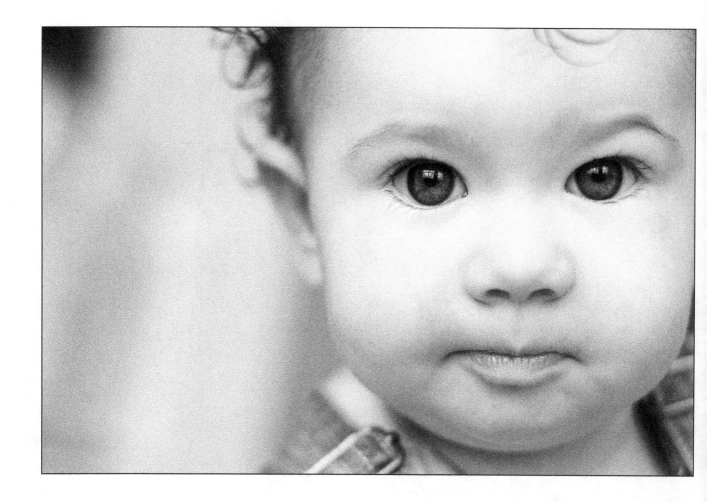

Baby eyes illuminate pureness of heart
Without the mind's defenses
That blind us from
The spirit that lies within.

May we experience life eternally through baby eyes.

Lesson 1
The Art of Meditation

> The Tao is called the Great Mother:
> Empty yet inexhaustible,
> It gives birth to infinite worlds.
> It is always present within you.
> You can use it any way you want.
>
> —Lao Tzu, *Tao Te Ching*

> Your spirit self is a "pregnant void" needing only direction.
> Intend a direction to create your life.
>
> —Tammy Wise, BodyLogos

Meditation as a Phenomenon

In Tao philosophy, nature is considered the supreme intelligence, the creator of all life. The ancient Tao sages recognized that nature supplied powerful imagery that connected them to the greater whole, to what they referred to as "universal spirit." Once you experience yourself as a part of creation, rather than separate from it, you experience yourself as an extension of nature, an extension of universal spirit.

Tao meditation was originally meant to help deepen understanding of the sacred and mystical phenomena observed in the universe. Still meditation practice is a quiet, mindful stretch to connect inwardly with the self. Active meditation practice is a quiet, mindful stretch to connect the self outwardly with the universe.

For example, the traditional Tao active meditation from the Han dynasty (206 BC–AD 220) of embodying an eagle offers a very specific union. The eagle within you surfaces. Then, as the eagle, you experience yourself as an integral part of a spiritual whole. In this way, all creation becomes a mirror, the teachers that reveal all aspects of being you.

A flying eagle represents the spirit self because of its holy, godlike qualities: silent, serene, and often hauntingly unnoticed. This exercise acquaints you with personal freedom. It gives you an experience of serene competence, helping you soar to the top of your game. It elicits in you independence, grace, and command. It is the only traditional Tao meditation in the BodyLogos practice.

Tao Eagle Active Meditation
Confidence. Perspective. Independence.
mindthebody.bodylogos.com/video1
(abbreviated description)

Ancient Taoists explore this eagle image by standing with arms outstretched. Feel your arms as wings, effortlessly holding you aloft, eyes open and attentive. Visualize your eagle self effortlessly soar to great heights, with sharp eyes keen to all details on the landscape below. You are intelligent and alert, gliding across the big-blue open sky. Enjoy the wind beneath your wings and the confidence of your mastery in the sky. You are one with spirit, untouched by insignificant matters, body relaxed, mind and eyes fully awake. Notice everything without focusing on anything. Connect to your independent sacred command and elevated yet piercing sight. Continue the exercise as long as the mind doesn't wander. If it does, stop and begin again.

Do you enjoy being an eagle? (Would you rather be a monkey?) Check in with yourself and discover your relationship with this angelic creature. Notice whether you were able to let yourself fully experience an eagle's flight or whether you were constantly wondering whether you were doing the exercise right. This kind of free association may feel foreign to you at first, but as you become more comfortable stretching your imagination, you will stop looking at the video and just fly.

Eagle Exercise Wish List

- Your mood and sense of personal value are more self-assured.
- You've separated from self-doubt.
- Your feeling of isolation has transformed into independence.
- Your experience of you is one of quiet competence.
- You perceive life from a newfound elevated viewpoint.

The Tao eagle active meditation is just one example. If there is a physical or emotional sensation you would like to transform, use that as the incentive for your meditation practice. To get you started, here are a few ideas:

- To feel more physically grounded, meditate on being a mountain.
- For more of a lightness of being, meditate on being the wind.
- To feel less emotionally guarded, imagine a beautiful flower blossoming from within.
- For less reactivity, imagine the loving eyes of your favorite animal softening your heart.

You are using your imagination to initiate a meditative state into being, because feeling whatever transformation you wish for is, at first, an alien feeling. But by setting an intention for your meditation—and drawing examples from nature to ground your experience—you can simultaneously connect with your spirit self and the world.

Today meditation is commonly used for its end result of relaxation and stress reduction as opposed to a journey toward resolution and connection. If your approach to meditation is focused on your desire to de-stress, your practice will become an escape from the world and bound by life concerns. It's true that retracting inwardly enables you to slow down and become curious about your spirit self. However, it will be difficult to deepen a relationship with your spirit self and integrate it into your life if it's not connected to your integral role as a part of universal spirit.

Exercise focused on tangible end results falls into the same trap. There's nothing wrong with wanting to look and feel good, but when a workout takes on an atmosphere of having to fix something broken or deficient, the practice becomes a place to compete for your own self-worth. A result-oriented practice, though it may be effective short term, sets up a haphazard experience that bounces you between two poles—one where you are enmeshed with life and one where you resent it. And though you are able to increase your physical strength and stamina, your strength is trapped behind your tension and cannot connect outwardly with the expansiveness of universal spirit. In BodyLogos, your workout resistance becomes a symbol of life's opposition, offering you a chance to practice connecting to resistance with curiosity rather than tension. Then your workout practice gives your mind and body an inward timeout from the tension of self-criticism, incorporating instead the poise of self-competence into the experience of your workout.

Meditative fitness is a quiet, mindful stretch that connects with resistance as if it were a connection with life. As you stretch away from what you know in yourself and toward what is less familiar in the world, you are awakening an innate trust in universal spirit. You are deliberately trusting that this connection will be one of safety, belonging, and awakening. Now your practice can do more than align your human self; it becomes the foundation for being your authentic, integrated, vulnerable, and bright spirit self in the world.

Active and still meditations are ways to intimately understand your own consciousness and fully use the power of a mind-body relationship. Active meditation specializes in transforming what your body is holding that encumbers your evolution, while still meditation specializes in expanding beyond your mind's limitations. The practice of meditation expands your perspective while calming your nervous system, which in turn gives you a sense of personal salvation and self-assurance. The sense of being supported unfolds as you deepen your connection to the universe and your certainty that it's for you, not against you.

Active Meditation

Meditation is a yin experience: contemplative, passive, and private. On the other hand, being active is the epitome of yang: practical, dynamic, and overt. Together, they create active meditation, a whole experience whereby your inner and outer lives thrive as one. Through your strength training, active meditation connects you to outside resistance with strength and sensitivity—a full spectrum of presence and potential. This connection awakens a central bond of oneness, whereby you connect yourself with the resistance as if it were an extension of you. The connection is made with care and concern. Your intention is to meet it, not beat it.

An active meditation posture requires the same focal point as still meditation. BodyLogos uses the framework of your bones to lead you to the tranquil stillness found in your body's center of gravity, known in Tao as your dan tien. Maintaining skeletal alignment feeds your connection with this central stillness and insists on a central bond of oneness. Any forced reps or reckless action that compromises your skeletal alignment compromises this central focal point. That quiet meditative presence that frees you from self-doubt and connects you to self-assurance is lost. Aggressive approaches to weight training walk this path and can weaken rather than strengthen you.

> ### What It's Not
>
> A common fitness mantra is "mind over matter," used to ward off physical laziness and discomfort. This mantra has motivated fitness enthusiasts to push past their previous physical limitations. When you look a little closer, there is a "matter of fact." Body limitations are expressions that are asking to be recognized. As an animated blueprint of your life story, your body's posture reveals who you are, what you want, and in what ways you are struggling with your present life. Your muscles hold the mysteries of past hopes and disappointments, good deeds and transgressions, accomplishments and secrets. Therefore, if you blindly push past or give up on your body's response to physical challenge without first considering its message, you actually disregard something your body is holding onto intently. That tension has morphed into the intention that is presently directing your life.

For centuries, Taoists have believed that our ability to listen to the body is as valuable as listening to the mind. Through the body's intelligence, we are informed and then inspired to create positive change, as opposed to simply exceeding our last performance. When we listen to—and then release—our pain and tension, we can steer our lives in the direction we want to go and build the real, relaxed strength required to get there.

~ feel into this ~
The Wisdom in Pain

Imagine, for instance, that every time you try to exercise, you develop lower back pain. You may begin your exercise pursuit with the belief that your back is weak and that once it is strengthened, the pain will subside. Through sheer will and determination, you limber up the back and exercise through the back's complaints. No pain, no gain, right? In time, physical exhaustion replaces mental determination, and your belief that strength is the answer dwindles, and confusion sets in. You may eventually come to believe that exercise is bad for you, so you avoid it. Mental supposition replaces physical freedom, because when you stop exercising, the pain subsides. But is the pain really gone, or is it just not being spoken to?

Engaging in a conversation with your lower back pain, which is the holding area for fear, means to systematically move with your pain rather than through it and allow it to express its various discomforts within a balanced, safe range of movement. Learning your external physical needs (limited range of movement) and internal emotional origin (what the fear is attached to) offers a holistic connection that addresses the root of your back pain. Once you are wise to the pain's nature, you can mentally resolve the conflict and physically let it go. You are able to exercise without constantly questioning whether it's good or bad for you.

Deeming exercise as good or bad is transformed into a willingness to take a closer look at your needs. In this way you begin to wonder, rather than fear, what else your physical needs have to teach you about yourself.

Tao practitioners understand that a balanced body supports a balanced mind—and vice versa. All Tao healing arts refer to these holistic relationships to understand the nature of disease. Inspired by this fact and using the principles of Tao, I have recognized the influence and analogous characteristics emotions have on the muscular system. Every muscle group corresponds to an aspect of the self and performs specific duties in regard to our survival. When isolated in a strength-training workout, that isolated emotion is stimulated. The BodyLogos psyche-muscular blueprint separates this understanding into psyche-muscular components.

Tammy Wise

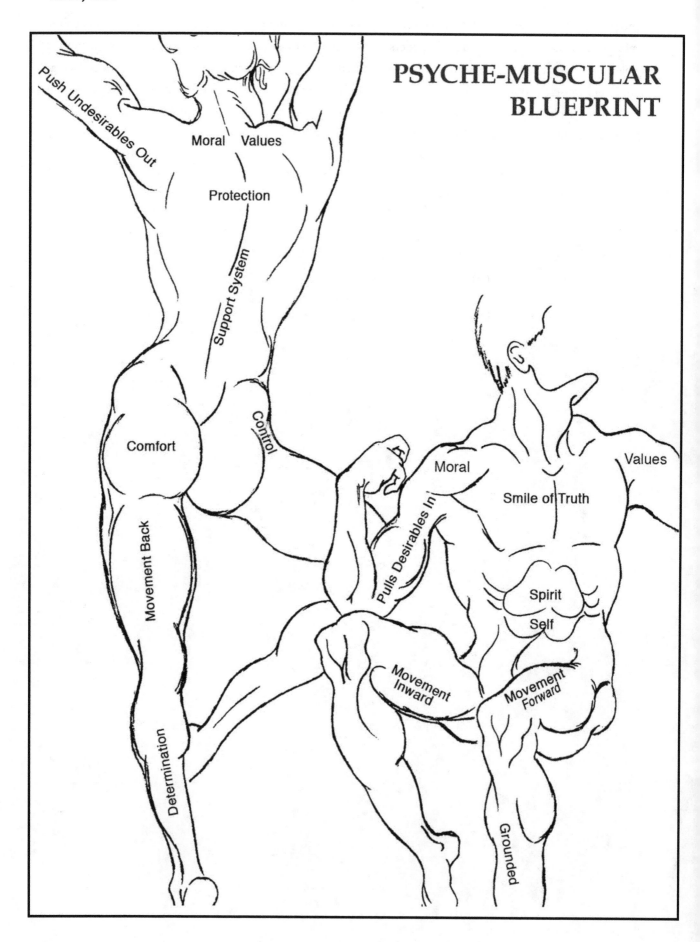

BodyLogos Psyche-Muscular Components

What follows is a simple explanation of the psyche-muscular components. These meditations will unite your mind and body on a common goal, creating the alignment needed for your spirit to awaken.

Abdominal Muscles: Spirit Self

As you observe your muscular center of gravity, challenging the abdominals is a time to focus inwardly on what is essentially you—to appreciate who you are now and who you are becoming.

Chest Muscles: Smile of Truth

Because they blanket the physical seat of your emotions, as you experience the strength of your chest experience your heart expanding and your dreams emerging.

Back Muscles: Protection

As your body's shield, back muscles give you a sense of safekeeping and courage as well as support for gentler heartfelt expression.

Shoulder Muscles: Moral Values

Shoulders frame your posture. Shoulder challenges frame the values presently being affected in your life to bring about clarity and authentic right action.

Biceps Muscles: Pulling Desirables Inward

Biceps' pulling action is an occasion to ask what you need mentally, physically, emotionally, and spiritually to create the life you envision.

Triceps Muscles: Pushing Undesirables Away

While working triceps' pushing action, integrate what you need to clear out of your life with a sense of personal responsibility and self-love.

Buttocks Muscles: Comfort

Because of the buttocks' strength and padding, keep the intention of buttock challenges connected to feeling comfortable with what's "within" and accepting of what's "without."

Quadriceps Muscles: Movement Forward

Motivate forward propelling quadriceps' activity by visualizing a goal, aim, or life purpose. Feel what motivates you.

Hamstring Muscles: Movement Backward

Consciously use backward-propelling hamstring movement as a time to reflect on your past. Experience the past neutrally, bringing more compassion into your present and future life.

Inner Thigh Muscles: Movement Inward

Use the inward movement of your inner thighs to connect you to your center. As you move in any direction, experience their constant inward commitment to stay aligned connected with your commitment to be authentically you.

Calf and Shin Muscles: Grounding and Determination

While challenging the spring-like levers of your lower legs, feel the grounded determination it takes to be your authentic self. Experience your tenacity.

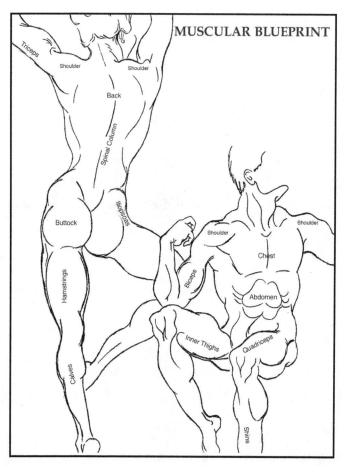

Iliopsoas: Control

When iliopsoas muscles (hip fold) are felt, they are generally being overused in a desperate attempt to control movement (and life). Let their voice lead you back to your central support and direct the flow of strength back to your primary supporting muscles (abdominals, inner thighs, and buttocks).

When isolating each muscle group, concentrate on the essence of its emotion. Allow the meditation to empower your physical abilities, while the physical action gives your mind focus. Moreover, just as in nature, everything in your body is interconnected, and every isolated action has consequences. By observing the response your entire physical body has to an isolated physical challenge, you will realize the response your entire being has to a specific emotional challenge. This is the process of uncovering unconscious muscular holding patterns.

Through specific observations, you learn to recognize the expressions of holding patterns. When you pair the expression of specific muscular holding patterns with their psyche-muscular component, you learn to decipher your body's posture and performance as a language and recognize that this language comes from the authority of your inner being. Strength training exercises are infused with emotional contemplation, and you find meaning that goes far beyond the size and shape of your muscles.

Five Forms of Expression

BodyLogos observes five forms of expression as they develop and change in workouts. Through them, you learn to recognize the body's messages in an exceptionally intimate way. Use these observations, in combination with the psyche-muscular blueprint, as a foundation to discern the meaning of your body's expression.

Posture: Balance

Observe how muscle groups relate to each other to see which psyche-muscular areas are dependent on each other. Excess muscle tightness illustrates the more aggressive (rescuer) muscle in the relationship; excess muscle laxity illustrates the more passive (abandoned) muscle in the relationship.

Ability: Weakness vs. Strength

Pay attention to which muscles fatigue easiest and which are your greatest source of strength. Muscles that fatigue quickly indicate which emotional aspects of your life need the most development, and your strongest muscles indicate your greatest emotional confidence and strength.

Size: Willingness

Pay attention to the size of your movements. Small, mindful motions show a willingness to explore yourself. Large, uncontrolled motions show where you haven't yet been willing to explore yourself.

Enjoyment: Comfort vs. Avoidance

The muscle groups you enjoy working show you where you are comfortable physically and emotionally. The muscles you can't really feel or dislike working show you where you are uncomfortable physically and emotionally.

Coordination: Reliability

Intellectually, you may understand what the exercise is, but your body isn't following—like a split between mind and body. This lack of coordination may be body wide or muscle specific, and it can be expressed in many ways. As you describe what you are feeling physically, recognize it also as what you are doing mentally and creating emotionally.

These basic expressions highlight and interpret the body's holding patterns. Once the pattern is identified, you can pinpoint the emotional tension that created the disruption through your meditative focus. Then, through precise mindful adjustments in skeletal alignment and muscular balance, you challenge your body to integrate those adjustments using strength-training exercises. In this way, strength training is able to unlock unwanted tension and establish a preferred pattern. Holding pattern by holding pattern, the energy system is restored to its original nature. These are foundational changes that reconstruct the underpinnings of habitual and unconscious ways of being.

To have the sensitivity to recognize these psyche-muscular expressions, you need to work from a place of neutrality. To do this, you need space for objectivity. The space I am referring to is internal—an inner space that decompresses the habitual ways you hold yourself together and the defenses that keep them compressed. This pregnant void of space within comes from exchanging your tension for your breath.

Connect to Your Breath

Life breathes. Breath connects your creative life force with the creative life force of the natural world. Creative life force is energized and exchanged by breathing. Exercising your breath builds up your energy reserve to realize personal potential.

> Creative life force
> Is
> The inception of being,
> Mysterious and organized,
> A force that creates passage and inspires life,
> Birthing a creation into a creator.

Though the lungs facilitate breathing, it's the diaphragm—a transverse muscle beneath the lungs—that enhances your lung's capacity. Greater lung capacity creates a surplus of energy that is then stored in your dan tien energy center, your physical center of gravity where *all* action is initiated.

The dan tien is located three fingers below the belly button, between front and back physical planes; it is nestled centrally within the body beneath the abdominal muscles. The lungs sit above the diaphragm, and the dan tien sits below the diaphragm. The rise and fall of your diaphragm keeps them communicating and connected. Think of your lungs as an energy generator and the dan tien as your energy storage tank. You can have a full tank, an empty tank, or anything in between. But it's up to you to manage it.

Managing your energy reserve means recognizing breathing as physical and mental respiration, because it affects physical and mental performance. Your creative life force is nourished by your body's inspiration and expiration, and breathing influences thoughts inspired and thoughts expired.

There are many breathing techniques, but there is a general principle that umbrellas the gamut of choices. Slow breathing relaxes the mind, and quick breathing excites the body. Be careful not to grasp for your inhale. Simply allow the breath to seep into your body. With your inhale, you are practicing the ability to receive energy from the universe with ease; with your exhale you are practicing the ability to release tension from your body with grace.

Breathing Exercise
Centeredness. Preparedness. Energized.
mindthebody.bodylogos.com/video2
(abbreviated description)

Like Buddha, fully accept all that is. Sit with your low abdomen completely relaxed and expanded outward. Breathe in to fill the abdomen like a billows. Then, like Gandhi, fully release all that is no longer. Gently contract the abdominal muscles to guide the breath out on your exhale.

Allow your expanding breath to guide the abdominal muscles to release on your inhale and the contracting abdominal muscles to guide the breath on your exhale.

Use slow breathing when you need to build up your energy reserve, your mind needs to focus its attention, or mental clutter is distracting you. Use fast breathing when you need to rouse the body's energy, your body needs to focus its strength, or you're preparing for a workout.

Give yourself some time to experience your altered state after the breathing challenge is over. You may experience dizziness at first, because you're not used to metabolizing so much oxygen. You may also notice that tension interferes with your ability to give and receive breath freely. As you practice, your body becomes more subtle and available to your wants.

Breathing Exercise Wish List

- Your mind becomes less anxious and more focused.
- Your body's tension releases and is free to receive new energy.
- An awareness of your senses is heightened.
- A dynamic presence in your center is realized.
- You become curious about giving and receiving.

Most of us can relate to sitting in the dentist chair and awaiting the next torture tool to scrape, poke, and drill into a tooth and pain that already exists. The contact can take your breath away.

Roberta, clutching the arms of the reclined chair and squinting into the dentist's spotlight, realized she had stopped breathing. After gulping air back into her lungs, she remembered the breathing exercise we had been working on. She quietly began breathing in and out slowly and consciously as the dentist continued probing. Not only did this full-bellowing breath calm her down and surrender her grip, but her focus on breathing redirected her attention onto something besides her pain.

> I felt empowered that I had a way of helping myself and relieved that I could focus on me instead of the dentist!
>
> —Roberta

Trauma Takes Your Breath Away

Trauma arrests breathing. It startles your diaphragm into spasm, restricting breathing mechanics. Shallow breathing disconnects you from your body, because it predominantly exercises and oxygenates muscles above the diaphragm. Your attention becomes heady; your voice becomes higher. *You stop feeling your feelings and start thinking your feelings.* We've all experienced this event at one time or another when we've told an emotional story. We start the story, wanting to share the heartache, but when we get to the emotional trauma, we change course and end the story in a tirade about how unfair the experience was. We went from feeling to thinking. By deepening breathing mechanics, you steadily relax the diaphragm, oxygenate your whole body, and permit pockets of locked-up trauma to loosen its grip. Not only will you take deeper breaths and begin using the lower register of your speaking voice, but you will feel more connected within yourself.

An external source causes trauma. You are psychologically or physically caught off guard or out of control. On the day I realized trauma was something that comes from outside, not inside, me, it was like the clouds parted, "Oh. Oh! This is not my fault!" What happened to me wasn't my fault, and the continued pain and tension weren't either. Once I recognized trauma for what it was, I recovered my power. I gained agency, the choice either to continue to let trauma sit in the driver's seat or to come back into my body and reclaim my worth, my sense of belonging, and the freedom to openheartedly share myself with the world.

Trauma can have serious long-term effects or be a vehicle for personal development. In the latter, you gain an internal perspective of something—a reference point for self-mastery. In the former, you remain outside the experience, unable to connect to the part of yourself that is traumatized.

To connect to your greatest joy, you connect by association with your greatest traumas. To summon one into existence is to summon the other. Your breath is the way into the places you are locked out of. These are the places where you freeze and feel self-conscious or defensive, the places where you're weak, rigid, or numb.

My introduction to this subject was through the coping skills my body exhibited through my repeated childhood traumas. A physical and mental disassociation would happen. Poof—I went from a curled up, terrified, tension-filled body in reality to being perfectly aligned between earth and sky, my body completely at ease in a mental separation from reality. I was totally conscious of my body's state in both universes, independent from each other, but unable to control which environment I was in. Disassociating is a natural strategy the mind uses to survive an event that is unmanageable or frightening. To have endured the incidents in my childhood, with a physical account of nature's way of protecting me, was a gift.

From my experience, I learned a reference point for strength and its distinction from tension. I was living tension but was rescued by strength. My work with BodyLogos has emerged from wanting to step into my strength at will, using the body as a gateway into physical and psychological grace, to supporting others in doing the same. At the root of stepping into my strength was a willingness to trust my breath—trust that where it would take me was in the best interest of creating my future story.

I believe we all suffer traumas that cause us to detach, and in these moments we establish beliefs that direct the course of our lives away from what is life sustaining and toward the very thing we are avoiding. Feeling the need to put on airs, for example, could come from the silent trauma of not hearing enough positive reinforcement about who you actually are and never learning that your unique way of being is valued.

What It's Not

"Keeping up with the Joneses." This phrase that refers to doing things to impress others comes from a cartoon strip of that name that launched in 1913 and ran for twenty-six years in the *New York Globe*. Rather than growing out of the need to "keep up with the Joneses," when the last episode of the comic strip ran, it seems we're trying twice as hard. Now, with the rise of social media telling us who we should be and what is relevant, we are more or less convinced we're not good enough. The need to impress others has been joined by a desperate chase to feel successful. We could blame the media for this epidemic, but the result of splitting our minds and bodies to the point of not knowing, valuing, or accepting who we are and what we deem relevant is the underlying grounds for self-deprivation. To experience ourselves with ease, we need to stop chasing success and stand in it.

My wish for us all is to be a neutral witness to our lives, have the courage to feel deeply—breathe deeply—and actively seek the stillness that preceded our traumas. I am committed to this because I believe the human body possesses divinity in the inner space our alignment and breath create and suffers terribly from the compression of modern-day norms: overstimulation, overreaching, and multitasking.

Active stillness is the practice of being successful moment by moment. Active stillness allows us to connect from the inside out rather than performing from the outside in.

Active Stillness

Active stillness is a period when reorganization of the nervous system is permitted. A transition from what was habitual to what is preferred takes place. Active stillness recognizes that to feel, experience, allow, align, and surrender is to take action. Although passive in nature, these requests require inner communication and diligence.

Only after mastering these actions in stillness can we become skilled at them in motion. Active stillness is first established in the BodyLogos practice between activities: the time between sets, the preparatory breaths before bursting into a challenge, and the integration of your active meditation insights at the close of a workout. These transitory times bring *clear intention* into alignment (mind-body relationship) and *focused attention* into posture (musculoskeletal relationship). As you develop the mind-body consistency to maintain what you prefer (physical alignment, emotional approval, and mental serenity) without constant scrutiny, relaxed strength will become your stance through workout transitions and activities.

Clear Intention

Clear intention is knowing what you want and stretching beyond what you know to get it. It is that gut feeling that says, "I know I want to get married and have kids—I don't know for sure if this is the guy to do it with." It is the ethereal work of active stillness. It is both the deepest and most expanded aspect of inner communication.

Clear intention connects you to the big picture of your efforts—why you are doing what you are doing. It connects you to your center of gravity as it relates to gravity itself, perceiving physical posture as an antenna that connects you to things that are intrinsic and eternal. Without bias, you connect equally to what is below and what is above; you surrender your weight into the earth and stretch relaxation up toward the sky equally and precisely. Through your commitment to posture, you are plugging into a celestial order of unequaled grandeur and elegance in which the body itself partakes and exemplifies.

This is the foundation for the more expanded alignment of mind and body. Mind-body alignment is established on clear intent to open you to subconscious insight. To be open to this deep, internal communication, you actively stretch relaxation outwardly through your alignment—beyond what you consciously understand into what you subconsciously know. You become a witness to the meditative journey your intention is taking you on from a blissful state in which the body is at its strongest—I call it "equipoise" (more on equipoise in chapter 5). From this multidirectional stretch of relaxation, you become liberated from tension, whereby your sense of separation between mind and body evaporates.

Clear intention helps you to receive what a challenge can offer you. It opens communication between the conscious and subconscious, past and present, mind and body, giving you direction in the following ways:

- A warning to descend into a protective posture
- Permission to expand outwardly into a provoking or arousing position
- Encouragement to ascend toward a loving connection
- Stability to withstand the added weight of being needed
- Or the freedom to contract inwardly and take a personal stand

Focused Attention

Focused attention is learning who you are and are not—and using what you know to create positive change. While clear intention is the motivating wind in your sails, focused attention is the anchor that keeps you from blowing off course. Your clear intention may be to get married, as above. But if you know a desire to give back to the world is one of your most strongly held values—and you're unable to respect a partner who doesn't share this value—you must keep your focused attention on that quality in every person you date.

Focused attention is the groundwork of active stillness. Focused attention is in service to clear intent, maintaining the central antenna of your posture as a *neutral* stretch between earth and sky. Focused attention makes you aware of the places you deviate from deliberate choice; instead, you unintentionally uphold the restrictive beliefs left over from trauma. It connects you to the subtle energy flowing between muscles and bones that keeps them related to the effortlessness of centripetal and centrifugal forces. You experience subtle energy as a powerful influence directing the quality of your inner relationships with your body, mind, and spirit.

This is the foundation for musculoskeletal posture. It aligns your bones and balances your muscles when on task. It is a conscious relationship with your mind to value what it is witnessing, a conscious agreement with your body to allow change to happen, a conscious direction of your breath to orchestrate deliberate posture. Giving challenge (physical, mental, or emotional), focused attention makes the body more useful to itself, more aware of its environment, more certain of its intolerances, and hence more adaptive to seemingly benign threats to itself (misaligning beliefs).

Focused attention opens communication between bones and muscles, head and heart, action and release, establishing what you need to give to a challenge, such as the following:

- A commitment to isolate a specific psyche-muscular component
- Mindfulness to surrender what muscles you don't need to engage
- Concentration to engage what muscles you do need
- A steady resolve to balance and align musculoskeletal integrity in the face of a challenge
- A deliberate awareness of your body's response to your meditative state

Active stillness teaches you to stay nonreactive in the midst of challenge, chaos, or confusion by aligning the focused attention of musculoskeletal posture with the clear intention of mind-body alignment. To practice active stillness, you use the challenge of physical fitness as your muse. This gives you an expanded viewpoint so you can step out of defenses that encourage you to over-exert or under-exert your life force. It also gives you the neutral attention to observe the emotional origin of an upset when it does happen. It connects your head and heart so "thinking" and "feeling" can work as a team and so you can respond to the challenge as a neutral witness.

Neutral Attention Offers Awareness

To be neutral is to allow possibility to develop naturally. To witness is to observe life. A neutral witness observes life's potential. Accurately aligning your head on your spine neutralizes your central nervous system to naturally become a neutral witness to life. You can imagine how many variables there are in your neck when aligning the crown of the head over the heart center. And let's say that the crown center influences your "thinking" and the heart center your "feeling." Accurate alignment offers awareness between your head and your heart so you can be in a state of "think" and "feel" simultaneously.

Your neckline oscillates between being a "pigeon" and a "swan," between being contracted in the neck, exhibiting nervousness, and contracted in the throat, exhibiting the quality of being stoic. To find center, we take from both sides of that duality.

- From the pigeon, we take the parallel roof of the mouth; feel for it being parallel with the ground and glide your head back into alignment, maintaining it.
- From the swan, we take the open occipital hollows at the base of the skull. You can massage them to become familiar with and relax them. Then adjust the roof of your mouth so it's parallel with the ground while you maintain the hollow's relaxed open state.

Let's explore this balance in movement. Feel for the relationship your head, neck, throat, and spine has with gravity to distinguish the subtle differences between "thinking" movement and "feeling" movement.

Neutral Witness Exercise
Compassion. Intuition. Objectivity.
mindthebody.bodylogos.com/video3
(abbreviated description)

Sit or stand erect. Gently drop your head forward, allowing the back of the neck to stretch. Take several deep breaths and permit the back of your neck to expand. Vertebrae in the cervical spine separate vertically, and muscles stabilizing the neck release horizontally. Maintaining the horizontal expansion in the neck muscles, lift your chin up through the crown of the head until your head is once again aligned with the spine. Don't contract the neck; rather, lift the smile of your jaw up through the tips of your ears and the crown of your head. Notice the widened-back space at the base of the skull coupled with a relaxed throat. Continue to magnify the space between head and heart. Experience the widened-back presence in mind and body, realize your expanded consciousness, and enjoy observing without judgment.

Take a moment to observe the quality of your attention. You may get restless during this exercise, your body wanting to go faster or feeling that it's wasting time. Or contrarily, you may drift off, your mind in a daze as your body stretches and rotates in a stupor. This is natural when you first start to align mind and body. They are learning each other's rhythm.

Neutral Witness Wish List

- Feel yourself building an awareness muscle.
- Permit time and space to control your attention and feel what is true for you.
- Experience a widened-back physical stance that connects you inwardly.
- Be in the moment rather than in your previous anxieties.
- Feel thoughts and emotions from your life story more integrated with your spirit self.

As a student of tango, my client Denise wanted to improve her balance, perfect her alignment, and build core strength. Her primary misalignment was in her neck and throat relationship; her neck was hyper-contracted, and her throat was hypo-released, causing neck pain and positioning her head in front of her spine. Initially, when lying supine, she couldn't rest her head on the ground; a pillow was necessary to support its forward assertion. As we released her neck and shoulder tension, and she began to feel her Adam's apple relaxing back into her neck and throat relationship, she began to neutralize her head's reach, and it could rest freely on the ground once again.

Gradually, her head aligned properly on a vertical spine. Her standing alignment and balance have greatly improved, as has her movement's grace—so much so that she encouraged her dance partner to consider adopting the same head, neck and throat alignment. She also realized that without proper alignment, she breathed directly into her dance partner's face—a factor that was taking the allure out of their tango.

> It takes two to tango, as the saying goes; however, the truth in tango is that each one is "on their own" in some aspects. Each partner has to take responsibility for his or her own balance, to remain on his or her axis, and not to rely on the other person to "do the job." Working with Tammy helped me to reach that goal. And more so I, with a better understanding of alignment, became more selective as to the dancers I choose to partner with.
>
> —Denise

In the BodyLogos practice, you are the neutral witness to your own experience. You recognize the resistance used in the strength-training exercises as the resistances being faced in life, and your commitment to alignment in the face of that resistance as your commitment to connect with personal integrity. This approach to physical movement starts from active stillness, and it sets up your exercise challenge with both personal integrity and universal alignment. You are connecting wholly—your body, mind, and spirit are integrated and connecting with the world—permitting the world to connect fully with you.

Active stillness—the ethereal work of clear intention and groundwork of focused attention—is at the heart of the BodyLogos active meditation practice. To master it, slow down. Use your time between challenges as time to organize your relationship with gravity, resistance, and yourself. Exercise active stillness before, during, and after each challenge. Use the time between sets to reorganize your body's posture and your mind's disposition, the starting position of an exercise as the calm before the storm of an energy outburst, and cool-down time as the integration of change. Choose a meditative intention intuitively (like those listed on p. 6). Allow the moment to move you.

To experience the deep connection of a meditative state in physical movement, breathe clear intention into your center of gravity (dan tien). Focus attention on how you connect to a resistance; be a neutral witness to your mind and body, and experience your three dimensions as they unite through active stillness.

BodyLogos practice uses the intention and attention of active stillness throughout a workout. Active stillness can be done outside your strength-training exercises in any position—perhaps seated on the floor or a chair, lying on the floor or a bench, stretching out on a gymnastic ball or a foam tube, or standing or holding a posture. What is crucial in activating meditative stillness is focusing your mind and body on the same intention at the same moment, with the same degree of curiosity attached to your mental and physical perceptions.

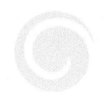

~ feel into this ~
Connected Transitions

Say you just finished a cardio warm-up and are about to jump into your strength-training series. Pause and experience the moment; celebrate the heart-rousing journey the mind and body just shared. Witness the mind and body shifting gears together and feel the shared shift as an intimate exchange. Sit, hydrate, or stretch and experience the reorganization happening between mind and body while you allow your heart and muscles to settle down; feel the weight of your bones ground you before embarking on another challenge. Observe your breath as it begins to deepen and slow down. Continue to zoom out—expand mind, body, and spirit—until you arrive in a quiet place of infinite possibilities, listen, and connect to the moment. Once your breath stabilizes, you are ready to continue with your next exercise challenge.

To create an environment where the insights found in your workout have an opportunity to integrate, pause between workout elements and finish with stillness. Let yourself feel change rather than think change.

The Self within the self

Meditation encourages "less is more." You experience this truth during your workout when your inward commitment to your alignment is more important than the number of repetitions completed with the chosen resistance. When quality goes up, quantity can go down. You will also experience this at the close of your workout when you choose to take time for stillness rather than squeezing in one more exercise. To relax with the metaphysical changes made through your workout is to allow the change to organically spill over into your life and integrate it into your consciousness. The awareness of newfound postural changes needs to be clearly felt; otherwise, you return to automatic reactive behavior in both your physical and mental stances. If you're working hard in your workouts and feeling no real improvements—or if you suffer from boredom—take time for still meditation or a meditative stretch at the close of your workouts. You will begin to see progress and recognize change; and what's more, you will feel the stir of inspiration. The greatest rewards are found in the subtle yet profound moments of your quietude.

~ feel into this ~
Trilogy of the Self

Visualize a speck of light at your physical energy center—dan tien, three fingers below the navel and centered between the front and back of your torso. Use your imagination to expand that speck of light throughout your being until you feel present in your body and time. This event is experiencing where you are.

As this central light emanates, allow your mind to relax into it until you're no longer an observer of your own light but rather the light itself. This is experiencing who you are.

Maintain this alignment until your attention stops trying to pull you out of it. You are experiencing the body, mind, and spirit as a united trilogy. This is experiencing the possibility—an expanding "pregnant void"—of creative life force.

Remember, you are a spiritual-physical being, managed by a mind. Your body feels, your mind listens, and your spirit expands. Expand your ability to listen, and you feel where you are. Keep expanding, listening, and feeling, and you'll experience who you are. Keep expanding your experience of you, and you keep expanding your possibilities in life. To realize your full significance, mastery of attention is essential. All three dimensions of the self—body, mind, and spirit—are attendees. Use this trilogy of self-experience as a way to explore being present in all three dimensions of the self at the same time.

Emotion Chapter

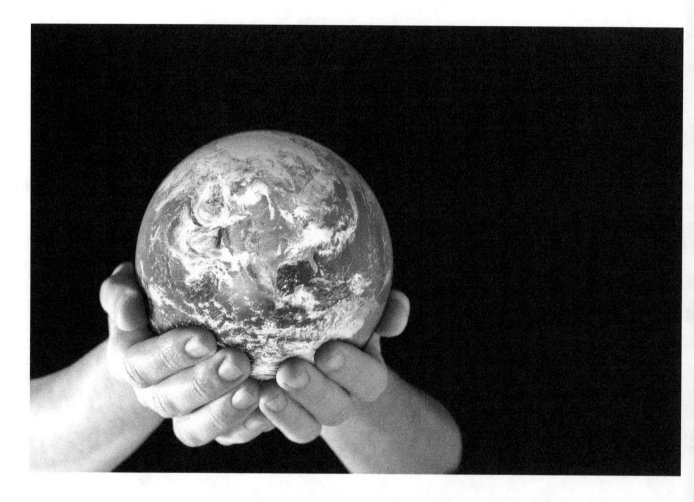

You are not the center of the universe,
But you are the center of your universe.
Together we, as a universal creative life force, co-create the world.

Lesson 2
The Practice of Meditation

Until you make the unconscious conscious,
it will direct your life and you will call it fate.

—Carl Jung, psychiatrist and psychoanalyst

The five elements of Tao recognize that the flow between elements creates cyclical patterns, and they observe five emotions that cycle routinely through human expressions.

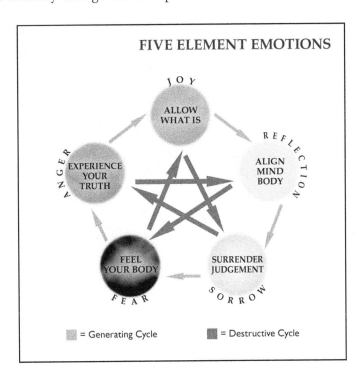

Element	Emotion	Direction of Mind
Water	Fear	Feel Your Body
Wood	Anger	Experience Your Truth
Fire	Joy	Allow What Is
Earth	Reflection	Align Mind and Body
Metal	Sorrow	Surrender Judgment

I'll depict this flow of emotion using the generating cycle. Human nature shows that the experience of *fear*, with its deep, piercing paralysis, brings forth the aggression of anger, which lifts us out of our temporary freeze.

Anger then explodes—be it toward another, toward oneself, or held tightly within, enraged by being disapproved of, disrespected, or disregarded. Once expressed, the flip-flop of fear to anger turns to the relief of *joy*. The conflict has burned itself out, leaving peace and hope in its wake. From this more stable position, one begins to *reflect* on the subtler aspects of an interaction and take some responsibility for its course. Then finally, through understanding an interaction, *sorrow* is inevitable in regret for one's own part or another's misfortune in the trials of living. The generating cycle imparts maturity and evolution.

And just as your emotions flow through the generating cycle to cultivate growth and maturity, each direction of mind flows from one to the other through the generating cycle in your meditation practice. Recognizing your generating cycle, created from these progressions, helps you to discover how a meditation design can best support your emotional development.

In our meditation practice, keep the following in mind:

- When you experience fear, you *feel your body* because it is the body that carries the emotional trauma of your life story, and the consequences of revisiting a trauma can feel frightening.
- When you experience anger, you also *experience your truth* because being a neutral witness to yourself is recognizing the good, the bad, and the ugly; we often are angry at what we see and need to be truthful about that disappointment to resolve it.
- When you experience joy, you *allow what is* because you have accepted that you aren't a perfect human being physically or mentally and can now focus on becoming happy.
- When in reflection, you *align mind and body* because an introspective awareness is revealed to create this alignment; and once aligned, a reflective connection to all you have been, are, and are becoming unfolds.
- When you experience sorrow, you *surrender judgment*. Sorrow is the lonely space left when we first surrender the beliefs that kept previous judgments going, beliefs that misled our judgments but kept us company.

When first considering the transition from bicycle to motorcycle, I would *feel my body's* fear overriding my excitement. This would then elicit anger, because to *experience my truth* was to experience myself as weaker than the traditional male rider. I felt I would blow the whole women's movement for equality if I cowered. I recognized the need to own my feelings and strengthen my faith in myself. This permission to *allow what is* brought joy back to my motorcycle idea, because I felt that if nothing else, I was strong enough to be honest with myself. Learning from bikers how to get started and *reflecting* on their counsel *aligned mind and body* on what felt like my pie-in-the-sky dream. I say "pie in the sky" because, although each action step got me closer to being a biker, there was sorrow attached to how far away actualizing the dream was. I managed to *surrender judgment* about the convoluted path required to realize my dream by remembering the rider's (very Tao) motto, "It's about the journey, not the destination." This generating cycle of emotions went around and around until my dream manifested with a Harley-Davidson 883 Sportster. That was twenty years ago. I now own my dream bike, a BMW 1200RC.

But there are times in our lives when the generating cycle's growth is detrimental to our meditative practice, and the destructive cycle is more healing.

For example, in our meditation practice, keep the following in mind:

- When battling a serious illness, to *experience your truth* is too disruptive; to *feel the body* and *allow what is* will give you a gentler path toward acceptance.

- The high-frequency energy of *allow what is* can often elevate you to *surrender judgment* toward those you love, but taking the time to *align mind and body* in between can diminish the necessary passion it takes to make amends.
- To *surrender judgment* is to create space and deepen your self-awareness on a particular subject; sometimes you need to *experience your truth* without *feeling your body* and the traumatic history it carries so you can just address the problem at hand.
- If you want to create major change in your life, sometimes to *allow what is* generates joy and gratitude for an untenable situation (ahem, a real crap situation). But if you *experience your truth* and *align mind and body*, you see the good, bad, and ugly for what it is—and you can act from a neutral and objective place.
- When you're processing a trauma, you may need to deliberately *align mind and body* to *feel your body* and unlock the fear you felt at that time without the regret or sorrow that comes when you *surrender judgment*. Sorrow and regret are tied to the aftermath, whereas sometimes you may need to heal by reexperiencing the moment itself.

Though it's a common belief that bikers are fearless, it's not true for me. I've spent twenty years in the saddle, and every time I *feel my body* getting on the bike, I experience fear. The anger of my truth would annihilate my ability to ride soundly (and any possibility of a good time), so I *allow what is* and let my joy of riding supersede my fear. The joy of the open road is great until something unexpected goes wrong—a mechanical problem, flat tire, or accident. There is no time for reflection in that emergency situation to align a better-laid plan. Allowing the sorrow of my plans to be disrupted and *surrendering judgment* about blame let me continue my journey efficiently and graciously. A biker's exposure and vulnerability make for inevitable mishaps; the journey is rarely a direct route.

Once an emergency is over, sorrow turns directly to an "I could have been killed" anger. I *experience my truth* regarding every aspect of the emergency with venom that I will never forget. But before returning to the joy of riding, I reflect on how to *align mind and body* to prevent a similar mishap in the future. This destructive cycle goes around whenever an unexpected situation threatens my soundness as a secure rider and quick responder. Even my protective brother-in-law, with a raised eyebrow, allows my sister to ride with me—without him. I take this permission as very high praise and attribute it to being aligned with the destructive cycle.

Each meditation breakdown offers a greater service to your personal development by omitting the result when navigating through high-intensity situations. The destructive cycle limits the scope of your focus to deepen your connection.

Meditation Breakdown

 Fear: Feel Your Body

The resistance to slowing down for meditation is often the resistance to feel. Fear about what you might find if you look too closely can unknowingly keep you on the outside of your own life experience and, even more unfortunately, keep you outside your greatest source of power—your spirit self. Meditation deliberately values "non-doing"—slowing down to cultivate genuine connection.

As you begin an inward journey, the first sensations are often physical and can be uncomfortable, annoying, or even painful. As you encounter an uninvited physical sensation, it is important to be present with it and carefully explore it. In so doing, you are allowing the source of your tension to express itself and be understood––yin. Once the physical expression is heard with neutral attention, you can successfully adjust your physical alignment or add necessary outside support, and then you can redirect your energy movement into a restorative direction––yang. You will instantly feel the discomfort dissolving.

Once the initial physical irritation quiets down, get really interested in the inner subtleties of an aspect of your physical body. In still meditation, focus on your breath, your alignment, the weight of your bones, or the space in your joints. In active meditation, your focus could be energy flow, a psyche-muscular holding pattern, or the stillness of your dan tien energy center. Study the psyche-muscular blueprint to understand the emotional component stored in your particular areas of discomfort. Use what you learn as a starting point for contemplation. Relax the area of discomfort as you focus on releasing the reactionary emotion attached to that subject. Watch for images of irritation regarding the subject pass through your mind's eye or witness a stir of emotions pass through as you experience the physical charge shifting.

The meditation will excite any physical areas that resist or impede your ability to relax and reorganize energy flow. As each tension surfaces, give its expression your attention. First, breathe into the discomfort and then direct its force outwardly through your energy flow. Send your energy in the direction that best eases the discomfort; energy can be directed up through the crown of the head, down through the feet, or away from your center (more on energy movement in lesson 2). Continue to focus on your energy's movement, flushing out tension until the uncomfortable sensation dissolves and your energy flows freely again. Then return to the intent of your original meditative focus. Once the congested energy is expressed and released, and energy is cycling, your discomfort and uneasiness will disappear.

Recognize your physical tensions and pains as areas that need your love and attention rather than judging them as weak, bad, or wrong. Self-judgment will escalate them. For example, your knees suddenly experience sharp pain. Your inclination is to feel agitated and blame them for holding you back. Instead, recognize their hesitation and move forward with curiosity. When you use this approach, their psyche-muscular hesitation has communicated successfully, hence bringing your attention to the pain's root cause. Deliberately direct your energy to move through painful areas, first in stillness and then in movement, to restore physical well-being. When you listen to your body's cries with curiosity and compassion, you soothe them and free up space inside you to create the life you want.

Meditation Guide to Feel Your Body

- Value non-doing as a means to cultivate genuine connection.
- Get really interested in the inner subtleties of your physical body. Be present with physical discomfort with neutral attention. Study the psyche-muscular blueprint to understand the emotional component of an uncomfortable area.
- Adjust your physical alignment or add the necessary outside support to encourage free-flowing energy.
- Direct the energy of holding patterns outwardly until they dissolve.
- Recognize that emotional holding patterns are co-created by mind and body; curiosity and compassion guide them back into alignment.

Anger: Experience Your Truth

Once you have become comfortable in your physical body, either in active or still meditation, you will encounter your emotions. The emotions you are uncomfortable with will be the first in line to get your attention.

In fact, you will likely come into contact with your resistance to having that emotion first, as opposed to the emotion itself. You may experience yourself hiding disowned, painful, or challenging emotions with angry-proclaimed defenses or excuses for their existence. Sometimes you can be more comfortable with your anger than with the true feelings beneath it.

You can identify resistance to genuine emotion by recognizing whether you are opposing or ignoring your experience. When you are in resistance to having an experience, you are in judgment of the experience; for example, *the anger connected to getting fired unfairly from a job is a constant distraction.* The anger will continue so long as you resist experiencing the deeper feelings of loss underneath. You may judge these deeper feelings as futile or senseless. You avoid the deeper emotional position when you choose to focus on controlling your appearance or throwing your arms in the air in defeat––yang.

When you are experiencing actual emotion, you experience the vulnerability, intensity, and truth of your internal state––yin. Mistaking your judgments for your emotions will create confusion and keep you from deepening your meditation and transforming your mental or emotional posture. That confusion exhausts your will and allows boredom or negativity to invade your meditation, workout, and life. Recognizing your resistance to emotion and your actual emotion as two separate phenomena creates the clarity you need to figure out what is genuinely taking place.

Let your meditative focus come from a phenomenon in nature that possesses what you are in need of (for example, a mountain or eagle) or use a word or phrase that can act as an anchor (for example, "I am loved"). Use your breath to continually direct your mind's attention toward the meditative focus and relax your body into the vision. Review the eagle meditation (p. 6). When meditating on an isolated psyche-muscular component, feel for emotional insights rather than asking for answers. Then recognize all insights as shared experiences in nature and with humankind. Realize, in a very real way, you aren't alone in the challenge of living. This intimate connection with what is natural then enables you to connect outwardly with greater honesty and self-assurance.

As you encounter the mishmash of resistances and emotions, experience them all with love and appreciation. No matter what you uncover, it's with you because there was a time when you needed it to survive. Your story is unfolding in front of you for your benefit. As you experience what you have resisted feeling and allow your consciousness to be explored, you will be creating a newfound intimacy with yourself and your life.

Meditation Guide to Experience Your Truth

- Find comfort in your physical body.
- Differentiate between your resistance to emotion and your actual emotion, then experience all expressions with appreciation.
- Choose a meditative focus and use your breath to direct your energy movement. Refer to the eagle exercise (p. 6).

- Observe emotional insights, then recognize these insights as shared experiences in nature and with humankind.
- Feel the self-assurance that comes with honest self-examination.

 Joy: Allow What Is

Once you have relaxed the congested energy within the physical and emotional bodies, you can simply enjoy being. You may not always like what you uncover in consciousness, but you are now freed from denial, confusion, and suppression. The joy of being honest and transparent with yourself can now assist your attention to experience life peacefully and freely.

For example, the anger and rejection experienced because of a neglectful parent can be crippling for a child well into adulthood. Let's say you begged your parent to play the drums as a child, and instead, he or she insisted that you learn bassoon. There was no compromise, no listening to your desire for rhythmic and percussive expression—just a foisting of his or her vision on you. While it's a small moment, it contributes to a larger feeling of never truly being heard or seen for who you are. Acknowledging that your parent was never aligned with you in the first place, though unfortunate, disentangles the parent's action from your feelings of rejection. Resolution around the abandoned feelings can now transpire because a deeper fundamental truth has been realized that neutralizes your reaction.

Pay careful attention to what happens when you sit with peace. Notice whether the inquiring nature of your mind—accustomed to analyzing, calculating, and interpreting everything you experience—interrupts this quietude. You may feel an overwhelming desire to do something, to jump up and convey your newfound clarity to the world––yang. On the other hand, when others aren't experiencing personal elation, you may feel guilty for being joyous and transparent, and feel the need to hide those emotions––yin. Whether your inclination is to do something about your newfound feelings or flounder in them, you aren't staying present with them. Meditation is a deliberate choice to be in the moment and appreciate the unique unfolding of your feelings without attaching to them. Use neutral witness (p. 19) to stay disentangled from mind chatter.

When your energy flows continuously, it stretches the body and mind to connect with nature. You begin to appreciate emotional states as natural experiences. With nature as an ally, the willingness to allow your own feelings to exist improves. As you allow your own feelings to exist and be counted, you start to allow the contradictory feelings of others to exist. And when you learn to appreciate emotional discomfort, it is allowed to change. You are expressing yourself without the defenses that keep you engaged in a fight.

Recognize that your mind and body don't know life's answers. This humbling mind-body position of "not knowing" is a position of wisdom and maturity. Allow the mystical intelligence of your spirit self to reveal its virtue through meditative insights. With these insights, you become more and more comfortable in each moment.

Meditation Guide to Allow What Is

- Relax the congested energy within the physical and emotional bodies.
- Quietly observe your encounter with peace.
- Notice whether your mind wants to do something or is overwhelmed by feelings. Use neutral witness (p. 19) to stay disentangled from mind chatter.

- Deliberately choose to be in the moment and appreciate the unique unfolding of your feelings without attaching to them.
- Allow the intelligence of your spirit self to reveal its mystical virtues through meditative insights.

Reflection: Align Mind and Body

You are an active observer passing through physical, emotional, and mental bodies—a witness to what excites and burdens you. As you relax, you become more able to channel your excitement and loosen the hold burdens have on your attention. Free attention allows for greater reflection. And to reflect you need distance—conscious space—for an objective viewpoint. From an expanded and organized alignment, regular viewpoint shifts can easily take place, so you can stay aligned with your development and growth.

There are two basic viewpoints to creating distance and space. One view disconnects you from the subject—indifference—yang; and the other connects you to the subject—non-attachment—yin. Indifference creates an environment of false disinterest and unresponsiveness that leads to more repression. Non-attachment creates curiosity and awareness, leading to discernment and self-discovery. While indifference is the action of pushing something away, non-attachment is an act of stepping back to get a broader perspective. With this broader viewpoint, you can see things in their entirety rather than in their parts. This holistic perspective enables you to comprehend the parts of something and experience the intimate, living weave that constructs a life's interconnectedness.

You will, at this point, be able to experience your physical, emotional, and mental bodies as separate aspects of the whole and experience these parts united as a whole being. Spiritual awareness reveals itself as lessons within life circumstances, a sense of purpose in your life's journey, or an essential belonging in the world. The way in which you arrange the parts of yourself within the whole may change as your spirit self is realized. Where you may have believed one thing at one time, you now may believe something quite different.

For example, perhaps you believed your body's outward appearance is what attracted love into your life; you may now believe your body's outward expression is what creates love in your life. While the former belief separated the body from the rest of the self as the love magnet, the latter connects the body to the self as a spirited expression that creates love. This inner reordering is an example of positive change being created in the foundation of your consciousness, bringing greater alliance and peace into your life and ultimately the world.

Alignment between your parts will be in constant flux as you develop. In fact, realignment defines growth. During still or active meditation, realignment is recognized as a celebration of personal growth, not an indicator of being imperfect. The quiet stillness found at the heart of energy realignment is experienced as a spiritual sigh of relief. Take regular moments to integrate changes in consciousness, use the trilogy of the self-experience (p. 21) for this purpose. The gift found in mind-body alignment is the ability to rest in the nurture of your spirit self. The nurture of your spirit self is the giving of sight—insights into your relationship with life.

Meditation Guide to Align Mind and Body

- Release congested energy within physical, emotional, and mental bodies.
- Recognize the process of realignment as an exercise in non-attachment rather than in indifference, leading you to a celebration of self-discovery.

- Create a broad viewpoint to experience mind, body, and spirit as separate aspects of a whole as well as an interconnected holistic trilogy.
- Realize the voice of your spirit self through insights, life lessons, and a sense of purpose or belonging in the world.
- Take a moment to experience a spiritual sigh of relief with each insight. And take regular moments to integrate changes in consciousness using the trilogy of the self-experience (p. 21).

Sorrow: Surrender Judgment

As you integrate a new-felt harmony in your life, it may be accompanied by an unexpected, concurrent sense of sorrow. The once-justified judgments that established your previous standpoints are surrendering and leaving an unknown and often lonely space in your consciousness.

Accepting change insists on letting go of a past choice or idea––yin––as well as conceding to your change of heart and the possible ridicule it might elicit from yourself or others––yang. What was experienced as a monumental personal truth in the atmosphere of meditation can crumble under the pressures of opposition or judgment. For example, it may become very clear to you during meditation that it's time to finally end things with your significant other; you may even imagine the entire conversation beat by beat. Brimming with confidence, you head to their place to have the big talk … and manage to get out only a few awkward vowel sounds before you have to bail. The tendency to contract energetically when up against contention can diminish the connections made in your more expanded meditative state.

Meditative insights are brought to your attention from an intuitive knowledge that prioritizes pure spirited intention. A thinking state that values conventional learned information or a defensive state that insists on being right might not be able to fully recapture the magnitude of a spiritual awakening. A reference point experienced at the time of your meditative insight can remain your anchor in spite of all the resistances to making change. For example, the sense of peace that rises with a meditative insight may accompany a release and drop in your shoulder blades. In real life, taking a breath and relaxing your shoulder blades will help cultivate that same sense of peace in meeting a challenge.

As you expand your consciousness, allow time to ground it. Prepare yourself to bring whatever illuminations you experienced in the intimate setting of your meditation into your life. Do this by observing the alignment distinctions and emotional qualities that accompanied an insight, particularly a newly expanded area in mind or body, a peaceful viewpoint, or a newfound appreciation for something or someone. While in the meditative state, your mind's management of energy established a new pattern in your body that positively guided your emotional response in a new direction. Coordinating the observations and energy alignment of this new direction offers you choices in life. Your old tensions, which have been unconsciously guiding your emotions, are one choice; the consciously created and meditatively inspired new pattern is a second choice.

Whenever you are triggered into judgment, first recognize you are in a psyche-muscular reaction. You are allowing an old pattern to interfere with your quality of life. Immediately surrender your muscular tension inwardly and mental attachment outwardly. For example, when engaged in a repetitive and destructive behavior, stop everything and breathe relaxation through your mind and body using the neutral witness exercise (p. 19). Rather than thinking about the judgment, illuminate the neutrality from the expanded viewpoint of a witness.

Feel the new pattern override the old pattern. Experience choice. With repetition, your new pattern will gain coordination and have greater success integrating a new behavior.

Cooperation between mind and body makes it possible to recognize and integrate insights. Deliberate realignment of your mind-body posture reshapes your consciousness to turn insights outwardly. Trust that what is illuminated through meditation practice is intended to accelerate personal development and maturity in your life.

Honor your intuitive nature. Meditation is worship of the divine in you. There is nothing more valuable to your sense of self than being in relationship with your spirit self, though it can initially feel like a lonely nothingness inside. This nothingness is the "pregnant void" Tao refers to as the "Great Mother" of all things. Surrender all judgments that keep you from exploring this place of personal integrity.

Meditation Guide to Surrender Judgment

- Use meditation to discover a harmonious way of being.
- Surrender judgment toward past viewpoints and empower any spirited change of heart.
- Bring whatever illuminations you experienced in the intimate setting of your meditation into your life by observing the alignment distinctions and emotional qualities that accompanied an insight.
- Recognize you have two choices, the unsuitable old pattern or the realized new pattern. Use neutral witness exercise (p. 19) to support coordinating the new pattern.
- Listen to the nothingness within you and hear the divine.

Your vision will become clearer only when you can look into your own heart.
Who looks outside, dreams;
who looks inside, awakes.

—Carl Jung, Swiss-born psychiatrist and psychoanalyst

Body Chapter

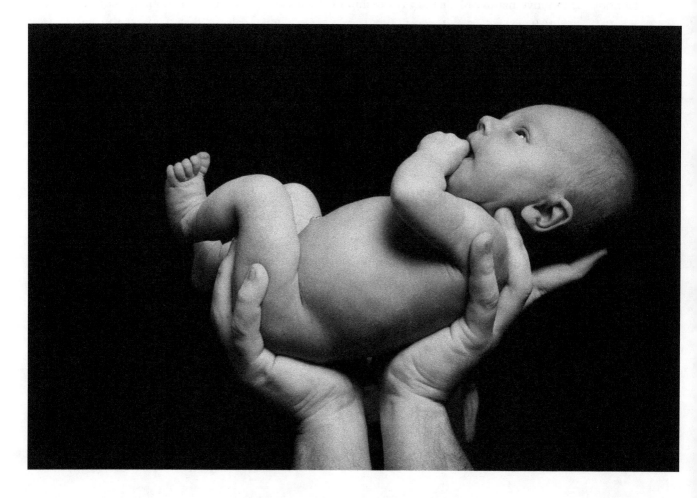

A newborn unable to hold herself up
Has no holding patterns.
As the demands to hold herself up increases,
Holding patterns develop.

May we learn the difference between the holding patterns that
Support us and those that defeat us.

Lesson 3
The Art of Strength

Learning consists in daily accumulating,
The practice of Tao consists in daily diminishing.

—Lao Tzu, *Tao Te Ching*

Align with a path
And mindfully eliminate obstructions.

—Tammy Wise, BodyLogos

Strength's Beauty

Like a fine artist sculpting clay or a dancer creating choreography, athletes lose and find themselves in their creative process. So why is conventional strength training presented so mechanically when its authentic nature is artistic? Traditional approaches to strength training can leave you feeling fit but empty. For a soulful fitness experience, yoga, tai chi, or dance classes have felt like the only alternatives that integrate a spiritual or artistic component into strength training.

Sculpting the body unites the artist and athlete within you, unveiling your inner beauty and connecting you to your own exquisiteness and virtuosity. BodyLogos brings you, the artist, into all strength-training workouts—be it in the gym, classroom, or a stay-at-home exercise program. Just as tai chi and chi gong are based on the ancient Chinese Tao principles, so is the BodyLogos practice.

In art and strength training alike, raw talent and power are meaningless without a sound technical foundation. Just as a sculpture's alignment and balance of weight give physical support to the artist's expressions, energy alignment and balance of force give your body's movement support for your expressions.

Alignment Flow

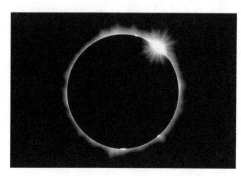
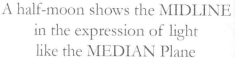
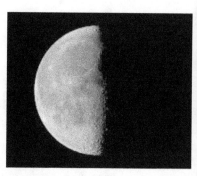

A CORONA eclipse radiates light like the CORONAL Plane

A half-moon shows the MIDLINE in the expression of light like the MEDIAN Plane

Imagine your body is divided head to toe by two planes. The coronal plane splits you into front and back halves. Imagine it splitting the top of your head like a crown and continuing down, right through your ears, and separating your chest from your back, your abs from your buttocks, and so forth. The median plane splits your body into right and left sides. Imagine it running from the top of your head, down the middle of your nose, along your sternum, and so forth.

The convergence of these two planes is the foundation of your body's three dimensionality, and it's called your "central plumb line." Your central plumb line vertically aligns your body with that of the earth's gravitational pull. It's the line that drops through the exact center of the internal cavity of your body, where your organs live, like the axis of your body from the north pole to the south.

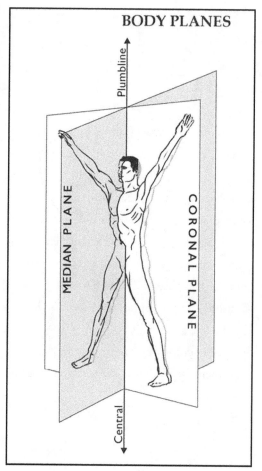

We are three-dimensional beings in every way. We have posterior, interior, and anterior sections of the body; we have past, present, and future phases of the mind; and we have universal, shared, and individual aspects of the spirit. All are inseparable and interrelated yet independent. By aligning our dimensions—physically, mentally, and spiritually—freedom of expression is permitted to exist.

By freedom, I mean we are no longer restricted by our own imposed physical compression, mental judgment, and emotional reactivity.

Neutral alignment brings you home to the center of your being's three-dimensionality by aligning your central plumb line. There are five energy centers that make up this vertical alignment. When aligned one above the other, you are aligned with gravity. This relationship with gravity finds the optimal positions for your energy, bones, and muscles; and it prepares you for physical or mental challenges.

In addition to aligning bones and muscles, giving you a sense of center in your own body, neutral alignment gives you a sense of center in the universe. Connecting your personal energy centers with universal energy opens communication between you as a universal creation and the creator of your life. In Eastern philosophy, they use the word *chi* for this life force, but BodyLogos uses the word *energy* (to make it easier for us Westerners).

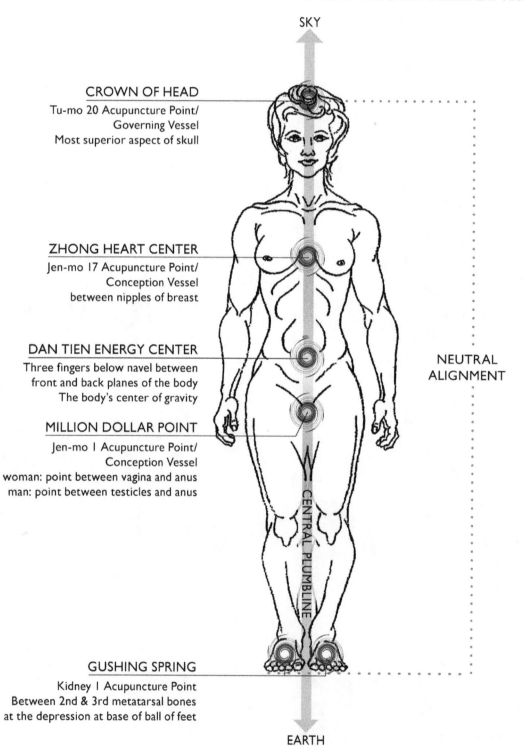

Neutral Alignment Reference Points

Gushing spring: This is at the base of the ball of the feet, between the second and third metatarsal bones, in the depression formed when the foot is pointed downward. Referred to as kidney 1 acupuncture point, it connects to and receives the earth's life force. Feel for an energetic current nourishing the body from this place.

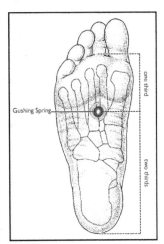

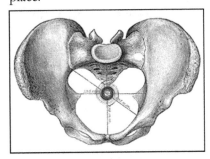

Million-dollar point: On a woman this is the posterior aspect of the vagina's opening; on a man this is the point between the testicles and the anus, placed directly between sitz bones. This conception vessel 1 acupuncture point is known as an energy gate that, when stimulated, prevents the loss of energy.

Dan tien energy center: This is located three fingers below the navel. This is one of Tao's "three treasures"—three major cultivating and storage energy centers in the body—and our center of gravity. All movement connects through this restorative physical generator.

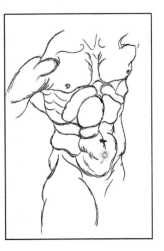

Zhong heart center: This is positioned between the nipples on the conception vessel meridian, a lifesaver acupuncture meridian that can give or take energy from meridians body wide as needed for homeostasis. It acts as the seat of our emotions.

Crown of head: This is the most superior aspect of a skull, positioned above ears on the top of one's head. This is the soft spot on a newborn, Tu-mo 20 of the governing vessel. It is the second of the two lifesaver acupuncture meridians that manage the excess or depletion of energy body wide.

Experience Neutral Alignment
Stable. Centered. Contained.
mindthebody.bodylogos.com/video4
(abbreviated description)

Visualize the crown of your head, centered between the tips of your ears and aligned above your zhong heart center; this is your heart center, placed between nipples and between sternum and spine, aligned above the dan tien energy center; your dan tien, three fingers below the belly button, centrally positioned, it is aligned above the million-dollar point. Your million-dollar point, the raised center between sitz bones, is aligned above and between the inner ankle bones. Your body weight is placed on your gushing spring points, the indentation between your foot balls and in front of their arches.

Body: Your energy centers are now in a relationship with each other. Experience their relationship as a central channel of life force, integrated and synchronized, passing through you.

Mind: Feel how your deliberate attention on physical alignment brings about greater calm and clarity. Experience the liberation that comes with the ability to soothe your own "dis-ease."

Play with deliberately going out of alignment and returning to alignment to explore the gamut of choices in each energy center. Notice what has changed in your body's aligned posture versus your default posture. Clearly define what the differences are in the relationships between energy centers so you can maintain these postural changes in your life. Also, notice what has changed in your mental disposition. Are there any new alliances you are experiencing? Aligning with gravity may feel unfamiliar at first, but your body instinctively wants to stay aligned. It feels good.

Neutral Alignment Wish List

- Awareness of subtle changes in physical posture improves.
- Unconscious tension becomes conscious.
- Concerns about being out of alignment with your world shift to creating alignment with it.
- Curiosity about misalignment inspires greater reflection on its psyche-muscular origin.
- A sense of being safeguarded by the strength of your own structure appears.

An eighty-nine-year-old-client, Elisa, had a severe spinal stenosis in her lumbar spine and alternated between a wheelchair and a walker. She worked diligently to relieve her pain with alignment awareness and strength. Our efforts enabled her to exercise without the need of pain medication and strengthened her ability to remain mobile in her life. My goal for her was satisfied beyond my expectations when she informed me that she used neutral alignment at meal times, and her digestion had greatly improved too.

> It is reassuring that, though my spine is weak, my esophagus is functioning perfectly. I grab all the little moments of comfort I can. Feeling the warm tea travel down through my digestive system is a daily comfort. I feel a cascade of sparkling water traveling through me.
>
> —Elisa

Adjusting Alignment

Because your body is three dimensional, alignment and stability come from understanding both your vertical and horizontal reference points in relationship to gravity. For your central plumb line to come into alignment and remain stable through movement, you need to recognize and use the horizontal couplings of alignment stabilizers.

Visualize two parallel lines running from the occipital hollows at the base of your skull all the way down either side of your spine, through your buttocks and legs, and into your feet. Your alignment stabilizers are equidistant pairs of reference points along those parallel lines that relate to each energy center and guide them into alignment. With alignment stabilizers, you can adjust your alignment and manage tension. Without alignment stabilizers, you would topple over when you try to use your body—like a table missing one leg.

The amount of tension accumulated in the muscles surrounding a pair of alignment stabilizers determines the degree of effectiveness they have in aligning their adjoining energy center. The compression of tension can freeze these stabilizing pairs into a pinch or an over-spread position, pushing their energy center into the anterior or posterior body. As you learn to release tension through these alignment stabilizers, muscular balance can be restored, and a free flow of energy can be reestablished through your central plumb line. The flow of life force through your central plumb line, or lack thereof, is what establishes your body's skeletal alignment as well as your mind's striving nature. Your striving nature, what Tao refers to as your "original nature," is the fundamental part of each human that wants to be good at what he or she does and be recognized for its universal significance.

The compression or freedom in your alignment stabilizers, as they relate to your three dimensionality, reflects your body's psyche-muscular freedom, which in turn affects your greater alignment with gravity through your energy centers and skeletal alliance. When your central plumb line is not in alignment with gravity, it's fighting gravity. Gravity's effect on misalignment goes beyond distorting the natural curves of your spine and constricting the central nervous system. Your striving nature is crushed, causing you to react to your life story and fight rather than align.

The free flow of life force, the porter of your striving nature, supports and balances the natural curves of the spinal column—central nervous system—and the inborn purpose of your striving nature to maintain relaxed strength in stillness and activity. Alignment stabilizers are the gatekeepers of that flow.

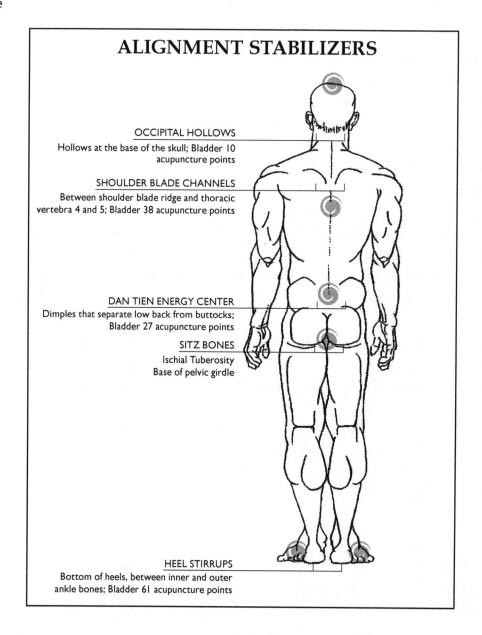

Alignment Stabilizer Reference Points

Occipital hollows: These correspond with the crown center and are felt as indentations at the base of the occipital bone, where the skull meets the neck. Experience their relationship by gliding your head forward like a pigeon and back like a swan. Notice how your crown center changes your relationship with the sky. Alignment in the crown center cultivates freedom to have your own mind.

Shoulder blade channels: Correspond with the zhong heart center and are located between the horizontal ridge of the shoulder blades and the spine. Experience their relationship by asserting your chest forward, like a soldier, and collapsing your chest backward, like you're protecting your heart. Notice how your heart center can change its placement within the chest. Alignment in the zhong heart center cultivates freedom to love.

Low back dimples: These correspond with the dan tien energy center and are felt as dimples just above the bikini line in the lower back. Experience their relationship by manipulating the waistline. Tip the pelvis back, like a baby-doll posture, and tuck the pelvis under like a punished puppy. Notice how your dan tien can change its placement within the torso. Alignment in the dan tien energy center cultivates freedom to move.

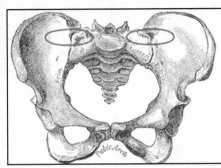
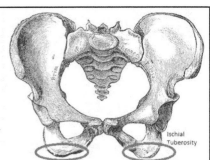

The sacroilliac joints are shock absorbing transfer stations between the sacrum and the hip bones.

The sitz bones--ischial tuberosity--are the weight stations stabilizing the sacrum and hip bones.

Their alignment with gravity assures our uprightness.

Sitz bones: These correspond with the million-dollar point and are felt when you sit as pointy bones in each buttock. Stand to experience their relationship by pressing the inner heels through the outer heels, causing the sitz bones to widen, and pressing the outer heels through the inner heels, causing the sitz bones to narrow. Notice how your million-dollar point drops and lifts the pelvic floor. Alignment in the million-dollar point cultivates freedom to surrender and trust in yourself.

Heel stirrups: These correspond with the gushing spring points and are between ankle bones on the bottom of each foot's heel. Experience their relationship by doing a relevé (heel raise) and placing the heels down close to the balls of your feet, then doing another relevé and placing the heels down far from the balls of your feet. Notice how your entire body's alignment changes over your gushing springs and your connection with the ground fluctuates. Alignment in the gushing spring points cultivates freedom to receive.

Each pair of alignment stabilizers will have their own unique characteristics and placement. Explore these pairs of reference points until you recognize their sometimes-subtle and sometimes-obvious abilities to move horizontally toward or away from their corresponding energy center. Their movement adjusts the placement of each energy center in your neutral alignment individually. Alignment between energy centers brings the alignment stabilizers into two parallel lines, one on each side of the spine's snakelike vertical alignment, supporting your central plumb line's movement in a fluid and expressive way.

Outside resistance challenges your central plumb line. When the combined resistance of gravity and outside resistance accumulates beyond your strength, it exhausts your muscles first. This mark of muscle failure is what ultimately produces an increase in muscle strength. If this marker is ignored and bypassed in the gym or life, then your energy reserve also depletes. As you become more and more exhausted, the curves of your vertical alignment become imbalanced and break down; your central plumb line becomes distorted by tension, and neutral alignment becomes compromised. When the gravity of life compromises neutral alignment, survival strategies are formed, reactive strategies that borrow energy from the emotional overflow of a situation. Emotional, fear-based energy is now supporting you. This temporary support can become your full-time support, creating psyche-muscular holding patterns. (Remember those from Lesson 1? They're back.)

A psyche-muscular holding pattern is muscular tension and psychological stress frozen in time. Although needed in a time of desperation or depletion, this pattern uses up a lot of energy because it distorts the flow of life force passing through your energy centers and compromises neutral alignment. This adopted energy use becomes so familiar that you carry on until pain or exhaustion forces you to stop. Physical discomfort and emotional sensitivity point out misalignments. But the hidden gift of this distress is that it points to the specific area or energy center that needs your attention to reestablish alignment.

Experience Alignment Stabilizers
Control. Empowered. Curious.
mindthebody.bodylogos.com/video5
(abbreviated description)

Visualize two parallel lines dropping down each side of the spine, each from the occipital hollows, the indentations at the base of the skull. Each line passes through the shoulder blade channels, between the ridge of the shoulder blades and spine; through the low back dimples, the indentations above each buttock; through the sitz bones, the pointy bones you sit on in each buttock; and then ground through the heel stirrups, the middle of your heels between inner and outer ankle bones.

Body: Now relate to the distance between corresponding points with the intention to align each pair of alignment stabilizers, one set above the other. Recognize how each pair of alignment stabilizers places its perspective energy center on your central plumb line, bringing the relationship between energy centers into absolute alignment.

Mind: Allow space within you; acknowledge areas that feel tight and stay with them until they start to breathe. Allow connection outside of you; acknowledge uncomfortable beliefs and stay with them until they start to shift toward greater alignment. Feel your life force free of impingement as your experience of being weighted lightens. You may feel as if you are drifting weightlessly. Experience the phenomenon of letting go of hardship.

Experience your search for alignment as a way of discovering misalignments in mind and body, which are blocking your energy. Allow this search to be an ongoing lifestyle, a fierce love for yourself. Learn the places in your life that need tenderness and understanding to relax and the places that need to be stimulated and strengthened to contribute.

Alignment Stabilizers Wish List

- Physical and mental alignment work in tandem.
- A sense of inner space becomes evident in energy centers.
- Confidence grows in your ability to turn off tension's grip with simple adjustments.
- Your specific misalignment tendencies become clear.
- A true sense of anterior, central, and posterior planes is experienced independently.

From Midwestern homecoming queen to high-powered management consultant, from mother of three to entrepreneur, Sandra is a type A go-getter. When she's not being challenged, she's thinking about her next challenge. Sandra's perpetual forward thinking and "take on anything" approach to life became embodied as a physical forward bend. Her iliopsoas muscles had shortened, causing discomfort in her hips and lower back, and her sitz bones tipped back, with her lower back dimples compressed. On top of that, her shoulder blade channels were overspread as if in a "ready to catch" position. We worked on muscular balance through strength training and relaxation techniques. But to bring these adjustments into her everyday posture, Sandra needed to understand and learn to feel the alliance between alignment stabilizers. Now, with a single breath of focused attention, she can release tension and call on only the muscular support needed along her central plumb line. This ability to quickly align many elements of posture has offered her a way to feel better (and look taller, slimmer, and more relaxed) with much more ease.

At first, I simply didn't believe that being more relaxed could mean having more strength. I had lost the ability to feel relaxed alignment in my body. Tammy (and BodyLogos) has given me a framework and tools to feel better and BE BETTER in body, mind and spirit.

—Sandra

Bones Don't Move—They're Moved

Neutral alignment is your starting position of stillness for any challenge. Finding your alignment starts in active stillness, and then the energy from your dan tien travels up and down your central plumb line. You feel like a balloon whose string is tied to the ground, connected to the earth but stretching and floating toward the sky. With energy centers and bones aligned, this foundational alignment can move fluidly to meet with outside resistance. Alignment isn't static—it's constantly in flow. In fact, the difference between tension and strength is that tension is static and strength is fluid. Your alignment should be able to stretch and move.

Here lies the challenge: Traditionally, we lift through the muscular system to find our alignment, enabling us to relate to the weightlessness of a balloon image. But without a proper downward influence—something tying the balloon string down—you can be knocked about by outside resistance. The muscular system is riddled with unconscious psyche-muscular holding patterns that are constantly reacting to gravity and will react identically to any outside resistance. To maintain alignment when up against outside resistance, you need to become conscious of the habitual ways you react to it. Bones meet gravity; muscles have the choice to react to gravity or work with it.

Bones and muscles have very different agendas. Think about it: Everything about your bone structure is energetically designed to help you expand and connect outwardly, whereas your muscles' literal energetic function is to connect inward—to contain and support that framework. In truth, many of us rely on our muscles to do the work of our bones; we ask our muscles to work overtime to ground us instead of finding our alignment through our skeleton's placement. This doesn't mean there's no muscular activity at all. On the contrary, your muscles serve a very important function in keeping you grounded and lifted. But when they're asked to do the bones' work, an ambivalent flow of energy is created, and that extra effort is transformed into tension.

To begin transforming this ambivalent flow of energy into a concise efficient flow, you need to separate your understanding and experience of bones and muscles. Experience the weight of your bones separate from the tension of your muscles.

To separate your feeling sense of the bones and muscles, you need to allow movement instead of forcing it. To allow movement is to control without being controlling, to surrender some authority and be open to your surroundings. When you surrender on purpose, you aren't giving up your power. Instead, you're learning to step up with confidence—the confidence that the universe is "for you," not "against you." And to micromanage every detail is to deny yourself the universal support and wisdom you have yet to behold.

Experience the Bone
Trust. Ease. Surrender.
mindthebody.bodylogos.com/video6
(abbreviated description)

Lie supine with arms and legs extended, hands lying palms up at your sides. Allow the weight of your body to relax into the ground. Pay particular attention to the weight of both shoulder blades and elbows as they drop equally toward the ground. Maintaining this groundedness, use as little muscular effort as possible to rotate the arms and reposition your hands palms down on your solar plexus, the soft spot where the rib cage splits beneath the sternum. Notice how heavy the lower arms are to move and how the weight fluctuates to weightlessness as it arches toward an alignment with gravity. Again, as easefully as you can, return your hands to their original position. Repeat this exercise until you can keep the weight of your shoulder blades and elbows equal as you move. The weight you are experiencing is that of your bones.

Body: Continue to surrender your muscle's tension so you can experience your bones' full weight.

Deliberately give the responsibility of holding your body up to the ground. Experience the earth as a trusted Great Mother. As you surrender the need to hold yourself up so diligently, recognize the earth's devotion. She is always there to nurture and nourish. The redundant tension you habitually used in the name of survival is, in fact, consuming you. Your life force is being used up in fear of being abandoned, in fear of neglect.

Mind: Realize that no matter what the challenges are before you, the earth is beneath you. As you begin to trust this newfound support from the earth's constancy and devotion, begin to trust your own constancy and devotion to support your spirit self. Allow yourself to feel loved by the universal Great Mother and you.

As you have just experienced, bones don't move. They are moved. Staying connected to the bones' stillness keeps you connected to both gravity and the internal quietude of your spirit self. You no longer need to choose between the world and yourself. You can have it all by simply meeting resistance rather than dominating it.

Experience the Bone Wish List

- The surrendering of your bones' weight teaches you to relax.
- Slowing down deliberately becomes possible.
- Your muscles build a relationship of trust with the earth.
- A weightless alignment with gravity becomes perceivable.
- A feeling sense that distinguishes between bone and muscle is awakened.

Susan sits at a computer, editing manuscripts and writing original stage plays. Her head and heart are drawn toward the computer screen, completely engrossed in an alternate world of words. Though she tries to break regularly to open the forward slump of her body, time slips away, and when she finally sits upright, her shoulders no longer return to their place of origin on the coronal plane. Her natural chest and shoulder openness has been replaced with an unintentional shutdown. Rebalancing the area muscularly with exercises that strengthen her posterior shoulders and upper back was needed; in addition, we needed to reacquaint her with the open space between her chest and shoulders, and re-establish a relaxed, narrower space between her shoulder blades.

Following her bones' weight, rather than her muscle's tension, relaxed this experience into being. Optimal posture is natural when lying supine; gravity blankets the entire body as the earth supports the entire body. Guiding her to recognize her arms' alignment with gravity while rotating the shoulder joint offered a direction for the habitual tension in the area to surrender. This awareness of shoulder placement allowed her to relax them into alignment while also outlining a range of motion that continues to keep her right shoulder from dislocating due to a past shoulder surgery.

> I look forward to this exercise because it's an expansion more than a strength exercise, giving me an effective visualization for sitting at the computer. And more profoundly, it gives me a feeling of acceptance toward my body, a shame free experience regarding my zaftig breasts.
>
> —Susan

Vertical Relaxation

By recognizing your connection with resistance as a balance between contracting and releasing, your movement always carries the potential for surrendering holding patterns a lifetime of unconscious pushback has produced. The phrase "That which you resist persists" is transformed into "That which you resist submits."

Neutral alignment is a foundational posture that positions your physical body to act as the alignment groundwork for an even greater alignment progression, one that expands you outward to experience a release that suspends you in gravity's force. That release surrenders muscular tension, perpetuates energy flow, and connects your bones to earth and sky. I call it "essential alignment."

Energizing neutral alignment elongates your central plumb line into essential alignment. Because gravity's grounding pressure on your physical body can now be experienced as the point between surrendering and awakening—what Lao Tzu so gracefully named Sweet Dew—you are conscious and simultaneously aligned with the needs of your environment and yourself.

Many of us associate the word *inertia* with apathy or lethargy. But I like to see it as that necessary pause before movement, a created space that is full of activity but no motion yet. If you pick up something heavy and just throw your weight around, you'll hurt yourself. You know you need to gather yourself.

I go one step beyond that. Once all your alignment stabilizers are aligned, elongate your alignment beyond your body. Do one lift without moving. Get yourself so grounded, so lifted, so under and over the challenge that by the time you move, there is no compression in your joints. You have so much energy moving through you, the integrity of your bones isn't disturbed. That requires a lot of the rocket fuel from the basic principles—rest on creation to keep energy true. It's like a rocket taking off.

Essential alignment is the foundation of active meditation (from Lesson 1). The vertical stretching of your central plumb line between the earth and sky draws you out of the comfort of your dan tien energy center to connect you with life in a new way. The multiple pairs of alignment stabilizers are like sets of wings extended horizontally to maintain your essential alignment in movement.

The more precise your neutral alignment is, the greater your ability to expand into essential alignment.

Neutral alignment creates the internal physical placement crucial for bones to support each other and muscles to relax, enabling your life force to stretch you beyond the compression that has become familiar.

> Life force
> is
> Life's greatest influence,
> Generating and inspiring,
> The driving force of evolution,
> Spawning the path of a creator.

When your universal parents—earth and sky—support and guide your life force, your energy centers regularly unite, causing an energetic stretch that liberates your striving nature. Your spirit energy is now free, able to extend beyond and connect you with resistance in an aligned and empowered way and in so doing gradually dissolve your psyche-muscular holding patterns.

Gathering Universal Energy

The rocket fuel needed to stretch your central plumb line from neutral to essential alignment is gathered from the earth through your feet. The opposing stretch between earth and sky, through your skeleton, lands your weight on the gushing spring points. This stimulates the gushing springs to receive earth's life force, feeding your life force. So although your weight is on the balls of our feet, the energy direction is upward. This can happen only when a downward pathway, which is also the pathway that releases your body's tension, drops through your heel stirrups. I call this the heel stirrup and gushing spring marriage. At once, we drink energy up through the gushing springs and release tension down through the heel stirrups. While the upward energy collects in the dan tien, the downward release of tension is channeled through the alignment stabilizers for the earth to transform. There is a perfect grounding and restorative triangle between gushing springs, heel stirrups, and dan tien. Then from the dan tien, the sky is the limit.

Gravity places you on the ground—earth—while at once beckoning your striving nature toward the outer limits of your potential—sky. Earth's upward rise of life force and the sky's downward force of gravity meet with your center of gravity—dan tien. Gravity is the resistance that makes your striving nature constantly rise to the challenge, and the earth supports you in that emergence. And it is in rising to the challenge that you find your purpose and triumph. Through alignment, you are energetically reconnected and recharged

The Art of Strength

Experience Essential Alignment
Safe. Strong. Full potential.
mindthebody.bodylogos.com/video7
(abbreviated description)

Use your alignment stabilizers to position your energy centers on your central plumb line until you feel the weightlessness of being in alignment. With all reference points aligned, recognize your steadfast relationship between earth and sky. Energize your alignment by stretching relaxation through your central plumb line from the dan tien energy center. Simultaneously breathe energy up through the crown of your head and down between anklebones. As your weight stimulates the gushing spring points, feel earth energy rise up to the dan tien and simultaneously release tension down through the alignment stabilizers, exiting through the heel stirrups. Experience an exchange of tension for pure universal energy, fueling your postures to stretch.

Body: This energy stretch may feel like a yawn that extends your linear plumb line or perhaps like an inchworm spreading outward from its center. Feel your unwavering position in space steadily elongating your physical body effortlessly. Experience an equal relationship with both earth and sky as you continue to stretch beyond your physical body and your energy body.

Mind: Feel your relationship with gravity, the total weight of your physical, mental, and emotional world. Feel the life force within you meeting that total weight and stretching with it. Feel your willingness to connect outwardly grow. Experience sensitivity, compassion, and stamina for your present circumstances. With this acceptance, your dan tien's life force becomes energetically unleashed beyond what you know to connect with earth and sky. Experience yourself as an interconnected energetic being rather than an isolated physical body; experience being an integral part of the world, unfettered by the gravity of your life story.

Your weight may adjust many times before settling into its rightful place. But once stretched into essential alignment, a portal that saturates your dan tien energy center with pure universal life force is in place, and your intention and attention become aligned with your being more significantly than on your doing. The amount of attention you give to balancing the stretch between earth and sky, opening this central portal to life force, will determine the available strength of your intention—striving nature—and dictate the degree of support you'll receive from it to guide your body and mind.

Essential Alignment Wish List

- Alignment feels life affirming.
- Energy movement and physical movement are recognized as separate movements.
- Your relationship with outside resistance takes on a perspective of inner receptivity rather than outward performance.
- The act of being is distinguished from the actions of doing.
- Your sense of time stands still.

Jessica stands in front of an easel, drawing and painting for five to seven hours at a stretch. The commitment to her skill began contorting her posture to a point of shrinking her height. Her postural developments made her feel weakened, and she knew they would worsen if she didn't intercede, and she didn't think the problem was visually becoming. We addressed the obvious condition of her hyper- and hypo-spinal curves by addressing muscular balance. But it was understanding the relationship her feet had with the earth that united these multiple muscular corrections into a single energetic adjustment. By directing a downward energy current through her heels, all the muscular tensions influencing her exaggerated spinal curves had a direction to release; and as a result, an energy current that could support this new alignment was allowed to pass upward through her body. Suddenly she was permitting the earth to hold her up. One postural energy correction now keeps her aligned rather than three muscular corrections. With this simplicity, her attention can be primarily focused on her art.

> The channeling of energy through my alignment takes me out of the destination of traditional strength training challenges—completing the number of reps @ x number of pounds—and instead, places me in the process of self-awareness and personal development. My workouts now have the creativity I am accustomed to living as an artist.
>
> —Jessica

Focusing on essential alignment organizes your spiritual-physical energy to transform your experience from surviving to thriving. As an aligned energy being, your physical body becomes open to the life-giving force of gravity. Your energy is no longer operating in survival mode, so you experience a surge of vitality and calm. This relationship shift with resistance synchronizes your spiritual and physical bodies, offering your mental body an opportunity to explore and evolve—and to change, if you wish.

The mind's need to understand and control can at times overpower its willingness to implement positive change. You may have noticed in these alignment exercises that the change being made in your alignment is one of releasing unnecessary tension that is throwing alignment off. Any change, no matter how beneficial, can inwardly feel like resistance. But it isn't. What you are experiencing is your resistance to change or flow differently within yourself. Your inward surrender to maintain status quo is what brings mind and body together anew. And once established, essential alignment itself inspires your mind's will to stay attentive to your newly aligned physical posture. Once your mind and body are synchronized, they develop as a unified team, giving your spirit self freedom to exist and thrive.

You will experience essential alignment as both weightless and grounded, both vertical (energy centers of neutral alignment) and horizontal (alignment stabilizers). It offers self-assurance and personal presence, placing you in the moment, your truth, and your power.

Movement Chapter

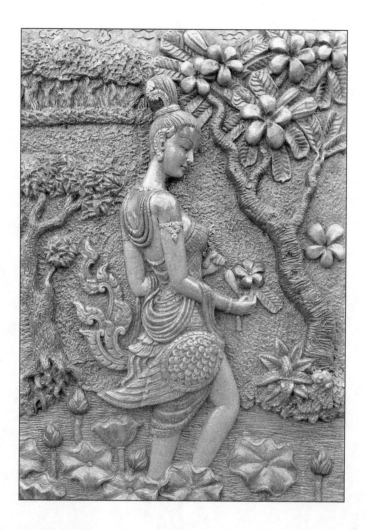

A masterful symphony lies within when mind, body and Spirit align.
A Master is unattached to what aspect of the self is leading or following,
Rather, she embraces the trilogy of her being.

To interact with the Universe, a cacophony of Life Forces,
The Master is asked to do without as she does within,
And remain unattached to who is leading or following.
She embraces her alliance with Nature.

—Lao Tsu, *Tao Te Ching*

Lesson 4
The Practice of Strength

> Many dancers today can do so much technically
> and they execute steps to perfection.
> But to do simple steps with a pure classical line,
> that is truly difficult.
>
> —Natalia Makorova, Russian-born prima ballerina

The five elements of Tao recognize that the relationships between elements are constantly in flux, and they observe five universal movements that facilitate this fluctuation.

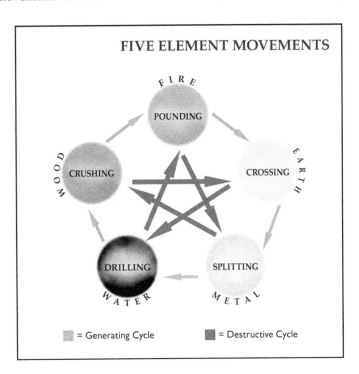

Element	Joint	Direction of Motion
Water	Wrists, shoulder blades, ankles, thumbs	Drilling
Wood	Elbows, knees, digits	Crushing
Fire	Shoulders, hips	Pounding
Earth	Head, spine	Crossing
Metal	Sternum, disks	Splitting

There are five Tao directions of motion:

- *Drilling* motions are circular in nature, such as water rings extending out from a pebble dropped into a lake.
- *Crushing* motions collapse in on themselves on a hinge, such as tree branches blowing to and away from the trunk.
- *Pounding* motions are explosive like fire. They have huge reach, impact, power, and range. They're 360 degrees like an explosion.
- *Crossing* motions are movements that cross over a line or plane, such as leaning over to the left or right.
- *Splitting* motions cut through or split something apart, such as an axe through a log or the ground in an earthquake.

In BodyLogos, we associate each of these motions with the joints most commonly used in strength training.

Drilling is associated with your wrists, shoulder blades, ankles, and thumbs because you can circle each of those joints—but you can't rotate them. For example, if you hold your forearm in place, your wrist can move your hand in a circle, but it can't turn your hand over. Similarly, you can move your shoulder blades and thumbs in circles, but you can't change the direction they face.

Crushing is associated with your elbows, knees, and digits because they fold inwardly and outwardly on a hinge—they go in only two directions.

Pounding is associated with your shoulders and hips because the ball and socket joints have the same three dimensionality of an explosion. They are far reaching and have the most power and freedom of motion.

Crossing is associated with your spine and head because these joints string together, and as a collective, they can cross over every plane of the body. The spinal column's balance of curves also crosses over the coronal plane at the central plumb line multiple times, creating the body's natural spring.

Splitting is associated with your sternum and the discs between your vertebrae. Because they are cartilaginous joints, their power lies in their pliability, which creates the padding between your bones and keeps them from fusing painfully or creating rigidity. So in a sense, the cartilage splits your bones to keep you mobile, such as an earthquake separating tectonic plates.

When becoming a bodyworker, I learned to penetrate my energy's strength beneath the surface of a recipient's tension. I discovered that contact using gentle cyclical movements, made with my thumb and wrist, coiled my energy's force for *drilling* down into their tense holding patterns. This coil set up a bull's eye for *crushing* through the surface tension with my weight. By simply extending my elbow straight, I could lean into their resistance. If my deep dive into the person's tension hit a plateau before surrendering, my shoulder's *pounding* jackhammer motion could penetrate my weight even deeper and also allow me to rotate my weight out of the full body lean without causing the receiver to recoil back into tension's persistent grip. These point-specific deep dives required whole-body integration. To actualize this integration, my spine's pivoting motion would guide their hips into a *crossing* over the midline stretch.

We experienced this as a full-spine stretch together, the final motion being the *splitting* karate chop into the client's softened tissues. This movement continues to draw tension out of his or her body, not from the downward chop but by the force under my sternum's limited mobility powerfully stretching upward toward the sky, as if extracting the tension out of his or her body with each chop's upward withdrawal. Each motion develops out of the previous, a generating cycle that encourages a penetrating touch. These intention-based motions, whose origins are, in most cases, not from the hand that touches but the entire frame of the giver, offer subtle yet deep changes in the receiver.

Every movement's limitation gives rise to another movement, meaning, while limitation describes an isolated joint's range of motion. Freedom of movement describes the transference between multiple joints. Healthy joints ask for healthy boundaries that seamlessly align through movement.

Now I'll depict the direction of motion in the body using the same generating cycle in everyday activity.

- While the revolving scoop of the drilling *thumbs and wrists* use their great dexterity to grab what you are reaching for, it is the crushing bend of the elbow that brings that item toward you.
- To put that item away in the cupboard, the crushing *elbow* then extends and calls on the pounding shoulder's full rotation to reach the top shelf.
- The farther back on the shelf the item needs to go, the more stretch and articulating strength are needed to move stuff out of the way. The pounding *shoulder joint's* rotation and shock absorption finesses this perfectly until you need to reach just one more inch, where the crossing rotation of the spine offers its support.
- The ability to rotate the *spine* and cross over your midline gives you that extra inch of distance to push the item to its resting place, where you need the splitting sternum's lift.
- As you retreat from this mega stretch, the splitting nature of your *sternum* stays in its upward thrust, keeping your posture lifted to soften the return of your muscles back to their neutral placement.

Each motion facilitates the need for the next motion, such as the evolution of a species. The generating cycle develops movement for survival and ease.

And finally, I'll depict the direction of motion in the body using the destructive cycle. Remember, use the destructive cycle to bypass one element for a specific goal.

- When you get tired of standing and lean on your hands, the weight through your wrists *(drilling)* connects directly with your shoulders *(pounding)*, keeping the elbows locked *(crushing)*.
- To type efficiently, your fingers and elbows *(crushing)* need to bypass your shoulders' involvement *(pounding)* and connect with the attention of your head and spine *(crossing)*.
- To kick a soccer ball straight down the field, your hip *(pounding)* sweeps through its full range of motion, using a lift through your discs and sternum *(splitting)* to stabilize the force, never needing to cross over the spine's *(crossing)* median plane.
- When your neck rotates your head *(crossing)*, the gliding dexterity of your opposite shoulder blade *(drilling)* provides the grounding balance for that motion. But your spinal discs and sternum *(splitting)* stay neutral.
- To sit down gracefully, you lift through the soft, pliable support of your spinal discs and sternum *(splitting)* as you fold your knees *(crushing)*, keeping the shoulder blades *(drilling)* neutral.

Each motion facilitates the need to omit the resultant for greater support or reach, each crafted for a unique purpose. The destructive cycle limits movement but offers specificity.

Movement Breakdown

 Drilling: Wrists, Shoulder Blades, Ankles, and Thumbs

All movement happens in a joint, the intersection between two bones. Bone is the underlying foundation for strength training and the overall body part associated with the water element. Bone movements that specifically relate to the water element are those that drill, such as the circling of the wrists and ankles.

Watch a river flowing between and around the protruding rock formations and root structures contained in them. Flowing in and around the crevasses of the riverbed, water manages to direct itself through this maze of formations with little conflict––yin. Imagine the water as your energy moving throughout the bones of your ankle. When aligned properly, your movement's energy flows in and around this maze of bones, keeping the flow of energy unified and directed.

We're most familiar with the muscles and bones at the exterior reach of our bodies. How often have you tried to lift something with your wrist before you've engaged your bicep? Trying to redirect the flow of your movement from the small muscles surrounding the wrist is like trying to redirect a river's current with a few pebbles––yang—a task that, though futile, the wrists, thumbs, and ankles are known to attempt. Your mission—should you choose to accept it—is to ensure that your drilling joints don't try to take on yang motions when yin is more appropriate.

When working with outside resistance, it's important to understand a joint's neutral position, the position that is optimal for energy flow and safety. In regard to the wrists and thumbs, it's easy to experience neutral when your arms are relaxed down at your sides. Gravity will naturally position your hand's weight in relation to the wrist and thumb, exactly the way you will need to maintain them throughout any lateral or overhead movement.

Ankles are a bit more complicated, since they need your body's weight resting on the gushing spring points for the heel stirrups to release ankle tension into the earth (gushing spring/heel stirrup marriage p. 48). In spite of this, once weighted properly, the ankles naturally neutralize for an easy relationship with gravity.

The shoulder blades, however, are a little more slippery—it's not quite as easy to recognize their neutral position. They easily glide apart and take away the backing for the chest to feel supported and lifted. Most of us recognize the computer crunch as our natural default in the twenty-first century. Once the chest is collapsed, it concaves into the back's musculature, and the shoulder blades will have difficulty collecting themselves into their tighter neutral position. To prevent this separation between shoulder blades, understand that the shoulders and arms reside on the coronal plane (remember lesson 3, p. 36) when one is standing upright.

Observe your profile: When properly aligned, your chest will appear in front of your arms, and your back will appear behind your arms. The shoulder blades will dictate where the shoulders and arms live in space. If they are too spread apart, and the shoulders shift to the anterior plane, hiding the chest; if they are too pinched together, the shoulders shift to the posterior plane, hiding the back. When successfully placed, the shoulder blades live directly behind the breasts and place shoulders and arms between front and back planes of the body.

The dexterity and cyclical movement the wrists and thumbs provide to a dancer in his or her expression or to a technician in his or her precision lie in their acuity. Their valued speed and dexterity are executed with little or no outside resistance. Therefore, in strength training the wrists and thumbs remain as a quiet support to simply help balance what you are handling. Remember that these joints, though exceptionally agile, merely align energy movement between the outside resistance and the muscle leading your movement—they aren't the leaders.

Shoulder blade and ankle movement, on the other hand, like a narrowing and widening riverbank, significantly leads energy movement toward the appropriate muscle group when handling outside resistance or managing posture. Their movement gives your energy clear direction. The shoulder blades' influential range of motion balances your torso's alignment, and the ankles' acute navigation to position weight properly on the feet influences the release of tension body wide in exchange for the earth's energy.

- Drilling joints have a reduced ball socket range where rotation isn't permitted.
- They rock, hinge, and slide to create cyclical movement in wrists, ankles, thumbs, and shoulder blades.
- Neutral position of the wrists, thumbs, and ankles feels like a stream of water flushing throughout and around the bones.
- Neutral placement of the shoulder blades positions them behind the breasts and places shoulders and arms on the coronal plane.
- The shoulder blades' range of motion manages your torso's alignment, and the ankles' acute navigation weights the feet properly to release tension body wide in exchange for earth's energy.

Wrist Roll

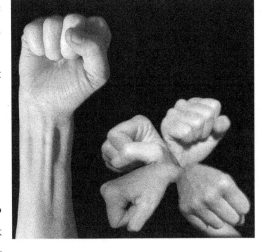

Wrist joints channel energy movement by aligning an outside resistance with the muscles leading your movement. Maintain a neutral position in wrists at all times when handling weight. Explore the full range of movement in this Wrist Roll without resistance to recognize its central neutral position.

 Crushing: Elbows, Knees, and Digits

The spooning configuration of a crushing joint is limited to two directions—flexion and extension. You can see this at work in your elbows, knees, fingers, and toe joints. Just as a secondary tree branch connects with its mother branch, the *C*-shaped connecting surface of a larger limb joins with the rounded attachment surface of a smaller limb. These wood element joints are crushing in nature, in that they can collapse in on themselves. As folding joints, they give great flexibility to a tree's branches and great mobility to your body's limbs.

The more distal musculoskeletal crushing joints provide the body's greatest mobility and dexterity and are, to a great degree, hinge joints. They are what make up much of the appendicular skeleton (the bones and cartilage that support appendages). The greatest danger to these joints is overworking their ligaments and tendons. This is done when the joint is your focus—yin—rather than the muscle creating the joint's movement—yang. If you are opening a door, your focus is on the door, not on the movement of its hinges. The same applies to extending an arm or leg. Your focus needs to be on the muscles extending rather than on the joints permitting the extension.

If the joint feels the brunt of your labors, it's a warning that you're working with too much tension, your resistance is greater than your muscular strength, or you're torquing your movement out of the two-direction limitation of these hinges.

To balance crushing joints at the onset of an exercise, you first square the flat supporting surface of your body's coronal plane and its active joint to the resistance, so as not to torque the joint outside its non-rotating folding motion. This aligns the motion safely. Second, you would connect to your abdominal strength to stabilize your energy's force and give your more distal crushing joints a secure foundation. Alignment and foundation are crucial to protect crushing joints from unnecessary wear and tear before they encounter an outside resistance.

- Crushing joints make up much of the appendicular skeleton and are limited to two directions, flexion and extension, in knees, elbows, ankles, fingers, and toes.
- Focus on the muscles creating a movement rather than on the joint permitting it.
- Square body and active joint to an outside resistance to align motion safely.
- Connect to abdominal stability to give the more distal crushing joints a secure foundation.
- When a crushing joint feels the brunt of your labor, adjust alignment or lessen resistance.

Prayer Position

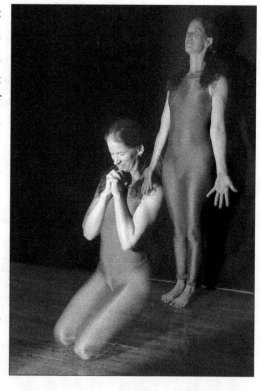

Explore your crushing joint's full range of motion without resistance throughout the appendicular skeleton. Do this as multiple stretches, one area at a time, to learn the range of motion in all the prayer position crushing joints. A range made without pain or discomfort in the joint is considered full. Full range of motion will stretch the surrounding muscles and is necessary to maintain joint health and agility. When challenging crushing joints with resistance, however, keep movements smaller than their full range and don't enter into the stretch zone.

 Pounding: Shoulders and Hips

Liberation defines these rotating joints. In a pounding joint, the ball-like head of one bone fits into the socket-like head of another, permitting a full range of movement, as in the shoulders and hips. They contain a lubricating fluid that protects bone integrity and absorbs the heat of friction. This lubricating fluid, known as synovial fluid, is contained in bursa sacs that can handle the pounding nature of fire element movements.

The excitement of watching a campfire is experiencing its wild, erratic movement. It flickers in every direction with far-reaching tendrils. Fire energy is enlivening, and when you direct its force, you can create comfort, safety, and artistry—yang. But when the force of fire is misdirected or unmanaged, it can destroy all in its path—yin.

Although the shoulder and hip joints have exceptional range of motion, the strength and flexibility of the muscles surrounding the joints determine how much of that range can be used. To determine your personal range of motion in hips and shoulders, move slowly through the strength-training exercises, paying attention to when you begin to feel a stretch or gripping reaction in or around the joint. Limit your range to what produces no stretch or gripping sensation. Without weight, you can extend farther into the stretch-producing zones. Like a crushing joint, the range of motion advisable for a pounding joint when in a strength-training exercise is smaller than the range of motion possible in normal day-to-day activities.

There is a complexity to pounding joints that is an additional reason for caution. These joints are a nexus of muscles, ligaments, and tendons coming together from every direction. The external momentum easily generated from these free-swinging joints can create a force that pushes through their infrastructure, akin to the force unleashed if you swung a punch. And as you may have learned on the playground, you can punch only as hard as you can sustain the counterpunch of that impact.

To manage this outward momentum, you need to organize stability, not rigidity, that equals the outward swing. Connect to your abdominal strength, feel the weight of your bones, and relax the joint when you connect with outside resistance. Without this organization, the muscle connections and sinews within these joints are easily inflamed, shredded, or torn. To protect the infrastructure of pounding joints, reduce range of motion and speed when handling outside resistance.

- Pounding joints are synovial joints with full range of movement in shoulders and hips.
- Strength and flexibility in surrounding muscles determine pounding joints' usable range of motion.
- Limit range to what produces no stretch or gripping sensation when strength training.
- To stabilize outward momentum, connect to your abdominal strength, feel the weight of your bones, and relax the joint.
- Greater range can be exercised without resistance in normal day-to-day activities.

Dead Cow

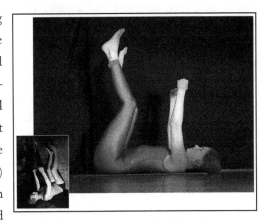

Clarify the bone placement of these flexible joints by lying supine and relaxing the bone weight of arms and legs through the ball aspects of hips and shoulders. While maintaining the natural curve of the spine—and keeping elbows and knees unlocked—position limbs directly over hip and shoulder girdles. Use a wall to support legs if needed. Once relaxed, observe the placement of hips and shoulders in relation to the spine. Notice that the spine between shoulder blades and the lower back (waistline) doesn't meet the floor. Instead, the shoulder blades and sacrum are meeting the floor. Compare this to your usual posture and exercise starting positions. Adjust your standing skeletal alignment using the bone placement found in the Dead Cow. When standing, imagine the floor at your back.

Crossing: Head and Spine

The axial skeleton is the principal support structure of the body, just as the earth is for humanity. It comprises your spine, ribs, neck, and head—oriented along the central vertical axis of the body, which possesses a series of thirty-one to thirty-three joints. Because this series of joints, which pivot and move around the axis of the spinal cord, connects the many bones of the upper and lower body via a single strand of vertebrae, a lot of muscular support is needed.

Taken together, your axial skeleton is associated with the Tao motion of crossing. Crossing refers to crossing over the line of resistance while turning over. This emphasizes a dominant and submissive role to its movement and is what you need to support the natural curves of the spine.

The crossing joints act as a spring for the body while simultaneously housing the central nervous system. The spring of the spine needs a blend of support––yang––and relaxation––yin––to be functional and balanced. If the curves of the spine become imbalanced, and the convex and concave curves aren't creating equilibrium along the coronal plane, there will be complications with the nerve exits between vertebrae. This lack of spinal equilibrium in time can develop into disc erosion.

The lower spinal column is actively supported by the abdominal muscles in the anterior body and the buttock muscles in the posterior body. Concurrently, for this support to be fully effective, the spine requires the lower back and iliopsoas muscles to loosen their grip. If we go back to the psyche-muscular blueprint, you can see that proper support comes from engaging your sense of self (abdominals), letting go of fear (lower back), releasing a sense of control (iliopsoas), and feeling comfortable enough (buttocks) to stand in your power.

The vertebrae-rib marriage of the upper spinal column responds to the relationship between chest and upper back muscles. The upper spinal column and connection site for the ribs maintain the integrity of your torso alignment. From a psyche-muscular perspective, this balance of support and relaxation is between your "smile of truth" (chest) and your "protection of self" (back), an impassioned relationship that is continuously exploring living your truth and ensuring survival.

This strand of thirty-one to thirty-three joints is dependent on equilibrium between anterior and posterior, and superior and inferior muscles of the torso. The opposition between dominant and submissive placement of the bones, and the active and counter-active forces in the muscles (more on this in lesson 5), are essential for fluid mobility. This equilibrium is the foundation for neutral and essential alignments.

Your greatest ally in establishing healthy alignment in the crossing joints of your spinal column is surprisingly gravity. Although lying horizontally decompresses the bones so the natural and correct curves of the spine can easily show themselves, bringing those same curves into a vertical posture gives the muscles an opportunity to establish a balance between lift and drop, contraction and release. This is your goal for optimum strength. Optimal alignment allows the spine's natural curves to snake upward on the body's axis in a fluid and balanced manner, permitting the compression-explosion sequence needed for its springing mechanism. Without these natural curves, rigidity creeps into your movement, and posture becomes frail and compromised.

- Crossing joints are the body's principal support structure, which houses the central nervous system. Vertebral junctures allow the head to pivot and the spine to move around the spinal cord.
- The spring of a spine needs balance between muscular support and relaxation.
- Engaging abdominal and buttock muscles while relaxing lower back and iliopsoas muscles balances the lower spine's curves.
- The upper spine's curves need balance between your chest and back muscles.
- Opposition between dominant and submissive placement of the bones and balanced muscular forces is essential for fluid mobility.

Supine Lie

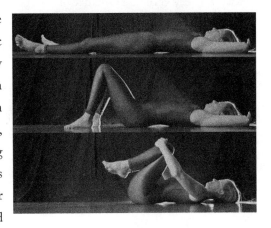

To experience spinal alignment, particularly for sitting, lie supine with legs extended and spine relaxed. Feel where the pelvic girdle begins to bear down into the floor, at the sacrum below low back dimples, and identify the lower back's natural arch. Maintain the natural lower back arch as you bend knees to place feet on the floor. Then, again maintaining the natural lower back arch, lift feet off the floor. Distinguish the difference between folding in the hip joints and folding at the waistline. Use this awareness of bone placement to inform your posture. Observe whether you are folding in your hips or waist throughout your day and what is required for a given movement. Sitting asks for folding at the hips with a quiet natural lower back arch maintained.

Prone Straight-Leg Lie

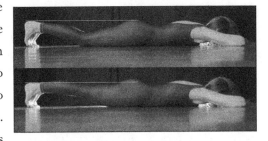

To experience spinal alignment, particularly for standing, lie prone with toes tucked under and knees bent while keeping spine relaxed, abdominals lifted, and hip bones weighted into floor. Push downward through your heels, keeping hip bones on the floor, to extend knees. Observe the placement of your pelvis in relation to your rib cage. Compare this alignment with your standing posture. You may notice your pelvis positioned much more forward than its usual position. Use this bone placement to inform your posture. Repeat this heel push several times to experience the pelvis's forward adjustment.

Splitting: Sternum and Discs

As you explore movement in the musculoskeletal system, you quickly become aware of where movement is limited. Splitting joints are cartilaginous connective tissue that makes up the discs between vertebral bodies of the spine and creates attachment between the three aspects of the sternum. These joints provide only partial mobility and are prominent in your upright posture and balance. The metal element's nature is to split. The ax goes in––yin, and the ax comes out––yang. Connective tissues—ligaments, tendons, and cartilage—have an inward focus to stay affixed with a stable reinforcement, to ground themselves like an electrical wire. This grounding alignment can draw the ax in, with little concern about its reemergence, leaving you with a collapsed posture. This obsession with fixed stability is what makes emerging from neutral alignment to essential alignment challenging. It involves an emergence into what is unknown.

A splitting joint is most easily felt when taking a deep breath. The swell of the chest gives rise to the sternum and brings a yawning sensation to the discs between vertebrae of the spinal column. It can be so subtle that you miss it. Imagine turning a light switch on at your tailbone, having the electrical current travel up the spine to the light bulb at your head's crown. Feel these attachment sites swell with vibrancy as if a soft light were emerging between every vertebral juncture of the spine. Give the central current that lives within the spinal cord the space to radiate.

This central current aligns you to both earth and sky, connects you to the ground, and inspires you toward spirit. This central current positions neutral alignment and is the source for expansion into essential alignment. Realize the importance of these stabilizing joints as the aligning segments that cushion and stretch the central nervous system. Before embarking on any movement, breathe life into these joints. Give them air.

Breath directs alignment and motivates energy movement. Use your breath to elevate the sternum and elongate the spinal column. Throughout an exercise, challenge splitting joints to connect upwardly and downwardly. Without this gentle encouragement, the limited mobility of these areas will turn to no mobility, creating shallow lung capacity and internal collapse.

- Splitting joints are stabilizing cartilaginous connective tissue with partial to no mobility.
- Splitting joints make up the discs between vertebrae and the attachments within the sternum.
- Experience these joints as attachment sites that swell.
- These junctures are aligning segments that cushion the central nervous system, position neutral alignment, and expand you into essential alignment.
- Use your breath to elevate the sternum and elongate the spinal column. Without encouragement to be in motion, limited mobility will turn to no mobility.

Supine Tube Lie

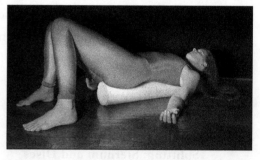

To experience the splitting joints of the sternum, lie supine with a three-foot foam tube or rolled-up beach towel supporting your pelvis, spinal column, and head. Surrender the shoulder blades on each side of the tube and relax arms on the floor, palms up. As you allow your arms and shoulders to fall beneath the level of the spine, the sternum will swell forward as if opening to the heavens. As these connection sites within the sternum gently stretch apart, feel how you are giving the heart center space and vitality. Use this stretch as a reference for keeping the heart center expanded.

Prone Ball Lie

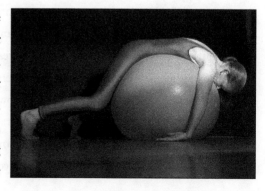

To experience the splitting joints of the spinal discs, lie prone over a large ball. Keep feet separated with toes tucked under for stability and allow arms and head to relax around ball. Soften knees, widen back, and allow the weight of your head to surrender muscle tension away from neck and spine. Feel expansion between vertebrae increase to a greater and greater proportion. As you relax, it will feel as if the central nervous system were yawning, allowing the discs to swell and giving greater space for nerve exits. Your spinal cord is sighing with relief as your body expands away from the need to grasp in on itself. Use this stretch as a reference for keeping the spinal column decompressed and disentangled with the central nervous system.

> The Universe lies before you on the floor,
> in the air, in the mysterious bodies of your dancers,
> in your mind.
> From this voyage no one returns poor or weary.
>
> —Agnes de Mille, American-born dancer, choreographer, and visionary

Connection Chapter

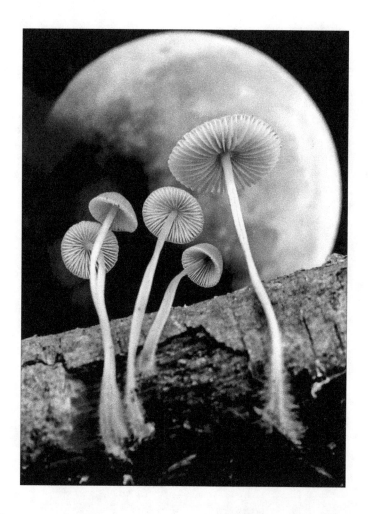

The reason why Heaven and Earth can endure and last a long time—
Is that they do not live for themselves.
Therefore they can long endure.

Therefore the Sage:
Puts himself in the background yet finds himself in the foreground;
Puts self-concern out of his mind, yet finds that his self-concern is preserved.

Lesson 5
The Art of Alignment

Tao produced the One.
The One produced the two.
The two produced the three.
And the three produced the ten thousand things.
The ten thousand things carry the yin and embrace the yang,
And through the blending of the material force they achieve harmony.

—Lao Tzu, Tao Te Ching

Universal energy produced the spirit self.
The spirit self produced mind and body.
Mind and body produced consciousness—a collection of beliefs.
Personal beliefs produced a psyche-muscular blueprint,
Psyche-muscular blueprints create myriad manifestations—a life and its creations.
And life is the opportunity to achieve harmony between one's self and one's environment.

—Tammy Wise, BodyLogos

Connect to Your Unique Purpose

The blanket response to the purpose of wellness initiatives is often "to live longer." But for what? What is the point? We need our strength to create a meaningful life and meaning in the world at large.

A fundamental principle of Tao is that every individual is a microcosm of the universe. What balances the universe also balances an individual life. Like the universe, you are an energy system composed of energy orbits and connections that keep you alive and in motion, no different than our smallest constituent the atom—the building block of every solid, liquid, gas, and plasma. The atom is composed of a nucleus, comparable to our dan tien; a nucleus has positive and negative charges called protons and electrons, comparable to our contractions and releases. When equal in number, that atom is electrically neutral; and when our forces are equal, we are neutralized. BodyLogos aims to align the inner momentum of our individual energy system with that of the outer universe, connecting to the spiritual meaning and purpose of each unique human existence.

> *Energy systems*
> *are*
> *Dimensions of empty space contained,*
> *Unparalleled and uncarved,*
> *A unique symphony of energy vibrations,*
> *Bringing an original nature into the light.*

Recognizing our individual energy system as a mirror image of the universal energy system helps us to acknowledge that every element, species, and manifestation is an integral part of the whole. And those individual contributions to the greater whole can—and should—vary widely from person to person. My mother was a participant at a personal development course where I assisted. The adviser asked her whether she had other children and whether they were alike. She said no.

"My oldest child, Sherry, is all about family and creating a nucleus. Tammy is all about the world at large."

Her analysis struck me as dead on. Neither of us has a grander or more important purpose, but we are both very clear on why we are here. But I also acknowledge that while our purposes may vary, our drive to contribute is the same. I never felt the urge to have children, but both of us were born to create. And in our separate micro purposes, we both perfectly reflect that macro of the universe.

To move with purpose in our lives requires us to accept that we have two aspects of our energy system to consider. While the theory of yin and yang forges a *spiritual* relationship between earth and sky through the bones' relationship with gravity, the five-element theory forges a *metaphysical* relationship between mind and body through the muscles' relationship with centripetal and centrifugal forces. Therefore, recognizing the difference between muscular balance and skeletal alignment is crucial to managing energy flow.

Balance versus Alignment

Alignment refers to the skeleton. Aligning energy centers organizes the bones optimally and creates space between them. Balance refers to the muscular system's symmetry between contracting and releasing forces. Balancing muscular activity maintains skeletal alignment.

Misalignment, in general, is the result of unbalanced strength or flexibility in the muscular system. That's because the muscular system is the easiest place for your body to retain tension. But the good news is that it's also the easiest place to relieve tension before it deepens its hold into the organ systems and becomes chronic illness or compulsive anxiety.

A balanced muscular system is divided into active (yang) and counter-active (yin) halves—one half contracts and the other half releases. To be balanced, the contraction of one muscle or muscular group has to be equal to the release of its opposite. Imagine two separate forces, one on the anterior plane (the front of your body) and one on the posterior plane (the back of your body), passing each other in opposite directions like the pistons of an engine.

You could compare this opposition to bicycle racing. Racers use pedal straps so they can simultaneously power down with one pedal and power up with the other. Every stroke, like the engine piston, has a spark firing its movement, and balancing those opposing strokes keeps the bicycle upright and its power twofold. Non-racers who cycle around without pedal straps have only the downward stroke of one pedal at a time to power the bicycle. It's as if half the spark plugs in the engine are burned out. The bicycle keeps moving but with half the power and futilely tips from side to side as you cycle.

In every muscular movement, there is a *plane* of stillness between the active and counter-active forces. This stillness lies in your skeleton's alignment. There is also a point of stillness in the muscle's and bone's common center—the dan tien—where you can gauge each force's level of intensity or speed. Once you recognize the stillness of your bones as separate from the movement of your muscles, you can begin to differentiate between tension and strength in your muscular activity and recognize balance as a spiritual state of quietude.

Mindfulness Delivers Equipoise

I call "equipoise" the spiritual quietude that lives in your dan tien energy center and bones. It is the eye of the storm, so to speak, the stillness in the middle of motion. You have experienced equipoise as a *point* of stillness in your dan tien. Remember, your dan tien is the center point of the stretch between earth and sky when you extend into essential alignment.

A plane of equipoise is sustained by balancing the two planes of muscular activity—every contraction has an equal and opposite release on its opposing plane. This can be true of isolated movements, such as balancing your biceps' contraction and your triceps' release, or of unified movements whereby the two planes of the whole muscular system are considered. Imagine the coronal plane splitting your movement between the front and back halves of your muscular system. You will find the stillness of equipoise in the dividing bones—the coronal plane—when muscular movement is balanced and skeletal alignment is present.

To experience this phenomenon, consider this: the duality of bone alignment and muscular balance asks your intention and attention to split. This split expands your consciousness between connecting inwardly and outwardly. If instead you feel tight and overwhelmed, stop thinking and *feel*. With this commitment to feel alignment and balance, you will create a foundation for dissolving the holding patterns that exhaust your energy. And this foundation develops the practice of active meditation, which resolves conflict, into a lifestyle.

Experience Equipoise Exercise
Serenity. Belonging. Hope.
mindthebody.bodylogos.com/video8
(abbreviated description)

Alignment: Stand in neutral alignment. With weight on the balls of the feet, drink earth energy up through the gushing spring points and release tense energy down through the heel stirrups. Balance the gushing spring/heel stirrup marriage, use alignment stabilizers to align energy centers, and stretch relaxed energy outwardly from the dan tien into essential alignment. Recognize your dan tien as a point of equipoise, the point of stillness between your upward and downward stretch. Feel for its quiet center as your energy keeps expanding. The more your energy radiates easefully outward, the quieter you feel inward.

Balance: Now imagine, without moving, you are about to take a step. Energy naturally ascends up the front of the body to propel you forward. At the same time, energy descends down the back of the body. Feel these two energies streaming through the muscular system, readying you for movement. The front and back of the body are energetically split, keeping your skeletal alignment centrally intact. As you balance the opposing forces of ascending and descending forces, your coronal plane—the plane separating the body's front sides from back sides—becomes distinguishable. Allow the quiet stillness of equipoise to spread through the coronal plane. Feel how the balance of forces in the muscles supports the bone's alignment, making the bones a tranquil plane of equipoise.

Action: Excite your energies' opposition until you are propelled into walking. Experience your skeleton traveling forward as a tranquil plane of equipoise. Keep feeling for the balance of forces that propelled you into movement, maintaining your movement. Keep breathing relaxation into the flow of energy; recognize you are continually releasing the stagnant energy of tension into the earth and restoring your energy from the earth.

Meditation: Experience the quiet equipoise of your bones as your essence. Allow yourself this meditative walk until you experience yourself present in time and space.

In this meditative state, you experience both who you have been and who you are intending to become. When these two perspectives meet, it's a sacred moment for positive change. It's the moment between what was and what will be. It's a moment of grace whereby your intuitive spirit voice can influence your way.

Experience Equipoise Wish List

- You experience an increase of free attention and release tension.
- Listening inwardly becomes easier.
- An inner awareness develops that offers meaning to strength.
- Contentment in being you emerges.
- You are introduced to greater and greater degrees of neutral attention.

After living in New York City for many years, where he raised a family and operated a demanding real estate business, Gene decided to take time to enjoy nature and the slower pace of life along the verdant Gulf Coast of Florida. After a while, he noticed he had established a calmer and more focused approach to living, with a deeper sense of natural rhythms, breathing, and body awareness—something he hoped to sustain and even augment after his return to New York. I was engaged to help him maintain flexibility, proper breathing, and body presence. I initially designed a stretching regime to release his impermeable hamstrings. The minute he hit the sting of his inflexibility, he experienced such unbearable pain that he instantly collapsed out of the stretch. He is an otherwise fit man, meaning good muscle tone and a healthy fat ratio. So I asked him, "Okay, you had to have worked through some pain thresholds to develop your muscularity. What makes the pain of flexibility training so unbearable for you?"

He's reply was, "It's never ending!"

I think what he was trying to communicate was, it's always there.

If you always react to life in a certain way, it's hard to separate it from who you are. The familiar sting he experiences, the pain of inflexibility, is a holding pattern he never remembers being without. To improve his flexibility, it was essential for him to recognize his tension as separate from himself. It was a limitation he took on. Just as the repetition of reacting with tension created the holding pattern, the repetition of balancing contraction and release also created change. Once he was free to penetrate his hamstring muscles, proper pelvic alignment was permitted. Body alignment led to the metaphysical state of equipoise, and Gene felt plugged in. His manner became more relaxed and trusting during our sessions as he learned to sit more quietly. He soon accepted one of the central principles of the BodyLogos practice: we are physically stronger, balanced, and in control of our bodies once we align with gravity, the quiet yet awesome force that regulates our existence. The ease of living he had found through his external environment in Florida was now becoming an internal environment. After sensing the presence of equipoise—an elevated force through the anterior body balanced with a grounded force through the posterior body—he experienced the coronal plane as an open "circuit" between earth and sky. He said to me, "This is a feeling of 'true strength.'"

> When I attain equipoise, I lose consciousness of gravity, of effort. My body is completely integrated with itself, strong and solid yet invisible to me. I need no longer think about it. My sense that there are body "parts" dissolves. The feeling of weightlessness born of balance and harmony is profound and liberating, and I experience physical and emotional tranquility.
>
> —Gene

The combined strength of bone stillness and muscular movement creates a heightened awareness of your energy's condition. You learn to gently steer your subtle energy with intention rather than demanding results with brute force. This sensitivity and experience of equipoise, in physical movement and mental discernment, conserve and respect your energy system. Developing equipoise staying power changes not only your physical and mental posture but also your life.

Replenish Your Energy

When your center of gravity becomes a microcosm of the macrocosm of the universe, your dan tien radiates an electrical current that makes your skeleton an antenna to spirit. You sense yourself as an integral part of the whole of creation. You know everything is okay because you have aligned the energy circuit of your body with that of the universe. You feel protected and plugged into nature's electromagnetic field. You feel content, fulfilled, and inspired all at once.

Let's review what you know to be true about energy as it relates to the body so far:

- Alignment is an opposing reach between earth and sky from the dan tien on a single plane. This opposition is experienced as a *point* of stillness—equipoise—between your bone's weight surrendering downwardly to the earth and relaxation stretching upwardly to the sky.
- Balance is an opposing force between active and counter-active energies, originating in the dan tien, traveling on two planes—anterior and posterior. This opposition is experienced as a *plane* of stillness between your body's two halves—the equipoise between a muscular contraction that moves you and its opposing release that stabilizes you.

While your skeleton's alignment with gravity houses and organizes your energy system, your muscles' relationship with centripetal and centrifugal forces cycles the life force of your energy system.

Due to the inherent momentum created as centripetal and centrifugal forces feed each other, their influence revitalizes your energy. Just like the balance between day and night, the balance between your muscles' contracting force and releasing force transitions into one another over and over again, renewing your energy.

In the experiencing equipoise exercise, you used the opposition of forces in the anterior and posterior body as a way to find the central stillness in your coronal plane, your skeleton. For the opposition of forces to generate energy anew, you connect them, creating an uninterrupted orbit of force that circulates through and around the muscular system. I call these "energy orbits," loops of internal momentum that rejuvenate your energy reserve.

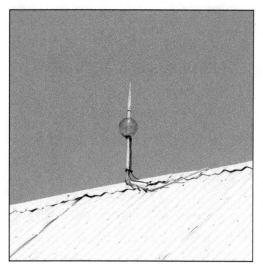

Imagine essential alignment (from lesson 3) as if it were the iron rod passing through the glass globe of a vintage lightning rod; only in reality, it is your energy axis passing through your movement's circular radius. Energy electrons are first drawn in through your skeleton's essential alignment (iron rod). The energy conducted is contained in your energy body (glass globe) to generate the muscles, using the principles of centripetal and centrifugal forces. When your bones are aligned with gravity and your muscles are balanced between contractions and releases, they coordinate as connected energy orbits and converge their strength in your dan tien.

In order for your bones and muscles to conduct energy efficiently, their alliance to the same center—your dan tien—must be maintained. In the complexity of aligning bones and balancing muscles in movement, this shared center brings order to chaos. When your muscles successfully come into balance with your skeleton's alignment, it's because the energy orbits successfully and freely cycled energy around the body and back to the dan tien.

The dan tien, your body's central energy source, is where your relationship with gravity and centripetal and centrifugal forces originates. All movement begins from and returns to the dan tien in the lower abdomen. When unimpeded, this creates organized energy orbits, whereby the whole body's alignment is in accordance with even the smallest muscular efforts. Feeling this uninterrupted current of energy cycling through the outer limits of our movement and back to the source power in the dan tien mimics the planets' orbit around the sun.

This circular pattern of force around your center of gravity will only generate energy if it is balanced; otherwise movement throws you off center, and you become energetically unplugged. Imagine if a planet's trajectory around the sun became unbalanced. It would be unable to regain its position in the solar system. Total chaos would unfold, and day and night, as we know them to be, would cease to exist.

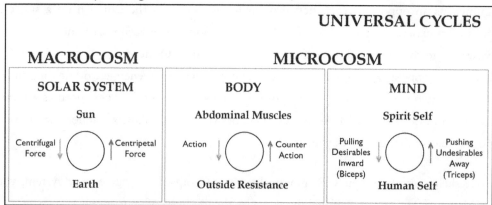

Just as the planets have outgoing and incoming energies that stabilize their center of gravity, so do we. In the above graph, the microcosm of our minds and bodies is compared to the macrocosm of the solar system. In the solar system, the life force is the sun; in our body, it is the dan tien energy center, found within the abdominal muscles. For this reason, every exercise can be considered an abdominal activity.

In my years of teaching group fitness, I've been known as the abdominal police. All I've had to do is look at a student, and he or she would be reminded to lift his or her lower abdominal muscles. My greater challenge has been getting students to release their lower backs with the same commitment in which they engage their abdominals. I have found that it's easier to get someone to do something than to stop doing something. For this, students need to realize less is more. They need a transformative experience that ensures them that releasing isn't lazy or slacking. Without my hands to position their pelvises into alignment, they often cannot experience the power of release. That's because it's the bones' alignment that ultimately leads to the surrender of the tension-filled holding patterns that block strength, not a mental command to your muscles to "release."

The BodyLogos technique considers the cyclical nature of energy when connecting to outside resistance. Outside resistance is anything that comes into our energy bodies, tangible or intangible, from our environment or our reaction to our environment. Active and counter-active forces mimic centrifugal and centripetal forces, and are the generators that give our life force movement—granting us the strength to direct our minds, bodies, external environments, and internal tension in the direction of self-realization.

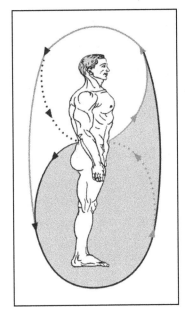

By orbiting the energy output of a movement back to its origin point—the dan tien—we are creating the same vital momentum observed in the solar system. This mindful approach to strength training naturally replenishes our body's life force and clears obstacles, supports a greater understanding of what is obscuring our life's alignment, and makes quality of life something we can manage with greater and greater effectiveness.

By connecting balanced energy forces into energy orbits, you are able to connect the relationship you have with yourself with your world, and vice versa. In this way, you can endure physical, mental, and emotional challenges with stability, strength, and endurance as well as with curiosity, contentment, and grace.

Expect to experience increased energy flow and unleashed emotional activity as you progress from this still meditation introduction to the video's active meditation.

Centripetal of Centrifugal Force Exercise
Protected. In control. Intelligent.
mindthebody.bodylogos.com/video9
(abbreviated description)

Alignment: Sit in neutral alignment, remembering to ground the million-dollar point through the chair and balance the gushing spring and heel stirrup marriage with the earth. Use alignment stabilizers to align energy centers and stretch relaxed energy outward from the dan tien into essential alignment. Again, breathe deeply and liberate any residual tension into flowing energy until you recognize your dan tien as a point of equipoise.

Balance: Visualize energy exiting the posterior dan tien sideways. This will create a posterior transverse plumb line. Your low back dimples will feel dilated, and lower back muscles will surrender more deeply. Now, visualize a similar energy pathway creating an anterior transverse plumb line. Your energy will converge in through the abdominal muscles toward the dan tien. Finally, allow the convergence of energy at your anterior center to pass through the dan tien to your posterior center and continue in two horizontal circular orbits again and again.

Action: Balance the expansion of outgoing energy through the lower back muscles with an incoming muscular attention through the abdominal muscles. Deliberately orbit your outgoing energy's release back to you as an energy resource. You are practicing giving and receiving simultaneously. You will know the energy orbit is balanced when you feel like you're sitting still in movement.

Meditation: Imagine your posterior body being spooned into a lover's body and his or her devotion; relax in the safety of a loving embrace. Then experience being cocooned in a constant current of your own care and devotion; relax in the safety of your own loving embrace.

Special Note: The adjoining video tutorial extends this foundation of transverse energy orbits. First, you'll sit with intention. Then you'll sit adding a physical movement with resistance. Lastly, you'll explore a balanced energy orbit from the perspective of mental movement. You will enjoy movement as receiving while giving. You'll experience connection with resistance as plugging into a power source; you feel an exchange rather than a drain of energy. You'll experience being recharged on the move.

As you balance energy flow and move from the aligned skeletal-plane of equipoise, you learn to feel the difference between static tension and flowing strength. You learn to differentiate between tension and strength as well as the pain of hard work and the challenge of working hard.

Centripetal of Centrifugal Force Wish List

- The ability to release tension in the lower back through energy movement is achieved.
- Abdominal support through muscular awakeness replaces muscular rigidity.
- A clear distinction between energy movement and physical movement is realized.
- Stability and coordination between your bones and muscles are improved.
- Energy is restored, and your vitality begins to rise.

As a finance executive, Sebastian's days are filled with analyzing information and managing high-performance analysts to assess the viability of our banking system. By the time he gets to the gym, he's mentally fried. By visualizing a release of tension that can balance the exertion of strength needed for each exercise, we connect him to his center quickly and efficiently. This balance of energy becomes an orbit of force that gives Sebastian access to his physical strength in and out of the gym whenever he takes a relaxing breath. This step has transformed his posture, giving his carriage a command and notability that matches his professional stature.

I have been working with Tammy for more than fifteen years, and the growth has been continual—but the real transformation came for me in the first two to three years, when I realized that we had retrained my mind and body to work together for the first time. I was never very athletic in my younger days, but I feel that through the BodyLogos approach, I have been able to reach back in time and correct that missing mind-body connection.

—Sebastian

Learning to Listen

We think we're so smart, but our bodies are smarter. To hear our bodies' inherent wisdom, we need to listen for the subtle energy that reflects our sensory perceptions. Subtle energy is sensed, not thought.

The central nervous system—our brain and spinal column—has motor nerves that transmit signals from the brain to the body to coordinate our movement. It also has sensory nerves that transmit information from the body back to the brain. They convey signals of pain and sensory perceptions, including the emotional undercurrent of unresolved personal conflict. The greater the conflict is, the greater the nerve response. Physical, mental, and emotional conflicts are the cornerstones of tension.

> ### What It Is
>
> Tension that is pain based is built on inflammation and nerve impingement; tension that is fear based is built on stagnant emotions. Either way, tension lives in your soft tissue—muscle—and narrows your nervous system's bandwidth for internal communication.
>
> Imagine trying to have an intimate conversation at a nightclub. The music volume saturates the environment, making it nearly impossible to discern what another person is trying to express. You can't hear, so you eventually stop listening. Tension is the loud voice that saturates your attention, making it nearly impossible to discern the tension-free soft voices that reflect your spirit self—your essential purpose. You can't hear what is tension free, so you eventually stop listening for it. You become numb to the ease of intuitive alignment. Potential becomes surviving the expectations of living rather than stretching toward personal dreams. You operate within the limited confines of your tension's convictions. You are blocked from recognizing the outward stretch of your life force.

If you have tools for discerning tension (static energy) and directing strength (fluid energy), you can navigate your attention toward equipoise—equipoise being the tension-free zone where you can experience your energy's full bandwidth. The intuitive alignment found through your internal communication can be heard. The softer, intimate voices that live within your sensory perceptions can connect you to life instead of your tension reacting to it. You stop chasing strength and realize the essence of strength already lives within you.

BodyLogos Orientations

Discerning between "energy" movement and "physical" movement is the first step to listening inwardly. Energy movement inspires physical movement with clear intention. It is a direction of force that adjusts your posture, and both precede and accompany physical movement. Physical movement motivates energy movement with focused attention on a single task. Physical movement is goal oriented and expects energy movement to support its drive and compulsions. To rise to the challenge of physical movement, we need to be tuned into energy movement and its needs—and that means cultivating our ability to listen to our body's more subtle communications.

Energy versus Physical Movement

To establish optimal alignment, the adhesions between "energy" and "physical" movements need to separate. Physical movement is easy to see and understand—the evidence is right in front of you. Because energy cannot be seen, it must be visualized and sensed. To visualize your energy, you direct your nervous system where it should place its attention. To sense your energy, you listen to the signals it's sending back. When energy and physical movement are separated, their relationship disassembles and transforms the habitual holding patterns you experience as limitations.

You want to stay awake and aware as a new alignment unfolds so you can recreate it at will. Only then are you free of the trauma that established the holding pattern in the first place. Awareness gives you the freedom to develop inward and outward strength. Explore these orientations to help navigate the nuances of "energy" versus "physical" movement.

Skeleton

Energy Movement

Visualize: Initiate the invisible radiance of energy from the dan tien energy center up through your heart and crown centers, and down through your million dollar and gushing spring points.

Sense: Central radiance could feel like it's holding you up, giving your muscles a respite. It could feel like time is standing still, and a sense of belonging in the world arises. The dan tien could feel like an internal "pregnant void" you experience as free attention. You may experience responding neutrally rather than defensively to challenge.

Physical Movement

Visualize: Energize the dan tien and stretch your central plumb line toward earth and sky as you begin walking. With each step, keep the million-dollar point aligned with the upper energy centers and facing the ground to pass between inner ankle bones.

Sense: The added internal stretch from your dan tien could feel like a caterpillar gracefully elongating its body through your body. You could feel more space between your bones, making each step feel cushioned; your spine could feel decompressed and elongated, or your skull could feel like its yawning. You may experience the world as a quieter place.

Muscles

Energy Movement

Visualize: Let an upward rise of energy pass through your anterior body, then balance this with a downward direction of energy through your posterior body. Feel these two opposing energies plugged into the dan tien and equalize in force until you feel them connect as an energy orbit.

Sense: Balancing energy forces may invoke an inner dialogue, asking you to listen for the sake of self-development. You may become aware of muscular tension or dominance. Curiosity about what is causing particular muscular imbalances may steer your attention. You may experience a renewed state of self-acceptance or a commitment to personal well-being.

Physical Movement

Visualize: Energize your dan tien; accelerate the force from above energy orbit to propel walking. With each step, allow muscle tension to release down the posterior body through the heel stirrups and muscle strength to lift up the anterior body through the gushing spring points.

Sense: Moving in your energy orbit through the world could offer a sense of purpose and importance. It could also expand your neutral attention to realize what triggers physical tension and emotional ambivalence. You could develop a better understanding of what is true for you in relation to the world around you—a sense of certainty or an allowing of uncertainty may unfold—offering relief from self-criticism. You may experience a sense of self-importance or self-care.

Balanced attention between thinking and feeling is also necessary to develop listening inwardly. The gray matter of the brain aids you in thinking or remembering your life story. The soft tissue of the body—organs, muscles, sinews—aids you in feeling your life story. Feeling combines physical awareness (the ability to recognize where you are in space and in your own body) and physical expression (the ability to recognize the emotional conviction or reaction your body is having).

Feeling versus Thinking

In a psyche-muscular approach to strength training, it's essential to think and feel each moment of challenge to develop physically, emotionally, and mentally. Mental managing uses thinking to sort through information and reason through problems without the reactivity of feeling; feeling is needed to realize the misaligning beliefs that create tension and drown out the softer voice of spirit. Separating thinking and feeling offers you the option to change your life by changing your body's position and your mind's disposition. Replacing what defeats you with what empowers you to build reliable strength and neutral attention.

Feeling: My chest muscles collapse when I feel unloved, and my upper-back muscles freeze in an over-expanded position. When I'm triggered, I feel a stabbing pain under my right shoulder blade.

Thinking: My upper back is protecting my smile of truth.

Feeling: When I feel accepted, my back muscles release their tension, and a surge of hope and open-heartedness opens my chest.

Thinking: Self-acceptance gives me the free attention to balance the descending energy through my back with the ascending energy through my chest. My spine elongates, and the pain I feel under my shoulder blade subsides. Awareness gives me the choice to react or respond to emotions.

Feeling: When my shoulder blade channels align between my occipital hollows and low back dimples, it feels like a silk robe draping through my central plumb line, and I experience an irrepressible space in my zhong heart center. Maintaining this when being triggered inspired an insight about why I feel the need to protect my smile—*I will be loved only if I can be whom the other person needs me to be.*

Thinking: Exploring the nature of free-flowing energy inspires me to delve beyond survival and pain management, and resolves the misaligning beliefs at the core of a holding pattern.

Energy movement pulses our life force through mind and body so our spirits can soar. The intention to connect energetically with our movement is to wholly unite mind and body to do the following:

- Improve physical awareness, free physical expression, and inspire physical movement.
- Structure a physical practice that provokes personal intimacy and builds vitality and strength.
- Bring confidence and creativity to a spiritual practice.

When all these elements are considered, our inner aspirations are permitted, delivered, and welcomed into our outer world. We experience life just as it is and personal disappointments just as they are. We believe in our own mastery and recognize our life story as an education rather than what defines us.

Life regularly challenges postural and movement integrity mentally and physically. Energy movement has deep roots; hence, it often passes through deep wounds. The goal of the BodyLogos movement is to continually explore these depths, develop a greater relationship with our striving nature, and infuse our spirit self into our lives.

May your body express as an artist and your mind direct with clear intent. As you experience greater depth within your own energy system, may you experience greater depth in your connection with the world. To know thyself is to free thy spirit.

Direction Chapter

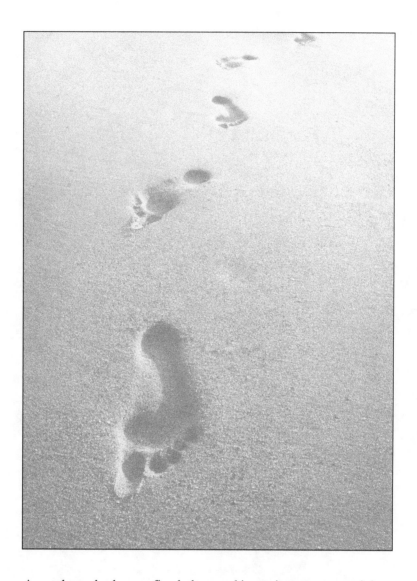

A good traveler has no fixed plans and is not intent upon arriving.
A good artist lets his intuition lead him wherever it wants.
A good scientist has freed himself of concepts
and keeps his mind open to what is …

He is ready to use all situations
And doesn't waste anything.

This is called "following the light."

—Lao Tzu, *Tao Te Ching*

Lesson 6
The Practice of Alignment

Obey the principles
Without being bound by them.

—Bruce Lee, Hong Kong-born martial artist and film actor

The five elements of Tao recognize five seasons, which ensure nature's life-sustaining development.

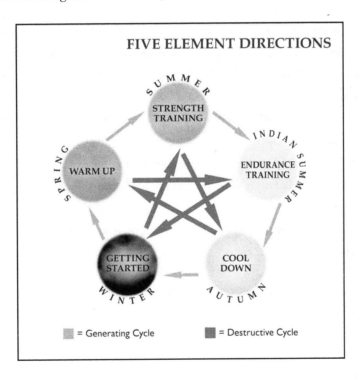

Element	Season	Direction of Body
Water	Winter	Getting Started
Wood	Spring	Warm Up
Fire	Summer	Strength Training
Earth	Indian Summer	Endurance Training
Metal	Autumn	Cool Down

Each season offers the next a starting point each season's unique characteristics can nurture, creating an entire life cycle. The generating cycle creates sustained well-being and growth through changing conditions.

In Nature:

- Hibernating in the freeze of *winter*, energy is stored, and a retreat to reorganize happens; preparations for a new cycle of life begin.
- Then *spring* brings fertility and vigor into existence, awakening fresh direction and hope, impregnating potential.
- This builds into the abundance of light offered by *summer*, inspiring newfound exuberance for growth and expression.
- And then the long drawn-out days of *Indian summer* push potential to its unrealized greatness.
- The cycle ends with the abundance of an *autumn* harvest, offering the reward of ripened emergence.

Similarly, there are five developmental stages in a workout structure. Each workout juncture, like the seasons, generates the next.

In Our Workouts:

- *Getting started* is associated with winter, a time of convalescence and reorganization. In it, you recall exercise preferences and organize a direction for your approaching resurgence.
- Your *warm-up* is associated with spring, a fresh start, a new day. A surge of energy moves you gradually into exercise anew.
- *Strength training* is associated with summer, a time of liberated enthusiasm, with a burst of energy you connect to each resistance challenge with passion and conviction.
- *Endurance training* is associated with Indian summer, extending your commitment and perseverance to the point of failure—muscle failure is success in the gym. It is then that your body builds muscle tissue and increased oxygen capacity.
- Your *cool down* is associated with autumn, the reaping of your labor and a satisfaction of efforts made, goals won, and positive change earned.

Now I'll depict the workout breakdown using the generating cycle. Like a bear hibernating in its *winter* cave, I stay tucked under my covers in the morning, gradually *getting started* with my workout plan. Once I know the plan, I'm ready to get up, choose a compatible outfit, and pack my gear for the gym. Upon arriving at the gym, I feel a bit like a *spring* awakening—organized and enthusiastic but still a little slow moving—so I climb aboard a cardio machine that will *warm up* the body parts I'm intending to work out. Once my body is warm and my mind is set to meet the challenges of *strength training*, my workout takes on the fun of *summertime* play.

Meeting the challenge of resistance has the same quality as my rollerblades meeting the boardwalk with each stride; I'm feeling for alignment and balance with each rep. As my body becomes fatigued, I lighten my resistance load and challenge myself with rehabilitation and balance exercises that focus my intention on *endurance training*. This step elongates my workout till I hit muscle failure. Satisfied weariness emanates from my being, like the close of an *Indian summer* day, as I collapse with delight, proud of my staying power. Melted onto the mat, muscles too tired to resist a series of deep muscular stretches, I surrender through my bones' alignment. As my mind and body become quiet, I begin to *cool down* as if the first breezes of *autumn* are relieving me from summer's heat.

The generating cycle shows that every action has its season, preparing my athleticism to develop in safety and recover with ease.

But per the five-element theory, sometimes the destructive cycle is more in line with your workout goals.

- Your *warm-up* can gently decompress tensions from the day. Sometimes you may skip that gentle decompression and jump straight from *getting started* into gentle *strength training* to get a stronger sense of where your tension is held and what psyche-muscular holding patterns need to be released.
- If your *strength-training* workout is preparing you for powerlifting, sumo wrestling, or bodybuilding competitions, where your weight and size are needed, skipping *endurance training* and going straight to a *cooldown* of stretching would suit your fitness goals.
- Going from the relaxed receptivity of a *cooldown* directly into a *warm-up* without the research and prep of *getting started* can teach or motivate you through doing—and embrace spontaneity.
- Going from your *warm-up* directly to *endurance training*, skipping *strength training*, keeps you light and flexible for running marathons and high-speed flexibility movements such as pitching a baseball.
- There's an endorphin high that comes with *endurance training* that can motivate you for *getting started* in something new and unfamiliar. Skipping your *cooldown* allows you to borrow energy from one activity and direct it toward another.

Workout Breakdown

Winter: Getting Started

Like the chill of winter, a static body is cold and dormant. An object at rest tends to stay at rest unless stimulated. Getting started requires incentive, organization, and willpower.

Incentive comes in two forms: motivation––yang, and inspiration––yin. Gathering data to decide how best to "get" what you want generates motivation; a creative insight or feeling that compels you to "give" something meaningful is inspiration. Motivation needs the promise of some reward. Inspiration itself is the reward. Motivation can lead to inspiration.

Recognizing what you want—a smaller waistline, popping biceps, a stronger core, a healthier heart, better balance—can feel daunting, but learning how to get it excites the body into action. Strength training will build bone and muscle strength, raise metabolism, increase muscular size, and sculpt the body. Endurance training will burn calories, increase stamina, improve agility, and strengthen the heart and lungs. Coordination training—your warm-up—will add grace, dexterity, and confidence. Flexibility training—your cooldown—will add greater speed and range of motion, and maintain healthy joint composition. Getting started is to choose what you want to build on. This is your motivation.

While the motivations to work out are plentiful, they're often not enough to excite you into action for long. You need an inspired outlook that gives meaning to life to commit to your fitness and well-being long term. An outlook like "I feel connected to the world when I am connected to my body" inspires exercise because it immediately "gives back." Review Experience the Bone (p. 46) to learn to connect deeply. The beauty of BodyLogos is that it involves you in an inner exploration of your own authenticity and specialty as it relates to the world around you. It inspires you to connect with a workout challenge to connect better with a life challenge. It builds a relationship with your spirit self that recognizes you are an integral part of all creation; so all effort to enlighten the self is considered an effort to enlighten the world.

- Recognize the benefits you want from a workout.
- Choose what kind of training you need or want to build on.
- Commit to what motivates you and connect deeply to it. Review "Experience the Bone" (p. 46).
- Be willing to explore inwardly and be inspired beyond your motivations.
- Realize how all efforts to enlighten the self are efforts to enlighten the world.

 Spring: Warm-Up

Springtime shows us that everything starts small: The brilliance of spring flowers emerges as tiny sprouts peeking out of the soil. After winter's rest, the bulbs are bursting with life, yet their outward expression is tempered. Without a gradual unfurling, new life can feel unstable and unprepared, assaulted by its sudden emergence into a new and unprotected environment. In the same way, your body requires a gradual progression to warm up and awaken its brilliance.

Taking time to offer warmth to the body gives it the opportunity to perform effortlessly and with greater intensity—yin. Expecting a performance on demand chills the experience and creates a forced effort and struggle—yang. Listening to your body's needs not only gives it the opportunity to lead your workout intensity but also allows you to appreciate the sacredness of both your body and the event. Expecting your body to perform at a predetermined ideal is forward seeking and absent from the intimacy and knowledge offered in the moment.

Exercise options that provide warmth include rhythmic movement, light stretching, isolated joint mobility, alignment, coordination, and balance challenges that progress into alternate quick and slow-twitch muscle activity. If strength training is your focus, prepare the particular areas being challenged: Warm up joint mobility to protect sinews, stretch for muscle availability, and practice slow and quick-twitch muscle isolation to penetrate the muscle belly. To focus on endurance training, build from smaller to larger rhythmic movements. Use posture and alignment challenges that stabilize your abdominal center, alternate traveling steps and jumps to challenge alignment, and add quick destabilizing movements to challenge dexterity. Connecting to your abdominal center and maintaining alignment are crucial to support the increase of intensity in all types of training.

A warm-up may last five minutes for a young fit person in the summer months. It may also require twenty minutes for an older, unconditioned person in the winter months. Understand the variables and observe what your body needs. Creating a warm-up is an organizational challenge. Spend time creating movement purpose. Review "Experience Neutral Alignment" (p. 39) and build your warm-up from there.

- Let your body lead movement intensity to warm up respectfully rather than expecting a performance on demand.
- Prepare muscles, joints, and alignment before increasing exercise intensity.
- Tailor warm-up movements for the type of workout you are going to follow up with.

- Connect to your abdominal center and maintain your alignment.
- Consider temperature, age, and condition to determine the warm-up intensity and duration. Review "Experience Neutral Alignment" (p. 39).

Summer: Strength Training

When you are warmed up, it feels like school's out for the summer and you're ready for fresh challenges. Both mind and body are fired up, and you're ready for action. Do you let the enthusiasm of your endorphin high lead your physical movement into attacking a workout—yang? Or do you use that high to fuel a mental attitude that connects you with your workout inspiration—yin? Blind enthusiasm, like a blazing fire, burns out mind and body—but using enthusiasm to boldly choose what you value in the world offers an eternal flame.

Let's be clear about it. Endorphins (your pain blockers) do liberate you to try new physical movements or mental identities without immediate concern of failure or judgment, and this liberation is important for exploring where your areas of competence or enjoyment lie. But becoming hooked on the domination endorphins offer you rather than on the clear intention they can lead you toward is hasty when developing a wellness lifestyle—and will cause imminent failure. The opium-like state of endorphins is short lived. Using your workout endorphins to recognize a life goal or interest connecting with your spirit self is conversely a connection with universal spirit and an inward feeling of pure intent.

Harnessing your fire is by no means putting your fire out. Taking action creates your life; considering a counter-action balances your life. By developing awareness around active and counter-active energies, you are essentially generating more heat from the fire with less wood. Approach your strength-training exercises with a pure intent to connect outwardly and inwardly. Review "Experience Equipoise" (p. 67). Energetic synergy aligns universal energies with the life goal you are working to manifest. There is no greater ally in the world to have rallying on your behalf.

Strength training is an opportunity to practice balanced energy, to lay a foundation to explore consciousness through active meditation, and to strengthen your understanding and commitment to creating the life you want. Balanced strength builds lasting vitality that can connect to the repetition of a discipline and the unpredictability inherent to living.

- Approach strength-training exercises with a pure intent to connect outwardly and inwardly.
- Use your endorphin high to perceive from your spirit self and connect with universal spirit.
- Develop awareness of active and counter-active energies. Review "Experience Equipoise" (p. 67).
- Align universal energies with the life goal you are working to manifest through your energetic synergy.
- Lay a foundation to explore consciousness through active meditation.

Indian Summer: Endurance Training

Our eternal Mother Earth teaches us endurance. Her ability to recycle, renew, and rebuild herself is a mirror of what is happening within our own existence, and this ability is again seen in the breakdown and rebuilding of a workout regimen. Like the earth, we flourish, collapse, mulch the experience, restore, realign, and do it all again to progress, revive, and survive. The unrelenting heat of an Indian summer, with its persistence and endurance, has a similar feeling as the endless circle of life.

To rebuild, we first need to break down. This is where the aches and pains of fitness training arise. There is the generalized post-workout pain associated with lactic acid build-up, muscular micro-tears, and inflammation. This generalized discomfort is found in the muscles, not the joints, and has a three-day recovery period. If it lasts longer, decrease your intensity. Three to six cardio workouts a week that last between twenty and forty minutes—maintaining optimal alignment—describe a general range of intensity. Should intensity cause you to stop when the going gets tough––yin––or forge on no matter how stressful––yang? How do you know when the discomfort of fatigue is helpful or detrimental?

When you approach training focused on alignment and balance, your movement simply discontinues when it is enough. You were moving in an aligned and balanced fashion, and then you weren't. Simple. There is no decision to be made in regard to "when it is enough." You simply can no longer maintain balanced alignment. This is why it's crucial to connect to and understand your neutral and essential alignment. The general rule regarding discomfort and intensity, however, is the following: sharp, cool pain is cause to stop; achy, warm pain is considered an expression of muscle activity. Your body alignment informs you when it is enough, so pay attention! Review "Essential Alignment Exercise" (p. 49). When you can no longer maintain essential alignment, you have hit muscle failure—muscle failure is success when training. The inevitable experience of muscle exhaustion is a celebration. The muscle is successfully connecting; be satisfied as opposed to irritated by failure.

Building endurance can be as basic as shifting your attention. Place attention on your active energy, and you connect with doing hard work. Place attention on your counter-active energy, and you connect with allowing hard work to happen. What you focus your attention on can change the whole experience. Be conscious of what inspires you on a particular day––action or counter-action––and balance your energy forces in consideration of any imbalance you may be having. This consideration will improve staying power through physical, mental, or emotional fatigue—it creates an interactive and resilient environment that maintains alignment and balance so you can reach your full potential.

With fatigue comes the tendency to throw weight around, be it the outside resistance in strength training or your own body weight in a cardio setting. Allowing outer momentum to complete your challenge disrupts essential alignment and implies distrust in your own strength and competence. Overriding trust in your abilities with recklessness also interrupts the mind-body connection and meditative experience. How you respond to muscle failure, moreover, mirrors how you respond to life when challenged. Where is your attention fixed—on the purpose of self-development or on your doubts about self-development? Recognizing the parallels your workout and life ethics share can inform you in how to adjust your intention to better serve your aspirations. Better to decrease intensity than to throw away integrity.

And when you truly can't do anymore, remember this: Muscle failure is magical. Muscle failure connects you to your striving, spiritual nature. Your willingness to fail is your commitment to evolve, and evolving confirms that you are living your potential. You can either experience your potential as worthwhile and vital, or you can feel threatened and defeated by present limitations. Endurance and strength training teach you that failure is the way to success. They celebrate your tenacity to challenge your potential.

- Be attentive to pain quality after workouts to discern whether it is generalized post-workout discomfort or reason to decrease intensity.

- Commit to three to six weekly workouts that last twenty to forty minutes.
- Balance active and counter-active energies, and maintain essential alignment to safely reach muscle failure. Review "Essential Alignment Exercise" (p. 49).
- Refrain from using external momentum and be honest about your abilities.
- Recognize the parallels your workout and life ethics share.

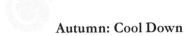

Autumn: Cool Down

Like reaping the harvest from an autumn garden, take a moment to reap the rewards from your workout. If you intend to inspire a lifestyle of self-development, it's crucial to celebrate the returns made from your commitment. In the recognition of your progress, you both celebrate your improvements and understand your shortcomings. You inspire greater commitment and deeper connections. Without this recognition of progress, it is all just empty, hard work.

One of the greatest rewards is found in your relationship with the psyche-muscular blueprint. Review the "Psyche-Muscular Blueprint" (p. 10). Recognizing the reactions that express in your physical body and analyzing their psyche-muscular meaning direct your meditation into the labyrinth of consciousness. Recognize that insights come in the form of a clear call to action, a feeling of clarity about something or someone, or in a feeling of assurance or shame about how you are being. Whether the insight is action oriented or a reorienting of perspective, it comes into being by feeling, not thinking. Insights are allowed to express themselves; they aren't reasoned into being.

The distinction between a "call to action" and a "reorienting of perspective" is that the former is nameable, and the latter is nameless. The nameable are specific things you are called to do, connect with, or disconnect from. Specificity satisfies all questions; thus nameable insights are easiest to identify and find rewarding and useful—yang. The nameless unveils the eternal, limitless, and primitive supreme intelligence that lives within you. Words aren't enough to define the nameless since its expression goes beyond words. A reorienting of perspective changes your life, and though an immediate action may not be required, its subtle presence alters your response to life's challenges and answers an intimate yearning that harvests undying rewards—yin.

The combination of being warmed up and worn down from your workout creates the perfect environment for heavy stretches and relaxation exercises. This is a perfect time to reinforce subtle postural awareness and allow further introspection of the psyche-muscular meditations. You are quiet in mind and body, and feel physically satisfied and mentally responsible, all of which surrender your obsession with "doing" to appreciate the "non-doing" aspect of a workout. As you relax, stretch, and appreciate your body, experience an expanding quietude in your dan tien energy center. Review the essence of your insights and allow the mind and body to be restored by the emerging creative life force of your spirit self.

Fully embrace the spirited connection of your workout before venturing into the distracting environment of the outside world.

- Celebrate your commitment to and connection with your workout as well as your improvements and new understandings.
- Recognize yourself as a psyche-muscular being. Review the "Psyche-Muscular Blueprint" (p. 10).
- Feel for a call to action or a reorientation of perspective.

- Reinforce postural awareness in heavy stretches and relaxation exercises.
- Relax, stretch, and appreciate your body as the emerging creative life force of your spirit self.

Ever since I was a child,
I have had this instinctive urge for expansion and growth.
To me, the function and duty of a quality human being
Is the sincere and honest development of one's potential.

—Bruce Lee, Hong Kong-born martial artist and film actor

Part 2
Our Life Practice: From the Outside In

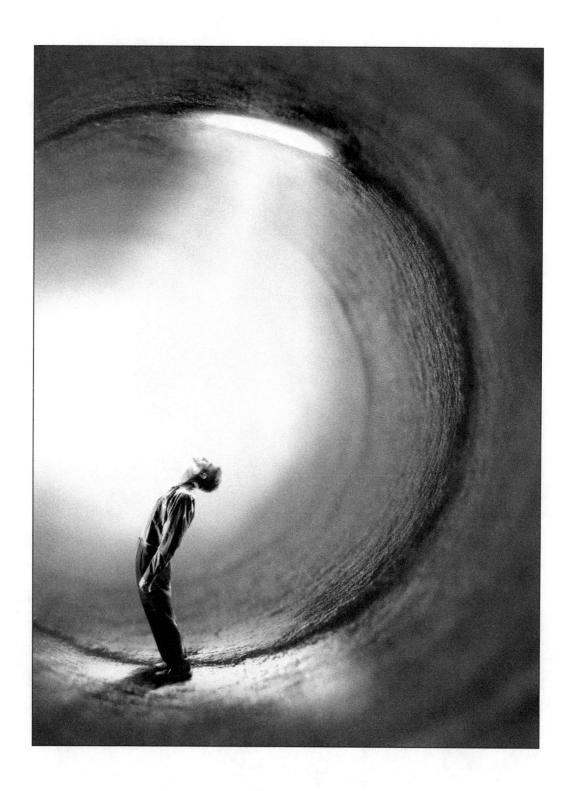

Overview

Lesson Chapters 7–12

> Your body is a walking, talking psyche-muscular blueprint of your life story.
> Every belief you have adopted in response to your life story is expressed
> Through your body's posture and its response to challenge.
> What is hidden in your silhouette?
>
> —Tammy Wise, BodyLogos

Part 2 brings Tao theory into a physical practice. You are studying the mechanics of energy in relation to your physical form and learning how to integrate deliberate energy patterns into your posture, movement, and relationship with outside resistance.

Part 2 is the breakdown of energy patterns as they relate to strength-training exercises. You are training to simultaneously pay attention to self (you) and others (outside resistance). This is a systematic and practical approach to strength that builds your ability to connect authentically with life.

Part 2 is divided into six lessons. Lesson 7 introduces the breakdown of each energy pattern, how they connect, and how to best utilize them in your workout. Lessons 8–12 present the five energy patterns. Each energy pattern supports specific muscle groups, and collectively they support all movement. It's going to teach you how to use the various energy orbits in strength-training exercises, how to implement active meditation, and how to analyze what you find in your body using the BodyLogos observations.

In "Our Life Practice: From the Outside In" chapters, you will experience your full potential multidimensionality. You will

- develop physical strength in your active muscles and release unwanted tension from your counter-active muscles;
- visualize musculoskeletal posture and sense mind-body alignment as it is challenged by resistance; and
- experience emotional frailty and spiritual stability.

Through this balanced and honest approach to strength, you experience newfound curiosity regarding your workout limitations and appreciation of your excellence. You create workouts that overflow into a greater relationship with your life.

Part 2 is the how-to for mastering your energy potential. It will teach you to create strength by closing energy leaks and increase flexibility by releasing energy congestion. This practice will also prove to you how much impact you have on your own state of health and well-being. Your attention to balanced energy leads to a balanced physical structure and an aligned psychological outlook.

Part 2 offers you a practice for gaining greater and greater mastery in directing your creative life force. Where you once felt unstable, you will find greater aptitude and new freedom. You will begin to dissolve chronic physical conditions and emotional complaints. You will stop operating from outdated habitual beliefs, imbalances, and judgments.

Part 2 offers you a practice for increasing energy equilibrium that dissolves feelings of physical detachment and emotional isolation, steering your direction of movement toward unity and connectedness.

Part 2 offers you a practice for creating peaceful relations with all you touch and the world at large.

> The Master views the parts with compassion,
> Because he understands the whole.
>
> —Lao Tzu, *Tao Te Ching*

Practice Chapter

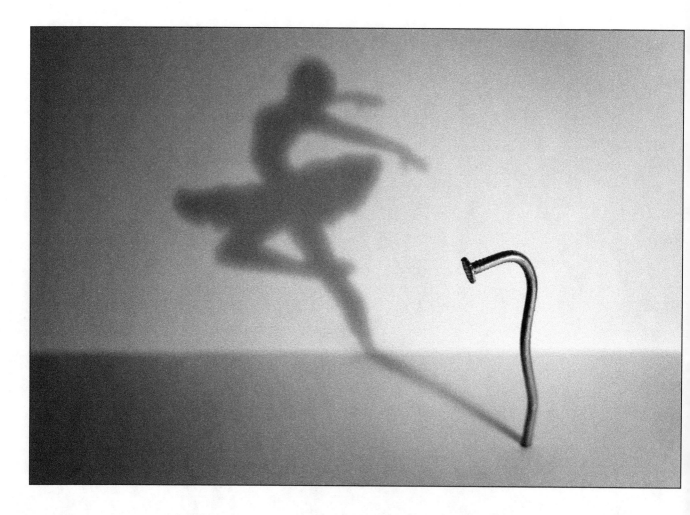

All things arise from Tao (nature). They are nourished by Virtue.
They are formed by matter. They are shaped by environment.
Thus the ten thousand things all respect Tao and honor Virtue.
Respect for Tao and honor of Virtue are not demanded.
But they are in the nature of things.

—Lao Tzu, *Tao Te Ching*

Lesson 7
The Art of Practice

The reason why I have trouble is that I have a body …

He who values the world as his body, (however)
May be entrusted with the empire.
He who loves the world as his body
May be entrusted with the empire.

—Lao Tzu, *Tao Te Ching*

To separate responsibility (mind) and environment (body) is troublesome …

When you are responsible with your environment,
You are entrusted with the universe.
When you are devoted to your environment,
You are entrusted with the universe.

—Tammy Wise, BodyLogos

A Current of Life Runs through You

In this lifetime, you have one body with which to develop nirvana—your promised land. With it, you create and develop the environment where you can find joy, pleasure, and enlightenment. This is a process of learning what you value and valuing what you believe, with enough conviction to face what is blocking its deliverance. This entire process of self-development lives within your energy system and your relationship with the energy orbits within that system.

You experienced energy orbits in chapter 5. Now you will develop that understanding and learn to apply them. This application is both a lifestyle and practice that guides your day-to-day posture and drives your strength-training workouts. Memorize and embody these concepts by envisioning your body as a vehicle for running currents of energy—your creative life force, the current that creates your life.

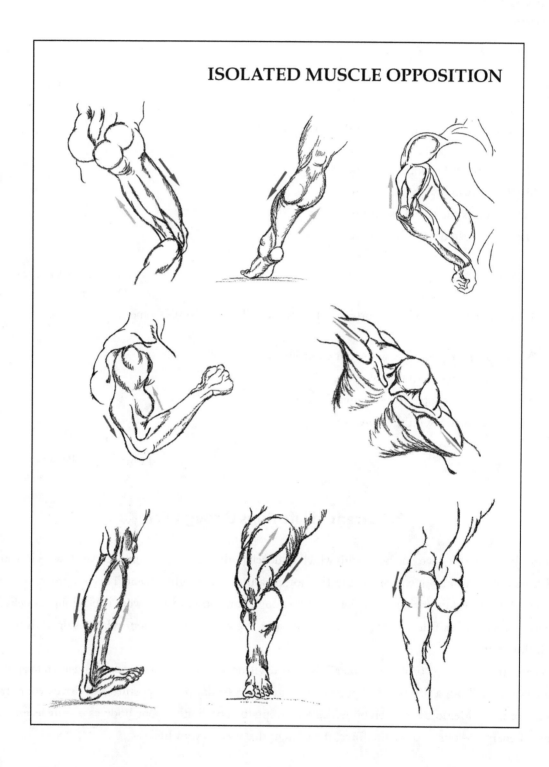

Isolated Muscle Opposition

Action/Yang	Counter-action/Yin
Abdominal Muscles:	
Upper Abdominal Muscles	Mid-Back Muscles
Lower Abdominal Muscles	Low-Back Muscles
Chest Muscles	Upper-Back Muscles
Upper-Back Muscles	Chest Muscles
Shoulder Muscles	Opposite Shoulder Muscles
Biceps Muscles	Triceps Muscles
Triceps Muscles	Biceps Muscles
Buttock Muscles	Iliopsoas Muscles
Quadriceps Muscles	Hamstring Muscles
Hamstring Muscles	Quadriceps Muscles
Calf Muscles	Shin Muscles
Inner-Thigh Muscles	Opposite Inner-Thigh Muscles

Isolated Connection

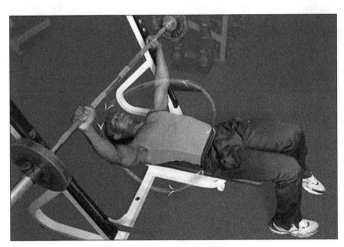

An isolated connection with outside resistance calls for a small energetic orbit, an opposition between the active and counter-active muscle groups being directly challenged. The action—a yang force—motors the movement by contracting; the counter-action—a yin force—allows the movement by releasing. An isolated plane of equipoise is found in the space nestled between these two opposing forces—the bone.

When the chest muscles contract upwardly, for example, the opposing upper-back muscles simultaneously release downwardly. With balanced forces in the contracted (chest) and released (back) muscles, the coronal plane between those forces where the spinal column resides becomes the plane of equipoise. If, however, you contract the back muscles to help the chest muscles in the challenge, equipoise cannot exist. Now tension develops between muscle groups, rather than the calm of equipoise. Be mindful that the opposing forces and muscle groups are independent aspects of a cooperative team. Their duality gives your movement two individual adjustment sources to create sustained equipoise. The dual function—theory of yin and yang—minimizes energy output by insisting on an equal degree of energy input. This teaches you boundaries, protects your joints and sinews, and creates movement control.

Mindful movement explores energy opposition as it applies to the muscular system. It allows you to experience a movement from the muscle powering it—action—as well as from the muscle allowing it—counter-action. Balancing these two influences produces a balanced muscular effort. Recognizing the various muscular oppositions in the body is establishing the various active and counter-active muscle groups that are always working together.

Unified Connection

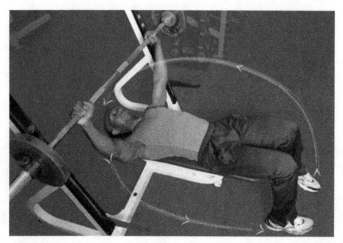

A unified connection creates a larger energetic orbit, which synchronizes these opposing forces with the whole body. A unified connection follows the same energy principles as an isolated connection while orbiting around the dan tien energy center. While the bone between an action and counter-action creates a "plane" of equipoise in an isolated connection, the dan tien energy center creates a "point" of equipoise in a unified connection.

To create this central equipoise using the above example, visualize a vertical force traveling upward through the entire anterior body supporting the chest's contraction. Then visualize another force traveling downward through the entire posterior body supporting the upper-back release. Both upward and downward forces are equal in intensity and arise from the dan tien energy center, producing an orbit of force around itself. This force has the potential to flush out stagnant tensions body wide that impede your energy flow. If upward and downward energy forces are unequal in intensity, however, stagnant tensions in the body remain unchanged, your force is inhibited, and your strength ultimately burns out and declines. The cyclical flow of energy—five-element theory—restores your energy system. This increases muscular strength, reduces stagnant tension, and centers you in your spirit self.

At first, the removal of tension––balancing energy forces––might feel like weakness. But that's because you've been overusing your energy to appear stronger than you really are, thus inhibiting the development of real, lasting strength. When you remove tension's energy drain and the muscles it holds captive, you give rise to rapid muscle maturity.

Unified connections direct your energy to connect an isolated connection with the dan tien energy center and with the outside resistance equally. These energy orbits and their variables will be clearly illustrated in the following chapters, but in the interim, understand that there are five energy patterns—unified connections—supporting twelve primary muscle groups—isolated connections. All energy patterns establish their cyclical orbits by charting how the dan tien can best support balance between the active and counter-active forces when challenged in specific ways.

Five Energy Patterns

The "coming home" energy pattern motivates abdominal, shoulder, and biceps exercises. When you are relaxed into your abdominal support, this energy pattern is like relaxing into your favorite chair; you regain balance to carry your intention to fruition. When you use this to satisfy your need to feel loved, the coming home energy pattern connects you to your spirit self.

The "determined power" energy pattern motivates back and triceps exercises. This energy pattern summons what is beneath the surface to rise, demanding beauty and rootedness to expand to the outermost limits of its expression. When you're feeling triggered, determined power helps you to summon the boldness to go beyond the limits of your fear-based tension and holding patterns.

The "creating forward" energy pattern motivates chest and quadriceps exercises. This energy pattern uses the embers that warm the heart, impassion the body, and ignite the mind to lift your creative life force and meet challenge with effortless wonder.

The "suspending judgment" energy pattern motivates hamstring exercises. This energy pattern opposes momentum, neutralizing the need for outgrown patterns that are distracting and destructive.

The "universal connection" energy pattern motivates buttock, calf, and inner-thigh exercises. This energy pattern morphs the body into an antenna that can pierce through misalignment and connect your physical center with gravity. Iliopsoas muscles (hip flexors) use this pattern to surrender their grip.

Special Note: Use your imagination to visualize the five energy patterns depicted throughout Part 2 while reading. You will then be creating the energy experience straightaway and learning postural reference points that will support the actual execution and challenge of exercises later in your workout. You can visualize the energy patterns as inside the muscles, on the surface of the body, or outside the body. The more expansive your energy pattern, the greater your force. The closer your energy pattern, the greater your control.

All energy patterns share the same orbit direction at the transverse energy orbits—expanding out of the posterior dan tien sideways and converging into the anterior dan tien in the same horizontal way. This continuous opposition at your vertical center makes for graceful transitions between the five energy patterns when combining movements. In BodyLogos practice, this constancy at the dan tien reiterates the steadfastness that every exercise is an abdominal exercise.

To experience this phenomenon, recognize movement is established energetically before it appears physically due to the orbiting pattern created by centripetal and centrifugal forces.

Meeting Resistance

Working with an appropriate resistance is essential. If an outside resistance is too heavy, you will be unable to release through the counter-action; if an outside resistance is too light, it will be more difficult to connect through the action. Strength is a combination of letting go of and holding on to our connections with life. *What inspires us is not the amount of weight we are muscling; it is the way we connect with that weight.*

Traditional strength training is disconnected from life's content and meaning—from any actual impact on our existence. This kind of sterile effort can become mechanical, done by route, and doesn't truly engage either the senses or the intellect. By connecting strength training to our ability to balance relaxation and hard work, we bring strength into the very center of our existence. It becomes what we are rather than what we are chasing after.

Back in the 1980s, at the forefront of group fitness classes and Jane Fonda workouts, I was teaching my first exercise classes. I marveled at how focused on alignment students were when involved in an exercise, but when I instructed them to get their mats to do floor work, almost every student's posture collapsed. The same would happen at the end of class as they were packing up their things. What they were working on in class wasn't translating into their lives. It was like they had an exercise posture and a life posture—and never did the two meet. The internal momentum generated by balancing energy patterns surrenders tension. With this setup, proper posture is made more useful to itself and its relationship with its surroundings. As students walk out of a BodyLogos experience, they maintain their alignment; I witness proper posture becoming the way they are meeting life.

The internal momentum being described in energy patterns is very different from external momentum. External momentum places your attention in the destination of an effort rather than in the movement's energetic and muscular origins. This external attention produces an external swing, whereby the momentum throws the resistance away from us rather than connecting us with it. External momentum is a more outward focus that can become reckless in strength training and obliterates any possibility of experiencing the meditative state of equipoise. The outlook of mindful strength training is to unite with resistance, where traditional methods strive to triumph over it.

The sensitivity to cycle energy inward through the muscular system is gained by controlling our expenditure of force. We start by meeting an outside resistance with the degree of force needed to create connection rather than movement. First, you calibrate how much release in a counter-active muscle is needed to connect to an outside resistance. Then you contract the active muscle to the same degree to which the counter-action is releasing. This focused attention to opposition creates an effective balanced energy orbit without over- or under-exertion. In so doing, we aren't giving our energy away to all we touch. Rather, we are deliberately practicing a skill whereby our energy output connects to an outside resistance and cycles back to us, so as we give, we simultaneously receive. The astonishing gift of this technique is that by connecting outwardly, we create intimacy inwardly. If, however, we pass through or fall short of the connection point—the point where counter-active energy transfers into active energy—we will disrupt the orbit of force and lose the balance needed to cycle and recycle our energetic orbit. When this happens, our energy system drains, our alignment is compromised, tension is employed, and our mind-body connection with the outside resistance diminishes.

When I was teaching my dog to play fetch, I threw a tennis ball against a wall just hard enough to establish the ball's return. This way the dog learned that the idea of the game was to return the ball to its starting place—me. Imagine the ball as energy, I'm the dan tien, and the wall is the connection point. If I threw the ball too hard, the ball's return would bypass my dog and me; I would have to chase the ball to continue the game. This energy exertion wouldn't connect energy back to the dan tien because its force overthrows the energy body's scope and ultimately exhausts the body's energy reserve. If I threw the ball too softly, it wouldn't hit the wall at all; it wouldn't establish a return, and she'd forget she was supposed to bring it back. I would have to chase her to get the ball and continue the game. This energy exertion wouldn't orbit energy back because its force never reached the connection point. It didn't extend its exertion to meet the intention and ultimately drains one's energy reserve. The degree of force that the ball hit the wall determined the outcome; the degree of force that your energy meets the connection point determines the movement's integrity. Through the years, this game brought my dog and me together because in no time, my dog became the connection point. We were a well-oiled team.

To practice this phenomenon, outgoing and incoming energies need to be balanced to generate an energy orbit, and an energy orbit is always established in your dan tien. Energy orbits will conform to your physical movement by recognizing the coronal plane as being flat, curved, or rotated.

Connection Point Exercise
Connected. Unified. Developed.
mindthebody.bodylogos.com/video10
(abbreviated description)

Alignment: Lie supine in neutral alignment with hands behind your head. Bend your knees and place your feet flat on the ground hips' width apart. Balance the gushing spring/heel stirrup marriage with the earth. Use alignment stabilizers to align energy centers and stretch relaxed energy outward from the dan tien into essential alignment. Feel for the point of equipoise in your dan tien.

Balance: To execute movement, visualize the two transverse energy orbits exiting the posterior dan tien sideways. Then add two more energy orbits exiting the same place upwardly toward the head and downwardly toward the ground between the feet. All four energy orbits make a circular trajectory through the posterior plan and around the peripheral body, and they reconnect at the anterior dan tien to pass through the body and begin again. This trajectory will continue throughout the exercise.

Action: Breathe deeply. With your exhale, release energy through the posterior aspect of the energy orbits until your head and arms are propelled two inches off the ground. Relax your head's weight in your hands, surrendering neck and shoulder tension. Notice how the abdominals spontaneously contract to the degree that the back expands, supporting the head's weight and readying you for movement. Stay mindful that you contract the abdominal muscles with only as much force as you are able to release the mid-back muscle. Breathe deeply, and with your exhale, motivate even more release in the back muscles and more contraction in the abdominal muscles. Inhale as your back is returned to the ground. Slowly repeat this up-and-down movement, keeping the contraction and release balanced at all times.

Meditation: Experience the coronal plane as a plane of equipoise. As your muscles' opposition rolls your skeleton up and down, recognize the coronal plane curving and uncurving, permitting the release of tension on its posterior side and the gathering of strength on its anterior side. At the outermost limit of the energy orbit, where it passes through the coronal plane, the release of tension transforms into strength. This connection point is where your essential alignment stretches through the upper and lower energy orbits. Witness and experience your movement from outside your energy orbit, then from the dan tien, then from the abdominal muscles creating the movement, and lastly from the back muscles allowing the movement. Explore the subtle differences.

> *Special Note: The adjoining video tutorial extends this foundation of identifying a connection point. First, you'll balance your energy orbits and identify the connection point when connecting to your own body's weight; then you'll balance your energy orbits and identify the connection point when connecting to an outside weight.*

By identifying the connection point, you can calibrate your force and produce subtlety in movement. The connection point mirrors back to you how you're acting and reacting in relationship to an outside resistance: aggressive, passive, neutral, uncertain, or disinterested. You feel self-possessed and informed to make decisions. Because this is where your energy's release has the potential to orbit back to you, it's important that you *give* with an intention to *receive* its wake. In this point, your mastery is realized. You feel fully connected to your strength.

Connection Point Wish List

- Your ability to transform tension into strength improves.
- The importance of moving with intent heightens as you begin receiving the quality of what you're giving.
- Balance improves.
- Movements become smaller yet more precise and effective.
- You master managing your energy level.

My client Judy successfully released a spasmodic lower back condition while also strengthening her lower abdominals, but she had trouble identifying the energy orbit these opposing forces established. The idea that there's a connection point where her outgoing lower back tension can orbit back around as incoming lower abdominal strength felt elusive to her.

"The connection point," I said, "is being considered whenever you test how heavy something is. You're calibrating the degree of force needed to manage a challenge and recognizing where tension could release to better get your force under the challenge."

"Like visualizing where my tennis racket will meet the ball?"

"Yes! The point of contact between racket and ball is the connection point."

She continued, "The shot is shaped by determining the amount of force I apply to the ball at the connection point. If there is too little release, the stroke will lack power. If there is too much contraction, the stroke will be too strong."

> I understand proper posture as a dynamic equipoise between the releasing of the lower back and the contracting of the supporting abdominals. As the body moves, so the releasing and contracting muscles adjust. The connection point is most relevant to me when determining how much force should be applied to perform a physical task efficiently, without tension and with neither too much nor too little force.
>
> —Judy

Our power to create the life we dream about, both physically and mentally, is in the subtle projection of our life force. Remaining conscious of the pattern of energy that exists in all movement, both physically and mentally, ensures our position on the planet and gives us a sense of belonging. The greater our command is of these forces at work, the greater our command is in creating our lives. How we carry ourselves energetically affects how we feel about ourselves and how the world feels about us.

Create the person you want to be in. Create the world you want to live in.

Visualize your energy system. See your cycling energy as pathways of force. As energy travels through these pathways, it asks the muscular system to follow its direction and degree of force. The muscles may or may not be immediately compliant, causing either a fluid or disrupted energy flow. Either experience needs your attention as it changes the degree of force needed to connect to the resistance. Disrupted energy (tension) adds weight to the outside resistance, reduces space in the joints, and inhibits muscular strength; fluid energy allows your effort to connect without distraction, lightens the outside resistance, restores space in the joints, and allows you to gain muscular strength. Disruption is felt as weakness, discomfort, or pain; and it indicates stagnant energy—a psyche-muscular holding pattern. Energy flow, though not dependent on the total absence of disruption (that would be unrealistic) feels like grace, coordination, or play. Energy flow simply requires that you use the degree of force needed for a connection point to be produced and maintained. The quality and degree of force used to support a connection can transform a psyche-muscular holding pattern into mind-body alignment.

~ feel into this ~
Relieving Lower Back Pain

For instance, if you feel pain and fatigue in the lower back during exercise, add support from the lower abdominal muscles, the lower back's opposing muscle group. The coming home energy pattern (more on this in the next chapter) does this by using the converging energy in your anterior body to draw obstruction in the posterior body outward. If you give your converging anterior energy too little force, it won't draw the obstruction out. If you give it too much, it can make the obstruction resist more. Coaxing the obstruction to shift is done by meeting the resistance of the holding pattern with the degree of force it is holding on with. Abdominal exercises are a wonderful way to care for and ultimately transform a disruptive holding pattern in the lower back muscles.

Your Energy Body Is the Container for Your Meditation

Once energy orbits can be cycled and recycled in our movements, we will be able to experience the stillness of equipoise within our strength-training exercises. Rather than the increase of resistance being the fitness goal, our goal will be to maintain balanced energy orbits as the weight of resistance increases or decreases. This is active meditation.

It's at this point that the clear intention needed to align the skeleton and the focused attention needed to balance the muscular system are integrated and can be put to task; and it's the point where the psyche-muscular blueprint can inform the ways we are feeding our tensions or strengths. By exploring this meditative dimension, an awareness of our present mind-body fitness can be sculpted into relevant resilient viewpoints that align our relationship with resistance.

Experience the energy body––the space the energy orbits occupy––as a sacred space where our human and spirit selves can communicate. The energy body is carrying the meditative focus (spirit awakening) and the response our bodies are having to our meditative focus (human awakening). This spirited communication fills the energy body with neutrality that allows a change of perspective to take place.

Maintaining equipoise within the energy body introduces us to a truthful and accepting relationship with our strength. Truthful strength asks us to constantly calibrate when the muscles need to assert or reserve their force. Stagnant energy (tension) in the muscular system is caused from over-asserting or under-asserting a muscle group's force, which disrupts balance in the energy orbit.

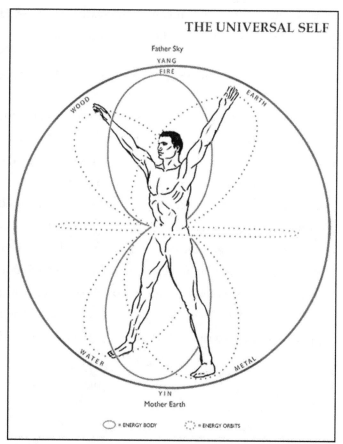

- Emotional reactions to life and working out with too heavy a weight over-assert the counter-active force, causing us to throw weight around.
- Emotional despair and misaligned posture under-assert the active force, causing us to give up prematurely.

The more congestion or imbalance that exists, the more our strength will be blocked.

~ feel into this ~
Experience Active Meditation

Body Alignment: Sit or stand in neutral alignment with feet hips' width apart and gushing spring/heel stirrup marriage balanced. Relax arms at your sides (with or without one- to three-pound dumbbells). Align and stretch your skeleton until you reach the relaxed stretch of essential alignment that extends beyond your energy body.

Energy Orbit: Now, expand through the posterior pathways of your energy orbits—a radiating outward star from the posterior dan tien. Orbit that expansive energy back in through the anterior pathways, an inverted star that converges in the anterior dan tien. Once the energy orbits are continuously cycling within your energy body, raise your arms sideways along the coronal plane, keeping palms down until they reach a horizontal position out from the zhong heart center (stay below shoulder height). Hold this position for three seconds, keeping the energy pattern in motion. Lower the arms to hip level and repeat the arm raise until you can keep the energy orbits constantly in motion or muscle failure. Be a neutral witness to the internal force generated from the energy pattern. And realize how essential alignment—the outward stretch between earth and sky that plugs you into universal energy—is the ignition for the energy pattern.

Mind: Transform any hyper-expressions to triumph over or judge the challenge into a deliberate intention to simply meet the challenge. To do this, keep your essential alignment stretching between earth and sky as you release existing tensions through the star-like energy emanating from your posterior dan tien (counter-action). And, as you orbit that energy back to the anterior dan tien through an inverted star (action), feel how the energy has transformed from triumphing over or judging resistance to connecting with it. As the orbits cycle and recycle your energy, feel your energy system simply meeting the challenge with only the degree of force needed to complete your movement. The balance you have created within your energy system is bringing balance to your body and mind.

Meditation: Summon up the psyche-muscular component of your shoulders—"value." Experience the "value" you hold of yourself filling your energy body. Witness the mind and body reorganizing as your mind-body relationship establishes its posture regarding your value. Refer to the psyche-muscular blueprint to recognize any mind-body area you are tensing when you are up against your relationship with value. Notice whether you've lost your connected stretch between earth and sky. What is your body expressing through its movement quality? Continually realign, rebalance, and recalibrate your energy until equipoise is reached—the emanating quiet center between your action and counter-action.

Special Note: Meet the challenge and aspire to maintain equipoise; finish the exercise when you can no longer continue. As you develop your ability to sustain equipoise in an exercise challenge, know you are developing your ability to sustain it through a life challenge.

In active meditation, you experience your spirit self and gain an objective perspective of your human self. You recognize the difference between your emotional reactions and mental beliefs (for example, when I react with impatience to a new challenge, I recognize it's coming from the belief that I'm going to fail), and how your body harbors these misalignments (for example, my diaphragm tightens, creating shallow breathing. My bones' connection to the earth is lost, and my shoulders creep up toward my ears). Allow this moment of self-awareness to be a moment of transformation, a bridge between where you have been and where you are going. Use the BodyLogos techniques to reorganize your energy system anew.

In doing so, you are deliberately asking your spirit self to witness your human self. This shifts you from a fixed stance to an evolutionary paradigm. You are no longer in the blame game or expectation chase; you are no longer in anxiety. You are an observer of the energy for your body.

Become curious about the array of emotions, identities, and influences that emerge around workout meditations. As a neutral witness of your emotional underpinnings, the messages found in your strength-training exercises become both meaningful and the opportunity to create positive change. Practicing mind-body alignment so your spirit self can express purely without conflict or obstruction is an example of that positive change. Recognizing and accepting your inborn intelligence and specialty are the result.

BodyLogos Exercise Structure

Each of the following chapters focuses on a different energy pattern: coming home, determined power, creating forward, suspending judgment, and universal connection. The chapter will begin with an overview that includes the following:

- A breakdown of each energy pattern's directionality
- A stretch to passively experience the energy pattern
- An outline explaining when to use the energy pattern
- And an in-depth exploration of the energy pattern's psyche-muscular role in your life

Then we'll focus on particular muscle groups. Each introduction will connect and apply the theory you learned in Part 1 to that muscle group.

- First, you'll use the theory of yin and yang to identify that group's active and counter-active muscles and the nuances of their psyche-muscular qualities.
- Next, you'll use the corresponding element from the five-element theory to explore the character and nature of that muscle group.
- Finally, you'll learn to isolate that muscle group through three to four exercises.

Each muscle group has a series of exercises that targets individual muscles within the group. Every exercise follows the same basic sequence.

- In your starting position, you establish essential alignment (p. 49). Visualize the energy orbit being worked.
- As you begin to move, you breathe movement through your counter-action to connect your releasing muscles to your dan tien and unlock tension (see "centripetal of centrifugal force," p. 71).
- Then you breathe movement through your action to connect your dan tien to the outside resistance (see "connection point," p. 99). That outside resistance could be a dumbbell, a band, or your own body weight.
- Once you feel connected to your resistance, you fully activate and stabilize the entire energy orbit to establish equipoise (p. 67).
- Finally, you use your active meditation to listen to and observe the targeted muscle group from the standpoint of the neutral witness (p. 19).

Part 3 will teach you how to customize your workout—from muscle groups to sets to reps—to release specific emotional, physical, and mental tension. Part 2 contains the exercises themselves but is not meant to be read straight through. For best practice, read the theory at the beginning of Lessons 8–12 for an introduction to the energy patterns and each muscle group; then go straight to Part 3 to customize your workout.

Creating Change Chapters

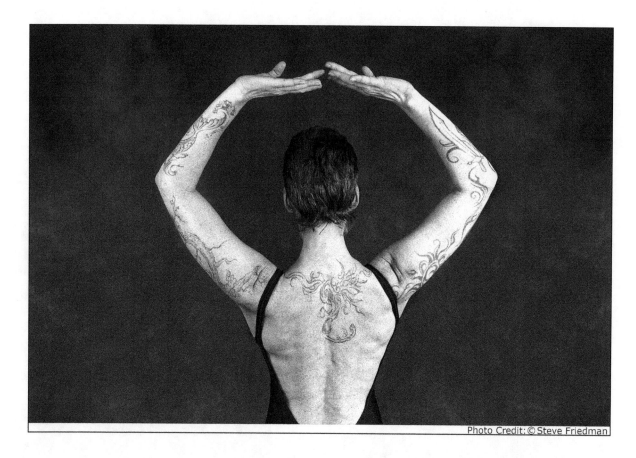

To yield is to be preserved whole.
To be bent is to become straight.
The movement of Tao consists in Returning.
The use of the Tao consists in softness.
Open yourself to the Tao,
Then trust your natural responses;
And everything will fall into place.

—Lao Tzu, *Tao Te Ching*

Open yourself to change;
Explore new beliefs and postures.
Present yourself to the world differently
To return to yourself anew.

—Tammy Wise

Lesson 8

Coming Home Energy Pattern: Abdominals, Biceps, Shoulders

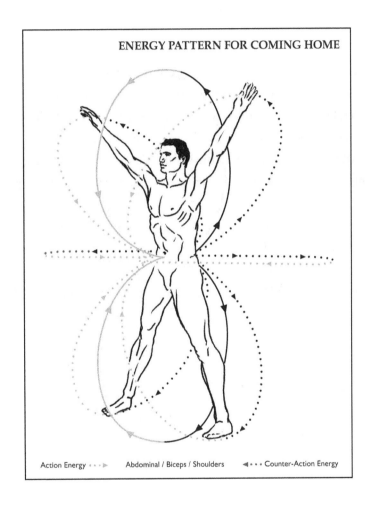

Imagine being curled up in a fetal position. Both upper and lower body hugs your center. Being tucked into your self feels safe and secure. This is the feeling of "coming home."

Directing your energy orbits as in a fetal position, while keeping your essential alignment intact, achieves the same coming home feeling but adds a dynamic and mobile posture. Coming home energy elongates your spinal column, alleviating back and neck discomfort. It powerfully connects you to your central abdominal strength for carrying heavy items and stabilizing your balance.

Coming Home—Seated Lap Lay and Active Meditation
mindthebody.bodylogos.com/video11
(abbreviated description)

To gain a sense of the coming home energy pattern, sit on a chair with feet flat on the floor, hips' width apart. Lay your torso over your lap with head dropped forward and sitz bones grounded into the chair. Take a few deep breaths, allowing the back to spread away from the spine in every direction. As you imagine this expanding star emanating from your lower back, allow all worry and concern to dissipate. Simultaneously, imagine an inverted star converging at your abdominals and feel connected with the self-care and confidence found in your dan tien energy center—spirit self.

Abdominal, biceps, and shoulder exercises all use the coming home energy pattern since they all serve you by connecting to what you need to survive and thrive—you. Abdominal exercises draw your body's weight into your dan tien energy center, bicep exercises draw your body's weight and an outside resistance into your dan tien energy center, and shoulder exercises draw your body's weight into your dan tien energy center while pushing outside resistance away. All these muscle groups gather your energy into the dan tien energy center, your center of gravity. This highlights what feels essential for survival and carries what you are presently holding sacred in your life.

Directing energy out of your posterior center and into your anterior center brings attention away from the fear stored in the lower back and toward expressing your spirit self through the abdominal muscles' support. This reorganizing of energy can change your relationship and connections. What once felt aggressive or arduous could suddenly be experienced as helpful, and what once felt familiar or soothing could suddenly be experienced as dangerous.

The Art of Strength

Practice Change

Henna tattoo of roots penetrating the **Earth**

Like the **Earth**,
Allow yourself to feel what is rooted within you.
When do you experience yourself
With the greatest integrity?
When do you feel your outward attention
Balanced with inward intention?

Coming Home
Is knowing what is true for you,
Honoring this truth,
And living your truth.

Coming Home Energy Pattern as It Relates to the Abdominal Muscles

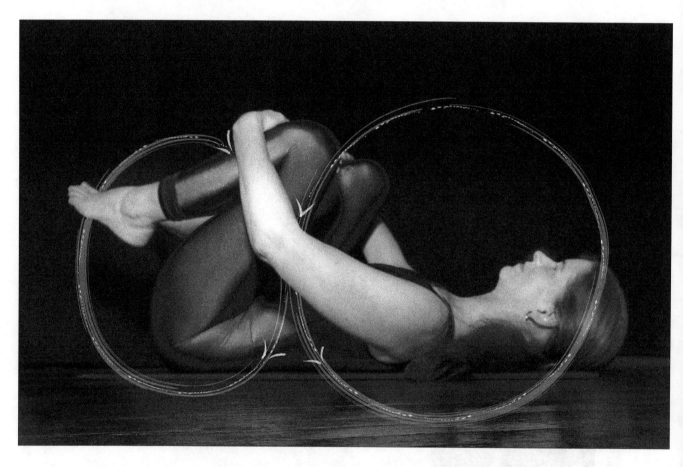

Visualize this energy pattern supporting all abdominal isolations:
Lower, upper, and oblique abdominal exercises.

Introduction to Abdominal Muscles

Theory of Yin and Yang

Yang: Active Muscle Group

Abdominal Muscles:
- Transverse Abdominals
- Rectus Abdominals
- Internal Oblique
- External Oblique

Yin: Counter-active Muscle Group

Mid- and Lower-Back Muscles:
- Latissimus Dorsi
- Trapezius
- Quadratus Lumborum
- Erector Spinae

Like a sneeze or cough, abdominal exercises contract both upper and lower abdominal muscles inward (action) while expanding the upper and lower back outward (counter-action). This phenomenon creates opposing energetic orbits that all converge in your abdominal center, separating the vertebrae of the spinal column and releasing the back's muscular grip on the central nervous system. Commit to motoring your movement from the abdominal muscles while permitting freedom of movement through the expansion of the back.

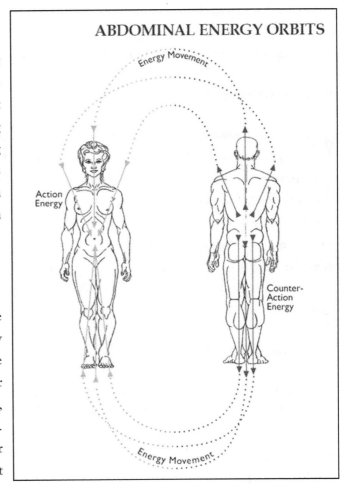

Action: Spirit Self

Challenging the abdominal muscles is a time to shift your focus to appreciate who you are now and who you are becoming. When contracting the abdominal muscles, meditate on creating a greater connection with all that is you—your body's weight, your mind's influence, and spiritual significance. Be with the weight of your power. Relax in your abdominals' command. Stay aware of each moment of movement. Notice that each moment of your life is yours to create.

Counter-action: Fear

When contracting the abdominal muscles, you can also contemplate expanding the psyche-muscular counter-action of your lower- and mid-back muscles. While the muscular stature of the middle back gives you a sense of protection, your lower back carries your fears. Notice how both of these qualities are mutable, both necessary and unnecessary. Be in the moment of movement and recognize what is true. Acknowledge the need for action or surrender, then quietly let the uncertainty of fear-based emotions melt away. Embody the essential power of your spirit self.

Five-Element Theory
Indian Summer, Crossing Joint, Reflection

Connection: Indian Summer

The inherent endurance of Indian summer parallels the commitment your abdominal muscles hold for you. Your abdominal muscles are part of everything you do. They are the manager of your energy, director of your breath, and the central muscular support for the whole body. They are the sun of your personal universe and an intimate ally. To set up abdominal exercises, concentrate on being the actual environment you feel supported and loved by. Be deeply engaged, connected to, and ever present with the purpose of your challenge and the condition of your self from the perspective of an active and trustworthy abdominal center.

Strength: Crossing Joints

There are twenty-seven to twenty-nine pivotal and axial joints that make up the spinal column—seven cervical vertebrae, twelve thoracic vertebrae, five lumbar vertebrae, the sacrum, and two to four coccyx vertebrae. Your spinal column serves as protector of the central nervous system and a bendable structure for the abdominal muscles' efforts. The inherent curves of the spinal column, which repeatedly cross over the coronal plane, produce a spring for the body to rebound and limit disproportionate ranges of motion that could impair your posture's uprightness. Abdominal exercises explore the range of your spinal column and the willingness of your back's muscular liberation. Experience the weight of your spine, neck, and head before contracting the abdominal muscles into motion. Breathe a relaxed central nervous system into being. Be resolved in the abdominal muscles connecting to and carrying the combined weight of your body and any outside resistance.

Meditation: Reflection

As the centerpiece of your entire musculoskeletal system, the abdominal muscles create alliance between upper and lower bodies. Additionally, they are the energetic convergence point—dan tien energy center—for the alliance between mind and body. Abdominal muscles have the potential to be the most outwardly active with, and inwardly reflective of, your character and temperament. This central responsibility of your mental and physical well-being can be daunting, causing neighboring muscle groups to automatically and unconsciously assist. This reflex to rescue can create over-extension and over-exhaustion mentally and physically if attention isn't placed on balancing your abdominals' demands with the release of your lower back. Create a peaceful reliance with your abdominal center and listen for its quieter spirit voice. Be mindful of your back muscles' trust, or lack thereof, in your spirit self, for this reliance allows freedom into your movement.

How to Isolate the Abdominal Muscles

Feel It Contract

Like Buddha, fully accepting all that is, sit with your lower abdomen completely relaxed and expanded outward. Breathe in. Fill the abdomen like a billows. Gently contract the lower abdominal muscles inwardly with your exhale, pushing the breath out. Allow the contracting abdominal muscles to guide the breath on your exhale and your expanding breath to guide the abdominal muscles to release on your inhale.

Abdominal Breathing Exercise

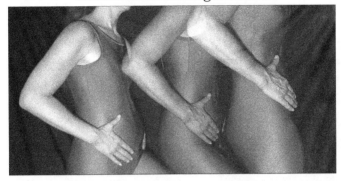

Exercise: Use four counts to inhale, expanding the abdomen, and four counts to exhale, contracting the abdomen. Then do two counts, then one count, and then one-half count, repeating each count several times. Be careful not to gulp your inhales as you increase the speed. Slow breathing relaxes the mind; quick breathing excites the body. Your capacity to fully expand and contract the abdomen will improve as your diaphragm becomes more agile. (Refer to breathing exercise on p. 14)

Feel It Release

As if floating on a lake's surface, surrender to the buoyancy of your environment and the suppleness of your body. Lie supine over a large GymnastikBall. Allow your body to conform to the ball's shape by relaxing the joints and opening the full length of your torso, particularly throughout the abdominal region. Focus on nothing but letting the ball support your weight and what it feels like to expand.

Supine Ball Abdominal Stretch

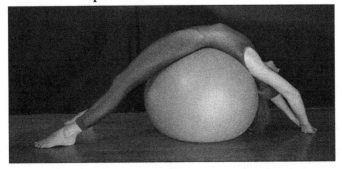

Exercise: Start by sitting on the ball with feet spread as wide as the ball's diameter. Walk forward, keeping feet apart as your buttocks roll forward on the ball. Allow the torso to roll back until your head is also placed on the ball. Once the ball is supporting your pelvis, back, and head with neck relaxed, gently stretch your arms

overhead. Be sure to position your body on the ball so your spine and neck are comfortable, and then enjoy the abdominal stretch. Bend knees more to lessen the stretch; extend knees more to increase the stretch. Hold for thirty seconds or until you're fully relaxed.

Feel It Fatigue

While upper abdominals burn when they are approaching muscle failure, the lower abdominals simply stop working. Both upper and lower abdominals, however, will resort to throwing the movement when they are feeling exhaustion. The neck and upper back will assist the upper abdominals; the hip flexors and lower back will assist the lower abdominals. When challenging the abdominal muscles, deliberately carry your body's weight through the concentric and eccentric movements, and look for a quiver in the muscle. This quiver is a sign of muscular isolation, not muscular exhaustion. As you approach muscle failure, the movement will get smaller until you can no longer manage movement or maintain good form.

Lower Abdominal Exercises

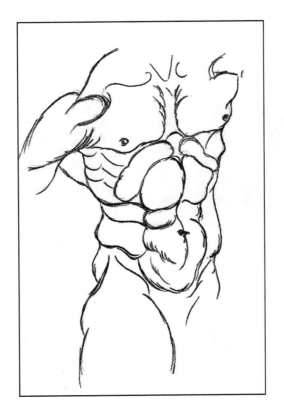

Lower Abdominal Muscles Embody Your Sense of Self

Spirit Self

Lower Abdominal Crunch

Flat and Decline

Starting Position:

- Lie back on floor, flat bench, or decline bench with head positioned above hips.
- Lift feet off the floor. Legs fold at the hips, relaxing quadriceps. Knees fold and point toward the sky (not your head).
- Relax lower back muscles, producing a neutral spine (maintain lower back curve),
- Commit to surrendering your body's entire weight. Let the abdominal muscles fully experience and guide the movement.

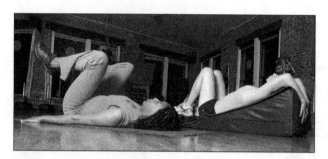

Starting Position

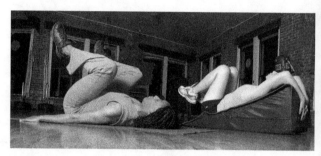

Action/Counter-action

Counter-action:

- Inhale: Visualize energy descend from the posterior dan tien through the tailbone.
- Exhale: Allow the tailbone to roll away from the floor, waistline to drop toward the floor, and lower back dimples to expand by relaxing lower back muscles around and between lower vertebrae of spine.
- Inhale: Return lower vertebrae and tailbone to starting position. Repeat.
- Be mindful of your lower back's expansion, giving your lower abdominal effort control of the movement.

Action:

- Inhale: Relax lower abdominal muscles.
- Exhale: Contract lower abdominal muscles to roll the pelvis and legs as one piece at the waist by visualizing energy rising through lower abdominals toward your anterior dan tien.
- Inhale: Use lower abdominal muscles to carry the pelvis back to the starting position. Repeat.
- Concentrate on connecting your lower abdominal muscles with your entire pelvic weight. Look for a subtle muscular quiver.

Energy Orbit:

- **Isolated Connection:** Visualize the counter-action before engaging in the action. Counter-action: Cycle energy down the lower back and under pelvis. Action: Orbit energy up past the pubic bone and lower abdominals.
- **Unified Connection:** Counter-action: Extend a symmetrical energy orbit up the upper back and under head. Action: Orbit energy down the chest and upper abdominals. Energize all eight energy orbits of the pattern through the dan tien. This adjoins active and counter-active energies associated with the whole body in support of the lower abdominal isolated connection.

Active Meditation—Spirit Self:

- Notice how you feel in this moment. Do you have pain in your body, clutter in your mind, or agitation in your heart? Be present with yourself. Experience what is taking place within your mind and body as unattached from what is essentially you. As if listening to a cherished friend, pay attention and appreciate who you are and release any fears about who you are not.
- Guided meditation: I am valued.

Lower Abdominal Touchdown

Flat

Starting Position:

- Lie back on floor or flat bench.
- Lift feet off the floor. Legs fold at hips, relaxing quadriceps. Knees fold and point toward the sky (not your head).
- Place hands under outer base of buttock muscles (not under tailbone), supporting abdominals in keeping pelvis stable.
- Allow knees to separate naturally while keeping feet together on median plane.
- Commit to maintaining equal weight distribution along spine as legs move.

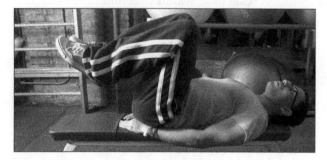

Starting Position

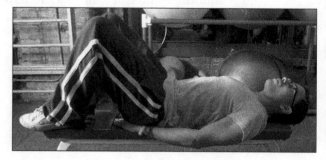

Action/Counter-action

Counter-action:

- Inhale: Visualize energy descend from posterior dan tien under tailbone and feet.
- Exhale: Maintain a neutral spine and relaxed back muscles. Do not allow weight to shift up and down spine as legs descend.
- Inhale: Continue to direct energy downward through lower back. Repeat.
- Be mindful of the quietude in the lower back when your lower abdominal muscles take full command of the movement.

Action:

- Inhale: Relax lower abdominal muscles.
- Exhale: Touch toes to floor as close to pelvis as possible as you contract low abdominal muscles and drop your legs away from torso. Visualize energy rising up through lower abdominals toward anterior dan tien. (Start without touching floor to build strength.)
- Inhale: Support legs back to the starting position using lower abdominal muscles. Repeat.
- Concentrate on lower abdominal muscles, catching the weight of your legs as they move to and fro.

Energy Orbit:

- **Isolated Connection:** Visualize the counter-action before engaging in the action. Counter-action: Cycle energy down the lower back under pelvis and posterior legs. Action: Orbit energy up the anterior legs, pubic bone, and lower abdominals.
- **Unified Connection:** Counter-action: Extend a symmetrical energy orbit up the upper back and under head. Action: Orbit energy down the chest and upper abdominals. Energize all eight energy orbits of the pattern through the dan tien. This adjoins active and counter-active energies associated with the whole body in support of the lower abdominal isolated connection.

Active Meditation—Spirit Self:

- Notice how easily you can unintentionally drop into the fear in your lower back, felt as tension or pain. By the same token, notice how easily you can intentionally stay connected to your center of gravity—spirit self—through your abdominal muscles. Feel the decision to stay connected with your spirit self. Enjoy your commitment to your own needs. Enjoy taking care of yourself.
- Guided meditation: I am worthy.

Lower Abdominal Leg Extension

Flat and Decline

Starting Position:

- Lie back on floor, flat bench, or decline bench with head above hips.
- Lift feet off the floor with a 90-degree bend at knees and hips.
- Place hands under outer base of buttock muscles (not under tailbone), supporting abdominals in keeping pelvis stable.
- Allow knees to separate naturally while keeping feet together on median plane.
- Commit to keeping your abdominal strength supporting your legs' weight at all times.

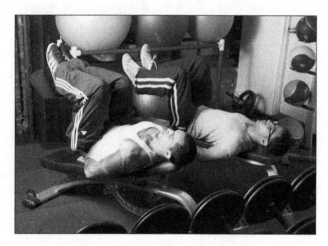

Starting Position

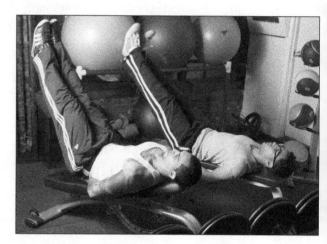

Action/Counter-action

Counter-action:

- Inhale: Visualize energy descend from your posterior dan tien under tailbone, legs, and feet.
- Exhale: Push heel stirrups out to extend legs, maintaining a neutral spine, equal weight distribution along spinal column, and relaxed back muscles.
- Inhale: Pull heel stirrups toward breasts as you continue to direct energy downward under folding legs. Repeat.
- Be mindful of your weight remaining unchanged as your legs travel in and out.

Action:

- Inhale: Relax lower abdominal muscles.
- Exhale: Contract lower abdominal muscles and extend legs toward ceiling-wall junction by visualizing energy rising up through lower abdominals toward anterior dan tien. Knees will stay slightly bent at full extension. (Lower leg extension to increase difficulty.)
- Inhale: Support legs back to starting position using lower abdominal muscles. Repeat.
- Concentrate on adjusting abdominal involvement to consistently support legs' movement.

Energy Orbit:

- **Isolated Connection:** Visualize the counter-action before engaging in the action. Counter-action: Cycle energy down the lower back under pelvis and posterior legs. Action: Orbit energy up the anterior legs, pubic bone, and lower abdominals.
- **Unified Connection:** Counter-action: Extend a symmetrical energy orbit up the upper back and under head. Action: Orbit energy down the chest and upper abdominals. Energize all eight energy orbits of the pattern through the dan tien. This adjoins active and counter-active energies associated with the whole body in support of the lower abdominal isolated connection.

Active Meditation—Spirit Self

- Notice how the farther away your legs get, the more easily you become an observer of your own experience. Stay an objective observer as the legs return in. Without judgment, recognize any adjustments you need to make to remain relaxed in your lower back. Be curious about your limits and challenge yourself by staying within them. Enjoy being in control of your movement.
- Guided meditation: I recognize and respect my boundaries.

Lower Abdominal Six-Inch Raise

Flat

Starting Position:

- Lie back on floor or flat bench.
- Place hands under outer base of buttock muscles (not under tailbone), supporting abdominals in keeping pelvis stable.
- Push through heel stirrups to extend legs toward ceiling wall junction. Keep knees slightly bent. (Lower leg extension to increase difficulty.)
- Keep feet together on median plane.
- Commit to maintaining soft hip and knee joints, keeping the quadriceps involvement reserved.

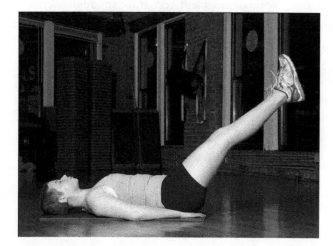
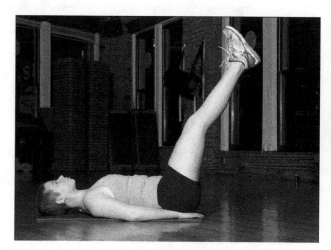

Starting Position **Action/Counter-action**

Counter-action:

- Inhale: Visualize energy descend from your posterior dan tien under the tailbone and through posterior legs and feet.
- Exhale: Allow pelvis to tip and legs to rise by relaxing lower back muscles around and between lower vertebrae of spine. Observe that the feet rise up to the same degree that your abdominals contract.
- Inhale: Return to the starting position, continuing to direct energy downward under legs' weight. Repeat.
- Be mindful of your pelvis and legs moving as one unit.

Action:

- Inhale: Ease lower abdominal muscles.
- Exhale: Contract lower abdominal muscles to tip pelvis and raise legs as one unit by visualizing energy rising up anterior legs and through lower abdominals toward dan tien.

- Inhale: Use lower abdominals to lower legs back to the starting position. Repeat.
- Concentrate on your lower abdominals' strength, giving your lower back permission to stay relaxed and elongated.

Energy Orbit:

- **Isolated Connection:** Visualize the counter-action before engaging in the action. Counter-action: Cycle energy down the lower back under pelvis and posterior legs. Action: Orbit energy up the anterior legs, pubic bone, and lower abdominals.
- **Unified Connection:** Counter-action: Extend a symmetrical energy orbit up the upper back and under head. Action: Orbit energy down the chest and upper abdominals. Energize all eight energy orbits of the pattern through the dan tien. This adjoins active and counter-active energies associated with the whole body in support of the lower abdominal isolated connection.

Active Meditation—Spirit Self:

- Notice how your abdominal connection to your body's weight has a greater value to your strength than the size of your movement. Experience less as more; experience self as enough. As your relationship with your own weight settles into unconditional appreciation, contentment with the present moment follows.
- Guided meditation: I am present.

Upper Abdominal Exercises

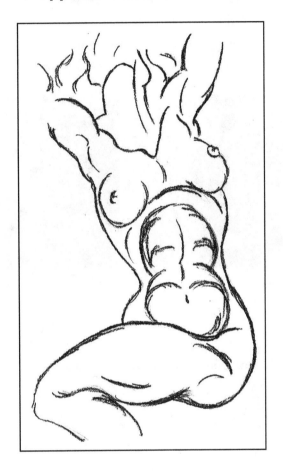

Upper
Abdominal Muscles
Embody
Your Sense of self

Human Self

Upper Abdominal Crunch

Flat and Decline

Starting Position:

- Lie back on floor, flat bench, or decline bench with feet above head.
- Bend knees with feet flat on floor or soft knees with feet hooked into equipment.
- Place hands behind head to fully support head's weight. Head placement should be two inches off floor.
- Place elbows as if they are an extension of the back's width.
- Commit to the back of your neck and shoulders, staying completely relaxed.

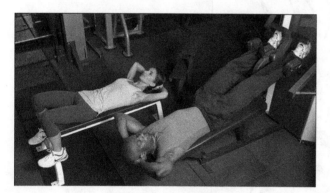
Starting Position

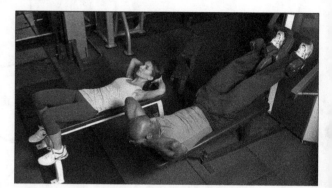
Action/Counter-action

Counter-action:

- Inhale: Visualize energy rising from posterior dan tien up back, neck, and head.
- Exhale: Allow upper-back vertebrae to roll away from floor by fully relaxing deep muscles around upper spine, vertebrae, and posterior ribs.
- Inhale: Allow upper torso to be returned to the starting position. Repeat.
- Be mindful to surrender muscles and relax nerves around upper spinal column to encourage space between vertebrae. Let your central nervous system yawn.

Action:

- Inhale: Expand upper abdominal muscles.
- Exhale: Contract upper abdominal muscles, moving head and torso as one unit, by visualizing descending energy passing through upper abdomen toward dan tien.
- Inhale: Carry torso back to the starting position using upper abdominal muscles. Repeat.
- Concentrate on connecting your upper abdominal muscles to the weight of your upper body and head. Look for a subtle muscular quiver.

Energy Orbit:

- **Isolated Connection:** Visualize the counter-action before engaging in the action. Counter-action: Cycle energy up the upper back and under head. Action: Orbit energy down the chest and upper abdominals.
- **Unified Connection:** Counter-action: Extend a symmetrical energy orbit down the lower back under the pelvis and posterior legs. Action: Orbit energy up the anterior legs, pubic bone, and lower abdominals. Energize all eight energy orbits of the pattern through the dan tien. This adjoins active and counter-active energies associated with the whole body in support of the upper abdominal isolated connection.

Active Meditation—Spirit Self:

- As the primary muscle group that gets you out of bed and unfurls you upright, your upper abdominals carry your life story into each movement. Move slowly and experience your body's weight from the perspective of the upper abdominals. Become curious about what motivates them. Rather than thinking of a motivation for an objective, feel for the uprising of your spirit. Let it inform and inspire you anew.
- Guided meditation: I am me.

Extended Upper Abdominal Crunch

Gymnastic Ball

Starting Position:

- Lie supine over a gymnastic ball. Place shoulders and hips at same distance from the floor, creating a spinal arch. Support arch with additional lower abdominal support.
- Keep feet flat on floor, as distant from each other as the diameter of the ball.
- Place hands behind head, fully supporting head's weight; position chin as if gently holding a grapefruit against the sternum.
- Place elbows as if they were an extension of the back's width.
- Protect lower back and stabilize yourself on the ball by committing to your lower abdominals' support.

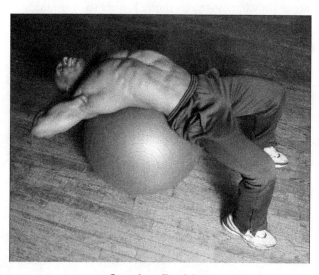
Starting Position

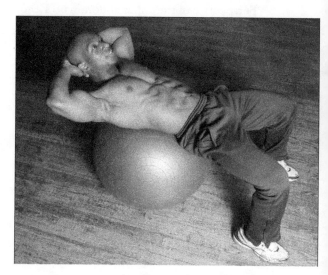
Action/Counter-action

Counter-action:

- Inhale: Visualize energy rising from posterior dan tien up back, neck, and head.
- Exhale: Allow upper back vertebrae to roll away from ball while keeping neck quiet. Fully relax deep muscles along entire spine, vertebrae, and posterior ribs.
- Inhale: Allow upper torso to be returned to the starting position. Repeat.
- Be mindful of how upper back and lower back expand away from each other in the crunch.

Action:

- Inhale: Hyper-expand upper abdominal muscles.
- Exhale: Contract upper abdominal muscles, moving head and torso as one unit. Visualize descending energy passing through upper abdominals toward anterior dan tien.

- Inhale: Carry torso back to starting position using upper abdominals. Repeat.
- Concentrate on the most superior aspect of upper abdominals, contracting toward the most inferior aspect of lower abdominals.

Energy Orbit:

- **Isolated Connection:** Visualize the counter-action before engaging in the action. Counter-action: Cycle energy up the upper back and under head. Action: Orbit energy down the chest and upper abdominals.
- **Unified Connection:** Counter-action: Extend a symmetrical energy orbit down the lower back under pelvis and posterior legs. Action: Orbit energy up the anterior legs, pubic bone, and lower abdominals. Energize all eight energy orbits of the pattern through the dan tien. This step adjoins active and counter-active energies associated with the whole body in support of the upper abdominal isolated connection.

Active Meditation—Spirit Self:

- Notice that the more you expand your abdominals, the more you arch and contract your back muscles. Explore allowing the back's arch to exist without contraction, without fear. Trust your ability to control your abdominal stretch into unknown territory with grace and intelligence. Feel grounded strength in your extended range.
- Guided meditation: I am confident.

Upper Abdominal Crunch with Crossed Legs

Flat

Starting Position:

- Lie back on floor or flat bench.
- Cross ankles directly over pelvis, knees slightly bent.
- Place hands behind head to fully support head weight. Head placement should be two inches off floor.
- Place elbows as if they are an extension of the back's width.
- Commit to keeping the knees, hip flexors, and quadriceps relaxed.

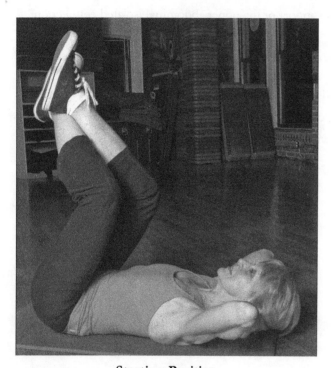
Starting Position

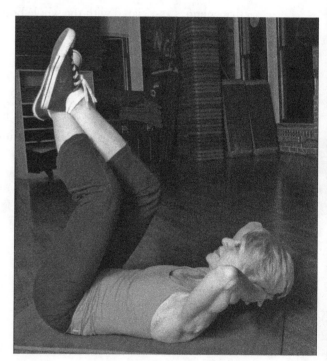
Action/Counter-action

Counter-action:

- Inhale: Visualize energy rising from posterior dan tien up back, neck, and head.
- Exhale: Allow upper-back vertebrae to roll away from floor by fully relaxing deep muscles around upper spine, vertebrae, and posterior ribs.
- Inhale: Allow upper torso to be returned to the starting position. Repeat.
- Be mindful to maintain an even distribution of weight along length of spine throughout movement to avoid disturbing the hip flexors and leg position.

Action:

- Inhale: Expand upper abdominal muscles.

- Exhale: Contract upper abdominal muscles, moving head and torso as one unit. Visualize descending energy passing through upper abdominals toward anterior dan tien.
- Inhale: Carry torso back to starting position using upper abdominals. Repeat.
- Concentrate on the stability your energy orbit provides—versus the typical tension your hip flexors create—to maintain this leg position throughout repetitions.

Energy Orbit:

- **Isolated Connection:** Visualize the counter-action before engaging in the action. Counter-action: Cycle energy up the upper back and under head. Action: Orbit energy down the chest and upper abdominals.
- **Unified Connection:** Counter-action: Extend a symmetrical energy orbit down the lower back under pelvis and posterior legs. Action: Orbit energy up the anterior legs, pubic bone, and lower abdominals. Energize all eight energy orbits of the pattern through the dan tien. This step adjoins active and counter-active energies associated with the whole body in support of the upper abdominal isolated connection.

Active Meditation—Spirit Self:

- Notice how you feel less grounded without your feet on the floor. Recognize the propensity to throw your weight, rather than fully connect with it, when you don't feel grounded. When meeting the resistance of your own weight, connect to the care and concern you would offer someone you'd like to know. Meet your weight with a wish to know yourself better. Enjoy your own care and concern.
- Guided meditation: I am love.

Upper Abdominal Crunch with 90-Degree Leg Raise

Flat

Starting Position:

- Lie back on floor or flat bench.
- Keep legs together with 90-degree bend at knees and hips.
- Place hands behind head to fully support head weight. Head placement should be two inches off floor.
- Place elbows as if they are an extension of the back's width.
- Commit to supporting the leg position with lower abdominals rather than hip flexors or lower back.

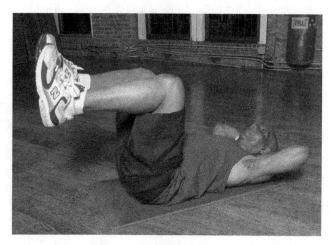

Starting Position

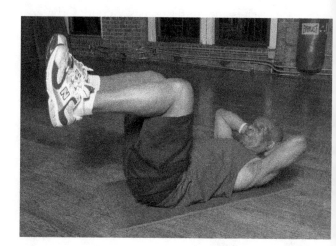

Action/Counter-action

Counter-action:

- Inhale: Visualize energy descending from your posterior dan tien under tailbone, legs, and feet to support leg position. Then visualize energy rising from your posterior dan tien under back, neck, and head to support movement.
- Exhale: Allow upper-back vertebrae to roll away from floor while lower spine (sacrum) stays placed by fully relaxing deep muscles around entire spine, vertebrae, pelvis, and posterior ribs.
- Inhale: Allow upper torso to be returned to the starting position. Repeat.
- Be mindful of the inner thighs and lower abdominals uniting to stabilize your position into your dan tien energy center.

Action:

- Inhale: Expand upper abdominal muscles.
- Exhale: Contract upper abdominal muscles, moving head and torso as one unit. Visualize descending energy passing through upper abdominals toward anterior dan tien.
- Inhale: Carry torso back to starting position using upper abdominal muscles. Repeat.
- Concentrate on distinguishing the lower abdominal muscles support from the upper abdominal muscles execution.

Energy Orbit:

- **Isolated Connection:** Visualize the counter-action before engaging in the action. Counter-action: Cycle energy up the upper back and under head. Action: Orbit energy down the chest and upper abdominals.
- **Unified Connection:** Counter-action: Extend a symmetrical energy orbit down the lower back, under pelvis, and posterior legs. Action: Orbit energy up the anterior legs, pubic bone, and lower abdominals. Energize all eight energy orbits of the pattern through the dan tien. This adjoins active and counter-active energies associated with the whole body in support of the upper abdominal isolated connection.

Active Meditation—Spirit Self:

- Notice how honest your movement feels when the support and execution of movement come from the same energy source. Experience your self-determinism and uniqueness in the world.
- Guided meditation: I am supported in being me.

Seated Combo Crunch

Machine

Starting Position:

- Sit on machine with torso against seat back; hook ankles behind supports.
- Hold handgrips with elbows positioned forward.
- Lean head back against headrest, relaxing neck and shoulders.
- Contract upper and lower abdominals simultaneously to position head and torso upright out of machine's resting position.
- Commit to simultaneously connecting lower and upper abdominal muscles with the machine as if becoming part of the mechanism.

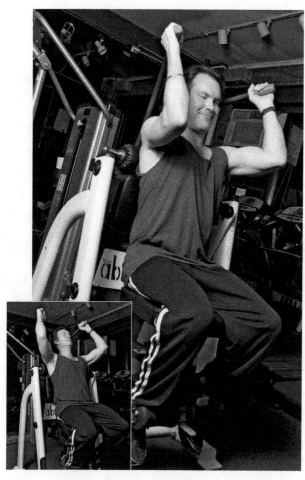

Starting Position

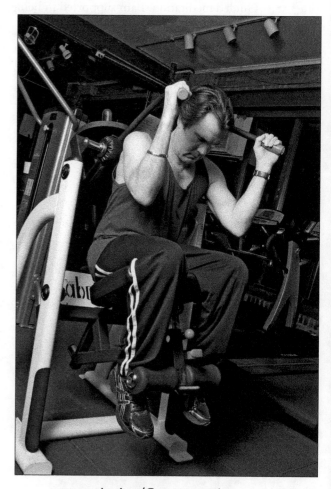

Action/Counter-action

Counter-action:

- Inhale: Visualize energy descending from your posterior dan tien under tailbone, hips, and seat to support lower abdominals. Visualize energy rising from your posterior dan tien up back, neck, head, and headrest to support upper abdominals.

- Exhale: Allow lower and upper vertebrae to expand while keeping head relaxed on headrest. Fully relax deep muscles around entire spine, vertebrae, and posterior ribs. Resist pulling with hands.
- Inhale: Move lower and upper torso with machine back to starting position. Repeat.
- Be mindful of upper and lower vertebrae energetically expanding, even as you return them back to the starting position.

Action:

- Inhale: Symmetrically connect to upper and lower abdominal muscles.
- Exhale: Contract lower and upper abdominal muscles, hinging lower and upper body forward as if one with the machine. Visualize ascending energy passing through lower abdominals and descending energy passing through upper abdominals.
- Inhale: Return to the starting position using upper and lower abdominals. Repeat.
- Concentrate on upper and lower abdominals carrying weight of machine and torso.

Energy Orbit:

- **Isolated and Unified Connection:** Visualize the counter-action before engaging in the action. Counter-action: Cycle energy up the upper back and under head as well as down the lower back under pelvis and posterior legs. Action: Orbit energy down the chest and upper abdominals as well as up anterior legs, pubic bone, and lower abdominals. Energize all eight energy orbits of the pattern through the dan tien. This adjoins active and counter-active energies associated with the whole body in support of the upper/lower abdominal exercise.

Active Meditation—Spirit Self:

- Notice how secure you feel when upper and lower abdominals are working equally toward a united goal. Experience hard work as different from suffering.
- Guided meditation: I have a purpose.

Oblique Abdominal Exercises

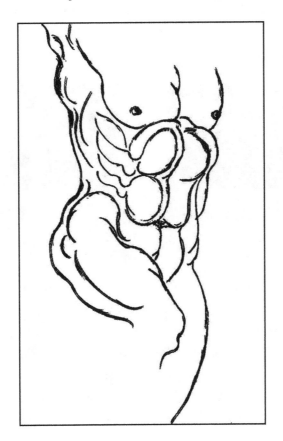

Oblique
Abdominal Muscles
Embody
the self relating with the Self

Spirit-Human Relationship

Oblique Crunch with Lower Torso Twist

Flat

Starting Position:

- Lie on back with knees bent and feet on floor, hips' width apart.
- Tip knees to one side while maintaining a square upper body.
- Place hands behind head, fully supporting head weight two inches off floor.
- Place elbows as if they are an extension of the back's width.
- Commit to supporting torso twist with lower abdominals rather than lower back.

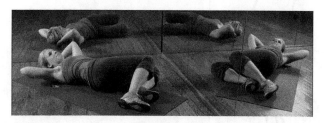
Starting Position

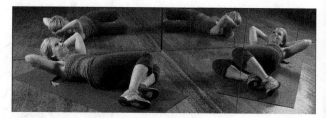
Action/Counter-action

Counter-action:

- Inhale: Visualize energy descending from your posterior dan tien under tailbone and feet to support lower body's twisted position. Then visualize energy rising from your posterior dan tien up back, neck, and head to support movement.
- Exhale: Allow upper-back vertebrae to roll away from floor while lower spine stays placed. Fully relax deep muscles around entire spine, vertebrae, and posterior ribs.
- Inhale: Allow upper torso to be returned to starting position. Repeat. Then repeat on other side.
- Be mindful of the upper back and shoulders staying square to the floor.

Action:

- Inhale: Expand upper abdominal and oblique muscles.
- Exhale: Contract upper abdominal and oblique muscles, moving head and torso as one unit. Visualize descending energy passing through upper abdominals toward elevated hip bone.
- Inhale: Carry torso back to starting position using upper abdominal and oblique muscles. Repeat. Then repeat on other side.
- Concentrate on maintaining the space between your feet and lining up elevated hip bone with your sternum on median plane.

Energy Orbit:

- **Isolated and Unified Connection:** Visualize the counter-action before engaging in the action. Counter-action: Cycle energy up the upper back and under head as well as down the lower back under pelvis and posterior legs. Action: Orbit energy down the chest and upper abdominals as well as up the anterior legs, pubic bone, and lower abdominals. Energize all eight energy orbits of the pattern through the dan tien. This step adjoins active and counter-active energies associated with the whole body in support of the oblique's isolated connection.

Active Meditation—Spirit Self:

- Notice how upper abdominals can disrupt your spiral's alliance with essential alignment when they're too aggressive. Overpowering your oblique muscles with your upper abdominals causes a loss of balance between upper and lower energy orbits. This can feel like losing your sense of self in the attempt to assert it. Feel the weight of your upper and lower body balance your spiral to connect you with your dan tien. Experience your physical weight actualizing the bond between human and spirit selves.
- Guided meditation: I am my own ally.

Oblique Crunch

Flat

Starting Position:

- Lie back on floor or flat bench, knees bent and feet positioned hips' width apart.
- Place hands behind head, fully supporting head's weight two inches off floor.
- Place elbows as if they are an extension of the back's width.
- Commit to the placement of your arms, shoulders, chest, and head.

Starting Position

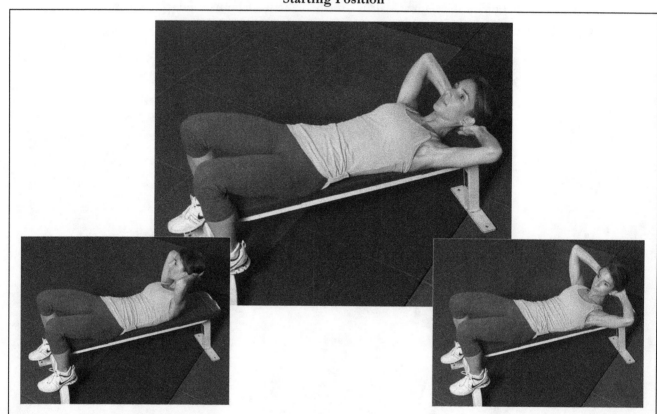

Action/Counter-action

Counter-action:

- Inhale: Visualize energy rising from posterior dan tien up back, neck, and head; overemphasize energy of posterior ribs spiraling up.
- Exhale: Allow upper vertebrae to roll away from floor, expanding and spiraling posterior ribs while lower spine and pelvis remain placed. Relax deep muscles along entire spine between vertebrae and posterior ribs.
- Inhale: Allow upper torso to unspiral and be returned to starting position.
- Repeat with opposite spiral and continue alternating.
- Be mindful to roll both sides of the rib cage off floor. Don't lean onto one side of ribs when spiraling.

Action:

- Inhale: Expand abdominal muscles.
- Exhale: Contract upper and oblique abdominal muscles to lift and spiral torso. Spiral chest, arms, and head as one unit toward opposite hip bone by visualizing descending energy passing through upper abdominals and spiraling oblique muscles toward anterior dan tien and hip bone.
- Inhale: Carry torso back to starting position using upper abdominals and oblique muscles.
- Repeat with opposite spiral and continue alternating.
- Concentrate on upper abdominals lifting you as your oblique muscles spiral you.

Energy Orbit:

- **Isolated Connection:** Visualize the counter-action before engaging in the action. Counter-action: Cycle energy up the upper back and under head. Action: Orbit energy down the chest, upper abdominals, and oblique muscles.
- **Unified Connection:** Counter-action: Extend a symmetrical energy orbit down the lower back under pelvis and posterior legs. Action: Orbit energy up the anterior legs, pubic bone, and lower abdominals. Energize all eight energy orbits of the pattern through the dan tien. This adjoins active and counter-active energies associated with the whole body in support of the obliques' isolated connection.

Active Meditation—Spirit Self:

- The ability to spiral and maintain essential alignment is artistry in motion. Connect to the belief you hold in your own grace and recognize your uniqueness. Choose self over fear.
- Guided meditation: I honor spirit through my commitment to my uniqueness and talent.

Hyperextended Oblique Crunch

Machine

Starting Position:

- Hook feet into foot platform with bottom foot forward and position side of hip on cushion just below hip bone.
- Keep legs straight and hips and shoulders square, with hands on the active oblique muscles.
- Place elbows out from center and keep head in line with spine.
- Commit to essential alignment while in an angled relationship with gravity.

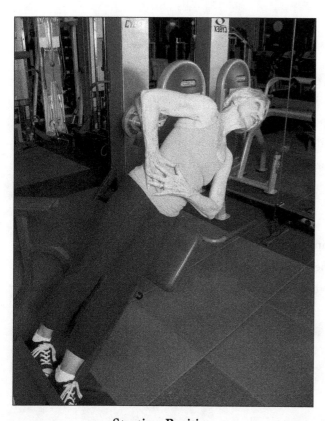

Starting Position

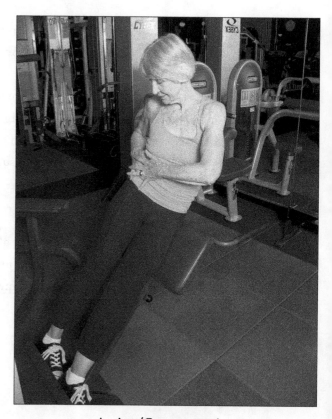

Action/Counter-action

Counter-action:

- Inhale: Visualize energy rising from posterior dan tien up back, neck, and head.
- Exhale: Leaning top hip back, allow lower spine and pelvis to expand downward while upper spine and vertebrae expand upward by relaxing muscles between vertebrae and posterior ribs.
- Inhale: Allow upper torso to unspiral and hips to realign as you return to starting position. Repeat. Then repeat on other side.
- Be mindful to isolate upper-body crunch while maneuvering lower back's expansion toward hip cushion.

Action:

- Inhale: Expand abdominal muscles.
- Exhale: Contract lower abdominals to stabilize pelvis, while upper abdominals and oblique muscles lift and rotate torso, arms, and head as one unit toward hip bone. Visualize descending energy passing through upper abdominals and oblique muscles toward anterior dan tien and opposing hip bone.
- Inhale: Carry torso back to starting position using upper abdominals and obliques, while lower abdominals stabilize the realignment of hips. Repeat. Then repeat on other side.
- Concentrate on upper, oblique, and lower abdominals, balancing their unique attributes.

Energy Orbit:

- **Isolated and Unified Connection:** Visualize the counter-action before engaging in the action. Counter-action: Cycle energy up the upper back and under head as well as down the lower back under pelvis and posterior legs. Action: Orbit energy down the chest, upper abdominals, and oblique muscles as well as up the anterior legs, pubic bone, and lower abdominals. Energize all eight energy orbits of the pattern through the dan tien. This step adjoins active and counter-active energies associated with an upper/lower oblique abdominal exercise.

Active Meditation—Spirit Self:

- You're out on a limb, relying on your ability to collaborate within your own center. Believe in what you know about yourself and be curious about what you don't.
- Guided meditation: I trust myself.

BodyLogos Psyche-Muscular Observations for Abdominal Muscles

Size: Release all expectations about the size of your body's movement. Allow the movement to be a truthful reflection of your abdominal muscles' strength and your back's limitations.

🛑 Large movement coming from external momentum. This leads you away from your abdominal center and indicates concern about not being good enough.

🛑 Small movement that doesn't sufficiently challenge the abdominal muscles. This points out the inability to find or an unwillingness to feel into your center or self.

🌀 Listen and lead with your abdominal muscles full strength. Literally experience the weight of your body solely motivated by your abdominal muscles. Meditate on the value of knowing your limits. Appreciate your physical limitation as a reference point as to how far you can honestly and realistically perform in all aspects of your life.

Posture: When challenging the abdominal muscles, you want to experience the work being done. If you are experiencing fatigue anywhere other than the abdominal muscles, it indicates feelings of insecurity regarding your present strengths and competence in the world.

🛑 Back fatigue points toward a fear of being honest with your authentic self.

🛑 Shoulder or neck fatigue is a sign of being judgmental with your authentic self.

🛑 Quadriceps or hip flexor fatigue shows a resistance to moving yourself forward.

🌀 Slow down and be present in your abdominal center. Exhale through the areas fatiguing you and recognize they're not needed to perform this exercise. Relax all extraneous activity. Trust in yourself.

Coordination: When done well, exercise looks easy. Putting it all together—mind, muscle, breath, movement, meditation—can overstimulate you to the point of checking out. It's important to build coordination one aspect at a time.

🛑 Holding your breath. When you stop breathing, you become inwardly out of alignment. You have created an internal freeze. This freeze is animating a mental or emotional freeze.

🌀 Consciously allowing your breath to flow during an abdominal exercise, through both the action of your abdominals and counter-action of your back, is a deliberate decision to allow yourself to grow.

🛑 Getting distracted. You make the same errors regularly; you'd rather be someplace else or use your abdominal workout as a time to chat. These are examples of disregarding your inner world. Your intention to work out is apparent, but you are compromising your efforts by making everything else more important.

🌀 Consciously focusing your attention inwardly on your abdominal performance is an action of believing in yourself.

Meet the Models

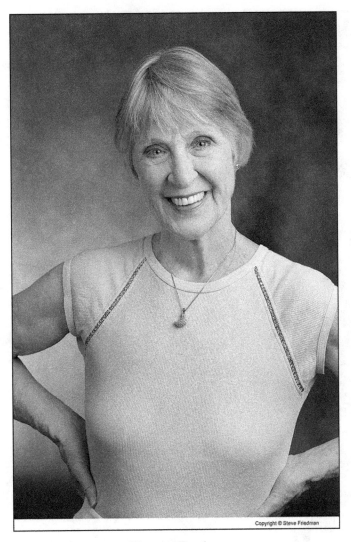

Yvonne Puckett

Dance. Dance. Dance! This seventy-five-year-old, all-American dancer has gone from beach go-go girl in the movies with Elvis to a classically trained dancer swinging in Fred Astaire films. Jerry Lewis, Debbie Reynolds, and Jonathan Winters are a few names included in her assortment of dance tales. After raising a family of two children and now enjoying being a grandmother, she still has the energy to share her passion for movement with others. Her present interests are in the fitness arena as a NIA and Zumba instructor. She and her daughter, Serena, are well known for their team teaching of NIA, a mind-body approach to aerobic dance. She says, "Strength training offers me a calming diversion from my fifteen to twenty aerobic dance classes per week." However, it is through playing singing bowls that she finds her greatest meditative retreat. If you wonder what this ageless woman does in her free time, Yvonne is an award-winning playwright for *Normal* and *Famous—A Hollywood Musical*.

Tammy Wise

Coming Home Energy Pattern as It Relates to the Biceps Muscles

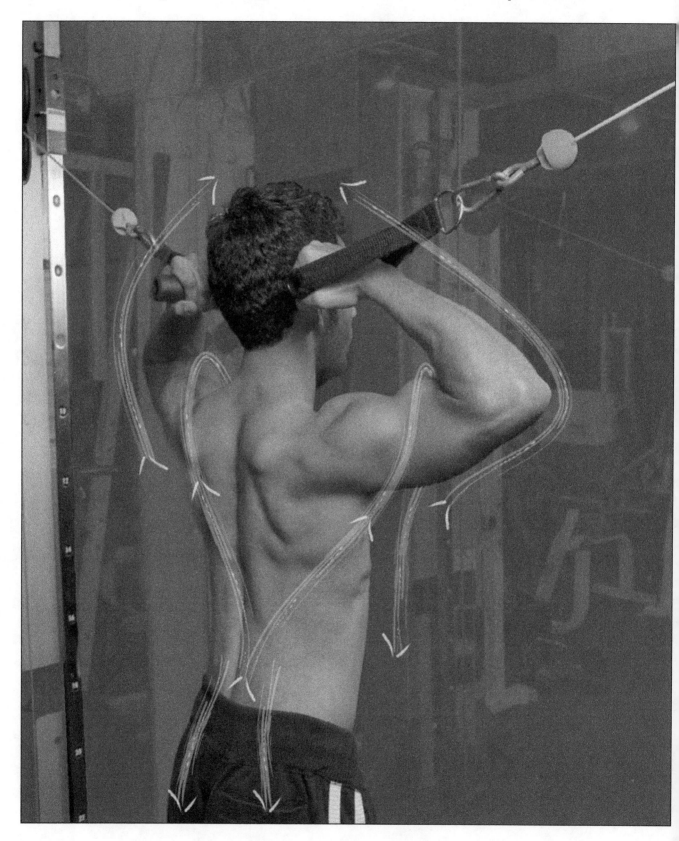

Visualize this energy pattern supporting all biceps isolations.

Introduction to Biceps Muscles

Theory of Yin and Yang

Yang: Active Muscle Group

Biceps Muscles:
- o   Biceps Brachii
- o   Brachialis
- o   Brachioradialis
- o   Pronator Teres

Yin: Counter-active Muscle Group

Triceps Muscles:
- o   Triceps Brachii
- o   Anconeus

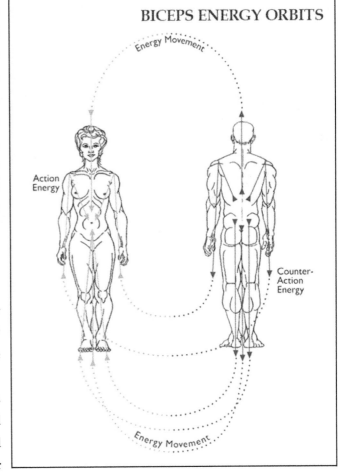

In a biceps isolation, the anterior side of the body is asked to contract while the posterior side of the body energetically expands. You experience this movement when shoveling. The triceps' expansive length (counter-action) scoops under the snow, placing the biceps' force in the most effective place to connect to the snow's weight (action). Meanwhile, the rest of the body's energy orbit is committed to cycling tension out of your lower back muscles and into your abdominal center to support the biceps challenge.

Action: Pulling Desirables Inward

This is a time to sculpt your inner and outer worlds. What do you want to bring into your life? Whether you can touch it or feel it, you have the power to create it.

Desiring big life changes or small nuances clutters the mind. Notice how an expanded overview of what you desire brings the personal priorities within that desired outcome into clear focus. When you channel desiring energy into an active meditation, a deliberate choice becomes apparent, and an organized intention is set into motion. Once energy is actively directed toward what you want in life, the mind quiets itself purposefully. Knowing your personal priorities makes choosing what you want to create a natural unfolding.

Counter-action: Pushing Undesirables Outward

When contracting the biceps muscles, you can also meditate on the expanding counter-action of your triceps muscles. As the primary muscles that push undesirables away, the triceps muscles create room for what you now want. Allow for change, new experiences, and growth in your life by letting yesterday's desirables, habits, and unneeded coping strategies go. It's a mark of maturity and evolution toward what you are creating today.

Five-Element Theory
Spring, Crushing Joints, Anger

Connection: Spring

To spring into action is the biceps' favorite calling. They are quick to facilitate you, grabbing what you want in life. Spring is a time to sow the seeds for tomorrow's harvest, and the biceps muscles are designed to gather what you need. Their sole purpose is to pull things closer so they can be nurtured. Celebrate being self-possessed. Recognize how you influence all you touch. As you set up for a biceps exercise, concentrate on your abdominal stability, aligning the dan tien for essential alignment; and on coming home energy supporting the weight of success. Experience the personal conviction connected to creating your life, acquiring reputation and lifestyle, since your abdominal center—spirit self—supports your biceps' effort to pull desirables inward.

Strength: Crushing Joints

The crushing wood joint of the elbows splits the action and counter-action—the biceps and triceps—when pulling in an outside resistance. Once the triceps' counter-action positions the biceps' action under a resistance, the biceps are fully connected to the challenge. Maintaining this connection point keeps the biceps' strength under the resistance, directing the resistance slightly away from the body in a circular movement. This circular trajectory moves the weight forward and then pulls it upward, pivoting at the elbow joints. After that, it's carried back to its starting position in the same circular path. Be resolved in keeping your elbows still, placing this circular pattern in front of you where you can see it rather than shifting elbows back, compromising the shoulders, and pulling the resistance into your body, where you can no longer maintain an objective viewpoint.

Meditation: Anger

As primary pulling muscles in the body, the biceps are used when you are in need of something. Pulling something inward is a worthy act of taking what is essential and getting what you need to survive and thrive. However, the need to need can feel offensive—even humiliating—and sometimes indignity slips in between the biceps and the challenge. Internal ambivalence about needing diminishes the biceps' connection with an outside resistance, and shoulder muscles will then, by default, step in to rescue the biceps. By focusing on the energy orbit and releasing your triceps and lower back, you flush out the anger related to needing and usher in a sound central support from your abdominals for your biceps' integrity. This connection to the spirit self inadvertently alleviates any overwhelming emotion related to needing and creates a mindset that can focus on what you deliberately want to pull into your life and how to do it. Be mindful of your abdominal strength supporting a stable foundation under the biceps' function to pull desirables inward. And appreciate the opportunity to sculpt your own life.

How to Isolate the Biceps Muscles

Feel It Contract

There are multiple joints and smaller muscles in the hands, wrists, and forearms that can initially interfere with a biceps exercise. It can be helpful to remove the effect of these other musculoskeletal elements so you can feel what an isolated biceps contraction feels like.

Supine Elbow Bend with Flexed Wrist

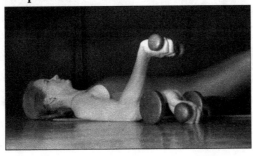

Exercise: Lie supine with knees bent and feet flat on the floor. Relax the back of one wrist over a large dumbbell (eight to ten pounds) while loosely holding a small dumbbell (two to three pounds) in your fingers. Notice the flexion in your wrist and relaxed hand and fingers. Feel the weight of your shoulder blade and elbow equally relaxed into the floor as you slowly lift the relaxed flexed wrist off the large dumbbells toward the sky three to six inches. By keeping the fingers, wrist, and forearm relaxed, your biceps muscles become the first contact with the resistance. This is an exploration to experience the biceps muscles without hand and forearm interference, and it is to be done only with light weights.

Feel It Release

Because the shoulder joints are so flexible, successfully stretching their neighboring biceps muscles can be tricky. When approaching this stretch, keep the shoulder joints aligned between the chest and arms.

Swan Dive with Flexed Wrist

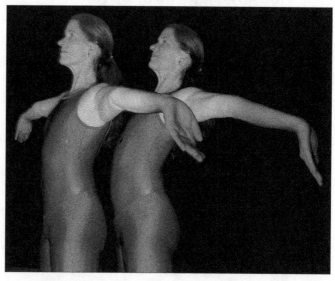

Exercise: Stand with feet shoulder width apart and knees slightly bent. Extend arms sideways, along the coronal plane, with flexed wrists and fingers rotated downward. Lift chest as in a swan dive, pushing strongly out through flexed heel of hands, then stretch outreached arms backward. Feel as though the biceps muscles were elongating between your chest and the heel of your hands.

Feel It Fatigue

Biceps muscles aren't big talkers. When they feel exhausted, they are exhausted. Rest when the biceps muscles fail. When the challenge starts to go into your shoulders and neck, or elbow and wrist joints, your body is telling you to stop. Once you are rested, return with a clean connection.

Biceps Exercises

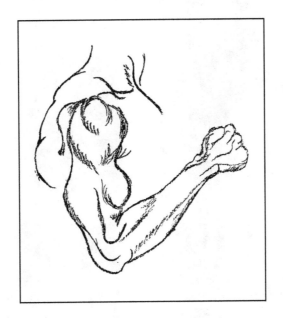

Biceps Muscles
Embody
Pulling Desirables Inward

Tammy Wise

Seated Biceps Curl with Hammerhead Grip

Dumbbell

Starting Position:

- Sit tall with feet flat on floor.
- Hold dumbbells, palms facing inward toward body.
- Connect to abdominal center. Relax weight of arms, shoulders, and outside resistance down through shoulder blades.
- Commit to keeping shoulder blades dropped.

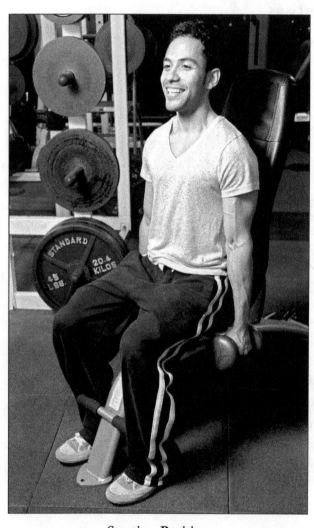

Starting Position

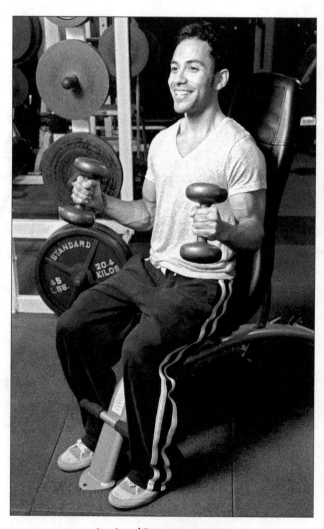

Action/Counter-action

Counter-action:

- Inhale: Visualize energy expanding outward from posterior dan tien through shoulders width, passing through elbows and under resistance.
- Exhale: Align forearm, wrist, and hand with resistance. Lengthen triceps, encouraging elbow to bend.

- Inhale: Keep length of triceps under resistance as forearm returns to starting position. Repeat.
- Be mindful to keep your relaxed elbow placement unchanged throughout the curl.

Action:

- Inhale: Establish the connection point between biceps muscles and resistance.
- Exhale: Contract biceps muscles to pull resistance through circular trajectory. Visualize energy drawn inward through anterior body—biceps, shoulders, chest, and abdominals—gathering energy in the dan tien.
- Inhale: Use biceps to carry resistance back to the starting position. Repeat.
- Concentrate on abdominals and biceps meeting the resistance as a dual force.

Energy Orbit:

- **Isolated Connection:** Visualize the counter-action before engaging in the action. Counter-action: Cycle energy up the upper back, posterior shoulders, and triceps past elbows, forearms, and hands. Action: Orbit energy through biceps, anterior shoulders, and down chest and upper abdominals.
- **Unified Connection:** Counter-action: Extend a symmetrical energy orbit down the lower back and posterior legs. Action: Orbit energy up the anterior legs and lower abdominals. Energize all eight energy orbits of the pattern through the dan tien. This step adjoins active and counter-active energies associated with the whole body in support of the biceps' isolated connection.

Active Meditation—Pulling Desirables Inward:

- Experience how the resistance travels forward before being lifting upward. This implies that pulling desirables inward is an act of initially gliding it forward, as if sharing it, then enjoying it. Feel the intimacy that comes with making your desires known.
- Guided meditation: I ask for what I need, want, and desire.

Standing Biceps Curl

Barbell and Dyna-Band

Starting Position:

- Stand with feet hips' width apart and knees slightly bent.
- Hold barbell shoulders' width apart or hold Dyna-Band ends while standing on band's center, palms facing forward.
- Connect to abdominal center. Relax weight of arms, shoulders, and outside resistance down through shoulder blades.
- Commit to the dual function of your abdominals, since they support alignment and empower the biceps action.

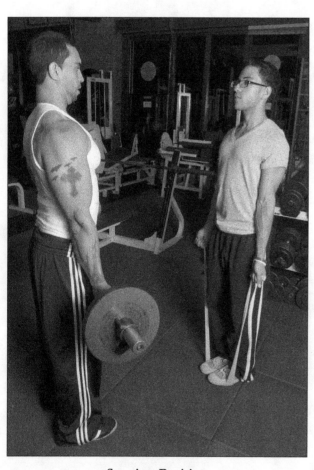

Starting Position

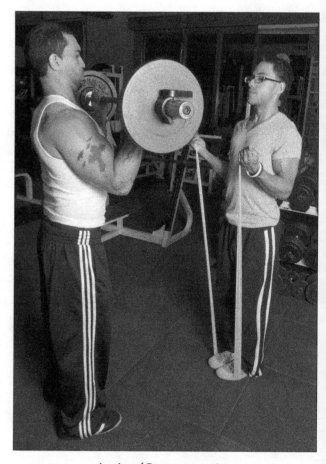

Action/Counter-action

Counter-action:

- Inhale: Visualize energy expanding outward from posterior dan tien through shoulders width, passing through elbows and under resistance.
- Exhale: Align forearm, wrist, and hand with resistance. Lengthen triceps to encourage elbows to bend and feel the back's width connected to your abdominal support.

- Inhale: Keep length of triceps under resistance as forearms return to starting position. Repeat.
- Be mindful to maintain space in the spinal column. From dan tien, elongate the spine both up through the crown of head and down through the million-dollar point and gushing spring points.

Action:

- Inhale: Establish the connection point between biceps muscles and resistance.
- Exhale: Contract biceps muscles to pull resistance through circular trajectory. Visualize energy drawn inward through anterior body—biceps, shoulders, chest, and abdominal center—gathering energy in dan tien.
- Inhale: Carry resistance back to the starting position using biceps. Repeat.
- Concentrate on biceps as a link between your abdominal center and the resistance.

Energy Orbit:

- **Isolated Connection:** Visualize the counter-action before engaging in the action. *Counter-action:* Cycle energy up the upper back, posterior shoulders, and triceps past elbows, forearms, and hands. *Action:* Orbit energy through biceps and anterior shoulders, and down the chest and upper abdominals.
- **Unified Connection:** *Counter-action:* Extend a symmetrical energy orbit down the lower back and posterior legs. *Action:* Orbit energy up the anterior legs and lower abdominals. Energize all eight energy orbits of the pattern through the dan tien. This step adjoins active and counter-active energies associated with the whole body in support of the biceps' isolated connection.

Active Meditation—Pulling Desirables Inward:

- Experience how your abdominals support your inner alignment while concurrently connecting your biceps outwardly with resistance. Acknowledge supporting your inward independence and outward interdependence simultaneously. Connect to the world from a truthful sense of self and a genuine motive to bond with another.
- Guided meditation: I connect authentically with life.

Seated Biceps Curl with Outward Rotation

Dumbbells

Starting Position:

- Sit back on a slight decline with feet on foot pegs or flat on floor.
- Hold dumbbells with arms rotated laterally at shoulders and palms facing slightly outward.
- Place backs of arms on or toward outer edge of bench.
- Connect to abdominal center. Relax weight of arms, shoulders, and outside resistance down through shoulder blades.
- Commit to the open space between chest and anterior shoulders.

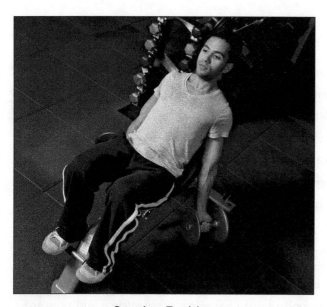

Starting Position

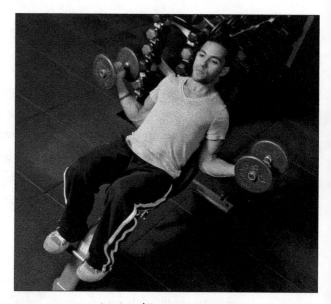

Action/Counter-action

Counter-action:

- Inhale: Visualize energy expanding from posterior dan tien through shoulders' width, passing down through elbows and under resistance.
- Exhale: Stabilize upper arm against or near bench edge to lengthen triceps. Relax head back against seat back as you encourage elbows to bend and maintain shoulder blade position.
- Inhale: Keep length of triceps under resistance as forearms return to starting position. Repeat.
- Be mindful to keep the shoulder placement unchanged throughout curl.

Action:

- Inhale: Establish the connection point between biceps muscles and resistance.
- Exhale: Contract biceps muscles to pull resistance through circular trajectory. Visualize energy drawn inward through anterior body—biceps, shoulders, chest, and abdominals—gathering energy in dan tien. (Curl is turned outward to the degree shoulders comfortably rotate outward.)

- Inhale: Carry resistance back to starting position using biceps. Repeat.
- Concentrate on shoulder blades sitting quietly behind breasts.

Energy Orbit:

- **Isolated Connection:** Visualize the counter-action before engaging in the action. *Counter-action:* Cycle energy up the upper back, posterior shoulders, and triceps past elbows, forearms, and hands. *Action:* Orbit energy through biceps and anterior shoulders, and down chest and upper abdominals.
- **Unified Connection:** *Counter-action:* Extend a symmetrical energy orbit down the lower back and posterior legs. *Action:* Orbit energy up the anterior legs and lower abdominals. Energize all eight energy orbits of the pattern through the dan tien. This step adjoins active and counter-active energies associated with the whole body in support of the biceps' isolated connection.

Active Meditation—Pulling Desirables Inward:

- Notice how challenging it is for the shoulders not to shadow the heart when pulling a weight inward. Experience heartfelt connection with the desirable, then allow your heart to expand so sincerely that the shoulders' defensive grip spreads effortlessly away from the heart. Pull your desirable into an open heart.
- Guided meditation: I celebrate the love in my life.

Crucifixion Curl

Double Pulley

Starting Position:

- Stand between opposing pulleys with feet hips' width apart and knees slightly bent.
- Hold pulley handles with arms extended sideways on coronal plane, palms facing up.
- Connect to abdominal center. Allow weight to draw arms away from shoulders to widen both chest and back.
- Commit to your torso's width and elbows' wide position in space.

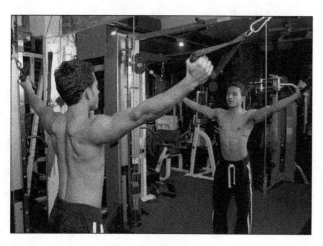

Starting Position

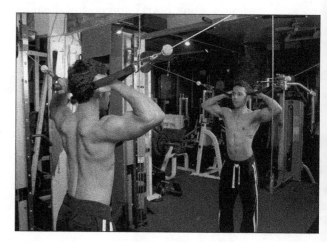

Action/Counter-action

Counter-action:

- Inhale: Visualize energy expanding outward from posterior dan tien through armpits, passing through elbows, wrists, and handles.
- Exhale: Direct back's width through triceps' length by releasing the triceps. Encourage elbows to bend and feel back's width connected to abdominals' support.
- Inhale: Keep length of triceps, elbow, wrist, and hand under the resistance as forearms return to starting position. Repeat.
- Be mindful to keep chest and back equally wide.

Action:

- Inhale: Establish the connection point between biceps' muscles and resistance.
- Exhale: Contract biceps' muscles to pull resistance through circular trajectory. Visualize energy drawn inward through anterior body—biceps, shoulders, chest, and abdominal center—gathering energy in dan tien.
- Inhale: Carry resistance back to starting position using biceps. Repeat.
- Concentrate on pulling the resistance in without pulling the elbows in.

Energy Orbit:

- **Isolated Connection:** Visualize the counter-action before engaging in the action. *Counter-action:* Cycle energy up the upper back, posterior shoulders, and triceps past elbows, forearms, and hands. *Action:* Orbit energy through biceps and anterior shoulders, and down chest and upper abdominals.
- **Unified Connection:** *Counter-action:* Extend a symmetrical energy orbit down the lower back and posterior legs. *Action:* Orbit energy up the anterior legs and lower abdominals. Energize all eight energy orbits of the pattern through the dan tien. This adjoins active and counter-active energies associated with the whole body in support of the biceps' isolated connection.

Active Meditation—Pulling Desirables Inward:

- Notice how narrow your torso becomes if the elbows drop. Feel your elbows' width give your back freedom to fully spread and experience your desirability expand to its full size and potential. As you connect to what you desire, believe in your potential to attain, achieve, and acquire it by way of your own appeal.
- Guided meditation: I am desirable.

BodyLogos Psyche-Muscular Observations for Biceps Muscles

Here are examples of how to interpret mind-body expressions.

Enjoyment: Biceps muscles are more superficial than the torso muscles. They are closer in proximity to the outside resistance held in hand. Hence, they tend to have the quickest reaction to any physical challenge.

🛑 Stop if you feel unenthusiastic, bored, or lackadaisical when working the biceps muscles. This condition implies that you don't want to pull anything toward you. Perhaps your life feels full enough, and the idea of inviting anything else in just causes stress. Or perhaps it feels time to clear room for new things to unfold.

🌀 Sometimes you are unaware of being so weighted down, but this response to an outside challenge confirms that you are overwhelmed. Your body is telling you to slow down, let go, or minimize your involvement outwardly. Work light and slow. Focus your meditation on the counter-actions—the triceps' release of stimuli in regard to pulling desirables inward. This is a time for maintaining or letting go rather than building.

🌀 On the other hand, when your biceps muscles are charged up and vigorously connecting with an outside resistance, they show an enthusiasm to create or develop something in your life. Your body is telling you that you are ready. Visualize the seed, the journey, or the outcome of creating your life. As you experience it fully, feel your workout motivating your life. As your biceps gain strength, so will your vision.

Posture: If your torso collapses downward when the biceps pull resistance upward, you are bringing the body toward the outside resistance rather than bringing the outside resistance to you.

🛑 Stop when you find the chest is collapsing to meet the resistance in a biceps curl. Recognize that you are shadowing your heart to pull desirables inward. This indicates a tendency to sacrifice yourself when pulling desirables into your life.

🌀 Maintain the openhearted chest placement of your starting position throughout the exercise. As your biceps muscles connect with the resistance, stay true to the connection point and feel your personal outside resistance—desirables you have yet to gain or assimilate—coming to you. Give yourself the experience of receiving what you desire.

Size: Swinging the arm in a biceps movement will create an outward momentum that takes the challenge out of the biceps muscles.

STOP Stop allowing the elbows to rock back and forth as you carry the resistance up and down. This situation indicates an unwillingness to control your relationship with the resistance—your desirable. You are essentially allowing the desirable to control you.

Stabilize the elbows by lengthening the triceps at the same rate of speed that the biceps contract. Once your movement is stable, experience the calm that accompanies self-control. Visualize yourself exactly where you want to be in relationship to your desirable.

Meet the Models

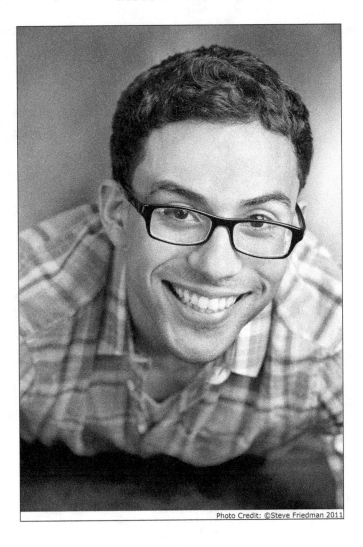

Photo Credit: ©Steve Friedman 2011

Michael Polanco

    A Dominican comedian, actor, and writer who has a love for personal training, Michael feels strength training has given his life an area where he has control, yet it also sheds light on the areas where he feels powerless. As a boy of thirteen, he decided that growing a mustache and "pecs" would attract more girls. As a grown man, he says, "Strength training puts me in a trance, a state of mental quietude, where all that I am aware of is my body and spirit; it gives me a drive to grow in my workouts and as a human being." The meditative aspect of strength training relaxes the unrelenting forward-leaning drive that he expressed. He lands in the present moment where he feels reintroduced to himself with each exercise. "My workouts help me learn about who I am and help to maneuver me through the obstacles of life."

Coming Home Energy Pattern as It Relates to the Shoulder Muscles

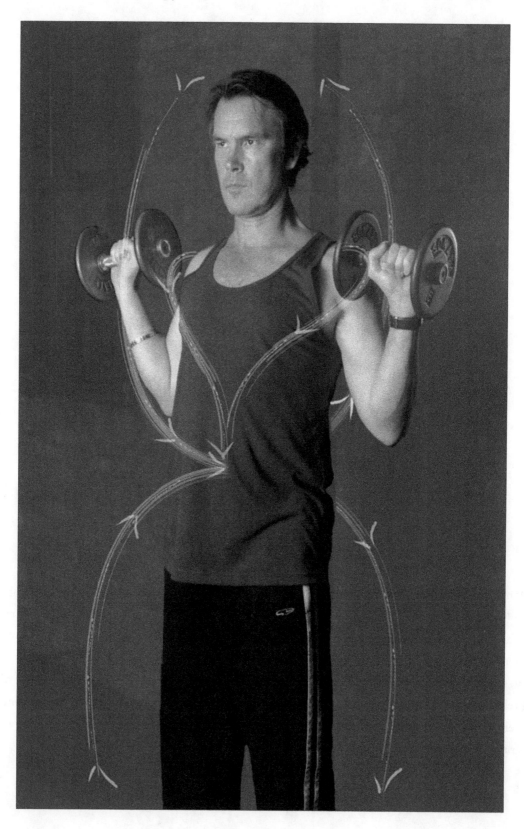

Visualize this energy pattern supporting all shoulder isolations.

Introduction to Shoulder Muscles

Theory of Yin and Yang

Yang: Active Muscle Group

Shoulder Muscles:
- o   Deltoid
- o   Supraspinatus
- o   Infraspinatus
- o   Subscapularis
- o   Teres Minor

Yin: Counter-active Muscle Group

Shoulder Muscles:
- o   Deltoid
- o   Supraspinatus
- o   Infraspinatus
- o   Subscapularis
- o   Teres Minor

The relief of a sigh is due to the added space created in both the mind and body. When you inhale, you expand all sides of the rib cage simultaneously and release physical tension. When you exhale, you release mental stress. Shoulder exercises create the same spaciousness. The outward posterior width (counter-action) balanced with the inward anterior stability (action) positions the shoulders on the coronal plane as the widest aspect of your skeletal frame. Essential alignment supports the shoulders' skeletal symmetry, while muscular balance dictates their expanse. Be your full size, commit to the shoulders resting on the coronal plane, and create the widest possible space between and within the shoulder joints.

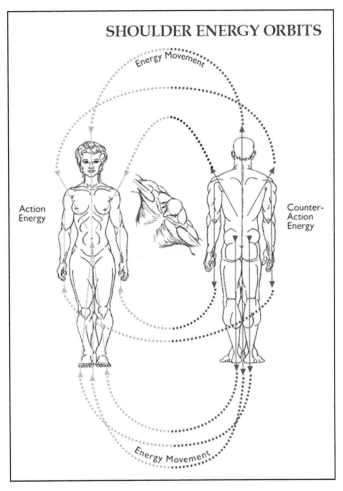

Action: Morals and Values

As your shoulder muscles connect with the world, you expand your sense of self. The more challenged you are outwardly, the more connected you need to be inwardly. Recognize what your beliefs are and how these beliefs have shaped what you value in life. Explore the moral guide from which you operate. Experience your posture and how it presents you to the world. How are you involved with and engaged in giving life to your beliefs? What you value in the world lives through you; its very existence is acknowledged and supported through your conscious or unconscious attention. Notice your sense of value being reinforced when you clearly feel what you are supporting and recognize your own confusion when your sense of value is feeling compromised.

Counter-action: Morals and Values

When contracting the shoulder muscles, you can also meditate on their expanding counter-action. Because shoulder muscles live on the coronal plane and encompass anterior, coronal, and posterior planes, they oppose each other. While their action is felt as an outward reach through the external aspect of the muscle, a meditative focus on how your values shape your life, their counter-action is the underlying inward stabilizer of the muscle that preserves the joint, a focus on how your values shape your beliefs. Your shoulder workout's counter-action meditation is a time to reflect on the morals and values being highlighted and tested in your present life. Orient and reorient your moral standards until you feel they align you peacefully with your life's challenges. Review who you are each day and allow your stance to change as you change. As your sense of center broadens out through your shoulder muscles' width, feel fully engaged by your deliberate internal stance. Feel your sense of value—not by a choice you have made but by the development of choices made through time. Experience your value as a developing reverence of self, other, and spirit.

Five-Element Theory
Summer, Pounding Joint, Joy

Connection: Summer

Like the long, sunny days of summer, the shoulders' unparalleled flexible width offers a lot of perspective with which you can clearly see yourself. Just as the shoulder's width presents the integrity of your posture to the outside world, its placement also illustrates the degree of integrity you enforce within yourself. Your shoulders' carriage shapes your body's stature just as standing by your morals and values shapes your life's status. Feel your shoulders' optimal position before connecting with a resistance. Recognize any physical adjustments needed to uphold this alignment as your amendments to uphold your personal integrity. Concentrate on preserving your shoulders' alignment with gentle insistence, as if their placement is what you value most in life. Gentle perseverance cultivates integrity, but demanding instant perfection fosters resentment and the progression of a holding pattern.

Strength: Pounding Joint

This pounding fire joint is freely mobile in almost every direction. This freedom offers movement in a myriad of ways, but with freedom comes personal responsibility. The extreme flexibility of shoulder joints comes with a price—great potential for injury. To heed this concern, connect your shoulder muscles to the outside resistance and connect the outside resistance to your abdominal center before you move. Gradually engage the shoulder muscles while paying attention to your abdominals' commitment to the resistance. Don't focus on the movement's destination. Be resolved in containing the challenge within a stable range of motion. This is not only safe—it's owning your personal responsibility. Feel the integrity of standing by your strengths and your limitations.

Meditation: Joy

Nothing generates more joy than freedom of movement. The shoulders deliver an incomparable free range of motion, yet a balanced connection with resistance needs to stabilize the joy of movement safely. Balance is preserved by the shoulders' counter-action matching your shoulders' action. If you find your joy turning to judgment or grandiosity, the balance between your counter-action and action is unbalanced. The uniqueness of the shoulder muscles is that action and counter-action coexist within the same muscle group. This is possible because the shoulders are multifunctional—providing extension, abduction, flexion, and medial and lateral rotation. Be mindful that the outward broadening of the shoulders expands from an inward connection with your dan tien, whereby multiple viewpoints are needed to be stable.

How to Isolate the Shoulder Muscles

Feel It Contract

In movement, attention can often be fixed on the destination rather than on where you are now. After all, the destination of any effort is where we collect admiration and praise. By using a reduced fixed outside resistance, you can recognize the opposing forces that broaden the shoulder muscles across the coronal plane and remove the distraction of a destination altogether. This approach connects you to the quieter inner life force—your spirit self—for recognition and awakens an inner source of admiration and praise for a new and personal sense of value.

Door Breaker Exercise

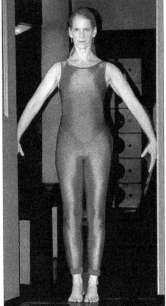

Exercise: Standing in a doorway with feet shoulder width apart and knees slightly bent, place the backs of your hands and wrists against the doorframe. Using the shoulder muscles, press against the doorframe with 75 percent muscle intensity. Hold this intensity for sixty seconds, being sure to keep your shoulders dropped and arms relatively passive. Distinguish between a desired isolated contraction that expands the shoulders and an over-asserted, antagonistic contraction that narrows and lifts the shoulders. When you have completed the time allotment, step out of the doorframe and relax the arms and shoulder muscles. Notice the weightlessness of your arms. They may even float up through the coronal plane with no effort or intention.

Feel It Release

The inclination to lift your shoulders toward your ears (a.k.a. to carry the weight of the world on your shoulders) adds tension in both the superior and posterior shoulder muscles. Deliberately rolling the shoulders forward disengages the defensive stance that keeps them desperately safeguarding and allows a calm restructuring.

Shoulder Blade Hug

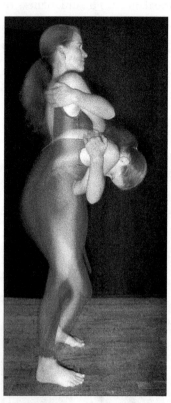

Exercise: Stand with your feet shoulder width apart and knees slightly bent. Wrap arms across the front of your body and grab opposite shoulders or shoulder blades. Take a deep breath. Release through your exhale by first rolling the nose toward the chest, then relaxing the tops of the shoulders forward and down, then directing the elbows to the bellybutton. Hold the stretch for another two to three deep breaths. Continue to relax the superior shoulders and neck as the posterior shoulders and upper back begin to roll up by dropping through the shoulder blades. As the spine and neck realign, the superior shoulders and arms drop down at your sides. Experience the chest's lift as prominent and the shoulder's width as natural.

Feel It Fatigue

Shoulders resist acting on their own and being their full size. The back and arm muscles are their favorite cohorts, and momentum is their favorite vice to employ to help in a challenge. Work with a reasonable weight the shoulders can manage solo and allow them to find their independence. As they resist, attempt, and ultimately succeed in working independently, you will witness how much courage it takes to be your own person.

Shoulder Exercises

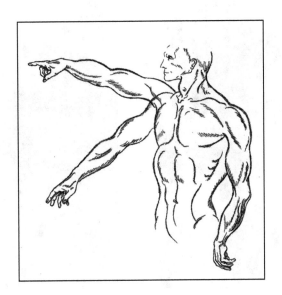

**Shoulder Muscles
Embody
Morals and Values**

Standing Side Lateral Raise

Dumbbells

Starting Position:

- Stand with feet hips' width apart, knees slightly bent, weight on the gushing spring points, and heel stirrups relaxed into the floor.
- Hold dumbbells at sides with backs of elbows rotated slightly outward.
- Commit to dropping tops of shoulders down through shoulder blades.

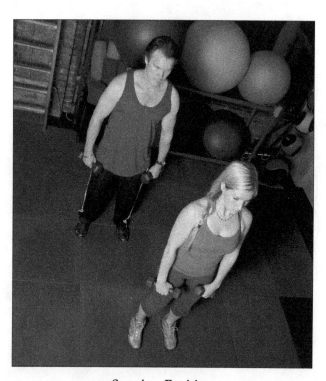

Starting Position

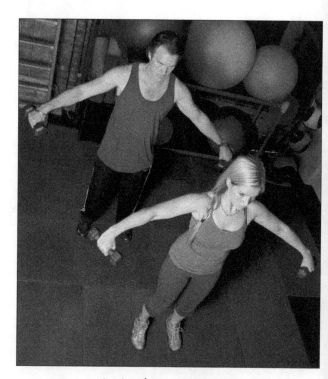

Action/Counter-action

Counter-action:

- Inhale: Lengthen energy from posterior dan tien up through torso, neck, and head as well as down through lower back and posterior legs.
- Exhale: Keep arms elongated sideways as they are raised laterally to nipple line. Energy travels from the narrow posterior waistline through a wide shoulder frame and posterior arms.
- Inhale: Maintain shoulder width and arm length as arms are returned to starting position. Repeat.
- Be mindful to expand posterior waistline energetically through transverse plumb line.

Action:

- Inhale: Visualize energy traveling up through lower abdominals as well as down through upper abdominals to establish a stable core.

- Exhale: Contract outer shoulders, pushing resistance laterally away from body to nipple line while pulling energy into your abdominal center. Movement travels out, not up.
- Inhale: Carry resistance back to starting position using outer shoulders. Repeat.
- Concentrate on elbows and wrists traveling outward with the same intensity as the outer shoulders.

Energy Orbit:

- **Isolated Connection.** Visualize the counter-action before engaging in the action. Counter-action: Cycle energy up the upper back, posterior shoulders, and triceps. Action: Orbit energy in through the biceps and anterior shoulders, and down chest and upper abdominals.
- **Unified Connection.** Counter-action: Extend a symmetrical energy orbit down the lower back and posterior legs. Action: Orbit energy up anterior legs and low abdominals. Energize all eight energy orbits of the pattern through the dan tien. This step adjoins active and counter-active energies associated with the whole body in support of a shoulder-isolated connection.

Active Meditation—Morals and Value:

- Notice how throwing the movement from your hands or weight can throw the torso backward, shortening the posterior waistline. Focus on leaning into your abdominal strength and steering the heel of your hands into the weight and through the coronal plane to keep the shoulders connected to the resistance. Allow the movement to pass through the often-weaker lateral aspect of the shoulders and experience their limited strength.
- Guided meditation: I appreciate having limitations.

Standing Anterior Lateral Raise

Dumbbells

Starting Position:

- Stand with feet hips' width apart, knees slightly bent, weight on gushing spring points, and heel stirrups relaxed into floor.
- Hold dumbbells in hammerhead grip against fronts of thighs, with folds of elbows rotated forward.
- Commit to weight staying forward on balls of feet while the heels stay grounded firmly into floor.

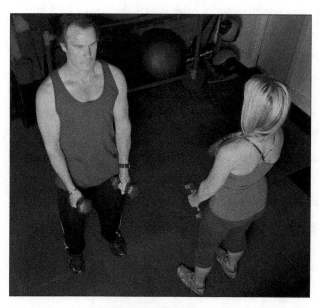
Starting Position

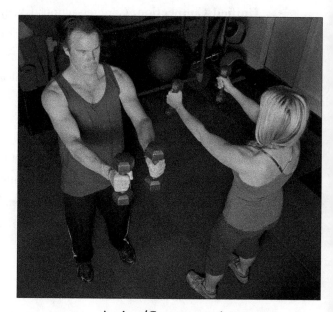
Action/Counter-action

Counter-action:

- Inhale: Lengthen energy from posterior dan tien up through torso, neck, and head as well as down through lower back and posterior legs.
- Exhale: Feel energy travel through a wide shoulder frame and down backs of arms to scoop under resistance while anterior shoulders and chest stay energetically connected to abdominals.
- Inhale: Keep shoulder blades stable as arms are returned to starting position. Repeat.
- Be mindful to stay as connected to the ground through your feet as you are connected to the resistance through the shoulders.

Action:

- Inhale: Visualize energy traveling up through the lower abdominals as well as down through upper abdominals to establish a stable core.
- Exhale: Contract anterior shoulders to push resistance away from the body to nose level, independent of the chest, while pulling energy into your abdominal center.

- Inhale: Carry resistance back to starting position using anterior shoulders. Repeat.
- Concentrate on keeping folds of elbows forward throughout movement.

Energy Orbit:

- **Isolated Connection.** Visualize the counter-action before engaging in the action. Counter-action: Cycle energy up the upper back, posterior shoulders, and triceps. Action: Orbit energy in through the biceps and anterior shoulders, and down chest and upper abdominals.
- **Unified Connection.** Counter-action: Extend a symmetrical energy orbit down the lower back and posterior legs. Action: Orbit energy up anterior legs and lower abdominals. Energize all eight energy orbits of the pattern through the dan tien. This adjoins active and counter-active energies associated with the whole body in support of a shoulder-isolated connection.

Active Meditation—Morals and Value:

- Notice how the scooping quality of your counter-action places the anterior shoulder muscles under the resistance, separating them from the chest muscles. Sustain this separation throughout the movement so the holding patterns between chest (smile of truth) and shoulders (morals or values) can disengage. Recognize that what is true for you can be different from what another deems valuable for the world. Experience having a choice to connect with or disengage from a resistance.
- Guided meditation: My heart is connected yet liberated.

Standing Posterior Lateral Raise

Dumbbells

Starting Position:

- Stand with feet hips' width apart, knees slightly bent, weight on gushing spring points, and heel stirrups relaxed into floor.
- Bend at hips, maintaining a neutral waistline; allow arms to hang over shoelaces from shoulder joints.
- Hold dumbbells with palms facing legs.
- Commit to a long, quiet waistline and square shoulders. No rounding of the back.

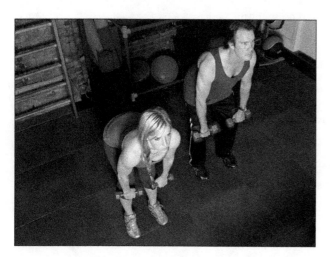
Starting Position

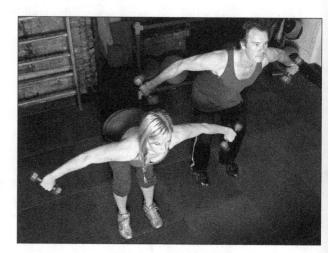
Action/Counter-action

Counter-action:

- Inhale: Lengthen energy from posterior dan tien forward through torso, neck, and head as well as back through lower back and tailbone.
- Exhale: Arms travel symmetrically outward. Feel energy travel from a wide shoulder frame through posterior arms and under resistance. Maintain opposition between head and tailbone throughout movement.
- Inhale: Keeping weight forward on gushing spring points, return arms to starting position. Repeat.
- Be mindful to keep shoulders wider than the back and the chest.

Action:

- Inhale: Experience energy convening in abdominal center.
- Exhale: Push resistance outward from body using the posterior shoulders while pulling energy into your abdominal center. As arms reach shoulder height, descend energy through lower back and posterior legs to keep position grounded.
- Inhale: Carry resistance back to starting position using posterior shoulders. Repeat.
- Concentrate on creating as much added width across shoulders as added length along spine.

Energy Orbit:

- **Isolated Connection.** Visualize the counter-action before engaging in the action. Counter-action: Cycle energy up the upper back, posterior shoulders, and triceps. Action: Orbit energy in through the biceps and anterior shoulders, and down chest and upper abdominals.
- **Unified Connection:** Counter-action: Extend a symmetrical energy orbit down the lower back and posterior legs. Action: Orbit energy up anterior legs and low abdominals. Energize all eight energy orbits of the pattern through the dan tien. This step adjoins active and counter-active energies associated with the whole body in support of a shoulder-isolated connection.

Active Meditation—Morals and Values:

- Notice that to create a greater degree of width in your shoulder frame, a greater degree of abdominal strength is needed. Appreciate your sense of value extending from your sense of self, with this connection with self having greater significance than your connection with the outside resistance.
- Guided meditation: My value is in my being.

Seated Overhead Press

Dyna-Band and Machine

Starting Position:

- Sit with feet flat on floor and body weight settled over million-dollar point. Relax upper back muscles into seat back if using a machine.
- Hold resistance on coronal plane outside shoulders and align bent elbows beneath wrists. Commit to a heavy elbow position and straight wrists throughout the movement.

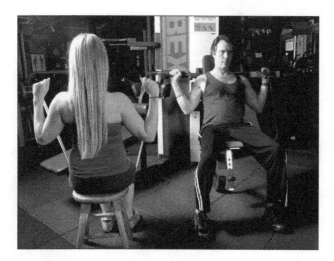
Starting Position

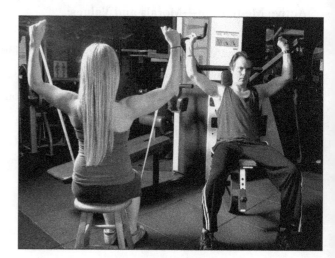
Action/Counter-action

Counter-action:

- Inhale: Lengthen energy from posterior dan tien up through torso, neck, and head as well as down through lower back and sitz bones.
- Exhale: As arms extend overhead, keep elbows slightly bent and, as elbows pass shoulder height, shoulder blades dropped. Feel energy travel from shoulder frame out through elbows, as if elbows were an extension of your back's width.
- Inhale: Keep elbows aligned under wrists as arms return to starting position. Repeat.
- Be mindful to keep elbows, shoulder blades, and sitz bones heavy throughout movement.

Action:

- Inhale: Visualize energy traveling up through low abdominals and down through upper abdominals to establish a stable core.
- Exhale: Push resistance overhead, using lateral shoulders without locking elbows. Maintain a neutral spine while drawing energy into your abdominal center.
- Inhale: Use lateral shoulders to carry resistance back to starting position. Repeat.
- Concentrate on arms and spine, aligning on same angle (in relation to machine or essential alignment).

Energy Orbit:

- **Isolated Connection.** Visualize the counter-action before engaging in the action. Counter-action: Cycle energy up the upper back, posterior shoulders, and triceps. Action: Orbit energy in through the biceps and anterior shoulders, and down chest and upper abdominals.
- **Unified Connection:** Counter-action: Extend a symmetrical energy orbit down the lower back and posterior legs. Action: Orbit energy up anterior legs and lower abdominals. Energize all eight energy orbits of the pattern through the dan tien. This adjoins active and counter-active energies associated with the whole body in support of a shoulder-isolated connection.

Active Meditation—Morals and Values:

- Notice how your arm's alignment can easily separate from your body's alignment. As you execute the rotation in the shoulder joints to align arms and torso on the same plane, experience yourself executing alliance between your values and what you choose in your life.
- Guided meditation: My life is aligned with my values.

Standing Overhead Press

Dumbbells

Starting Position:

- Stand with feet hips' width apart, knees slightly bent, weight on gushing spring points, and heel stirrups relaxed into floor.
- Hold resistance on coronal plane outside shoulders and align bent elbows beneath wrists.
- Commit to connecting your abdominal support with the outside resistance.

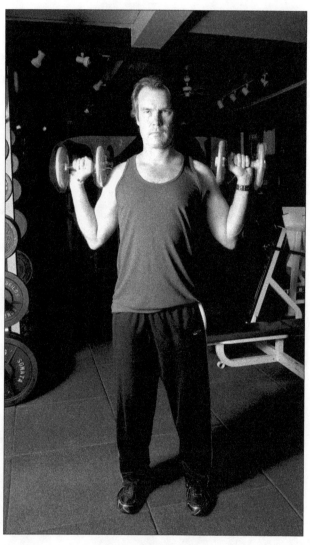

Starting Position

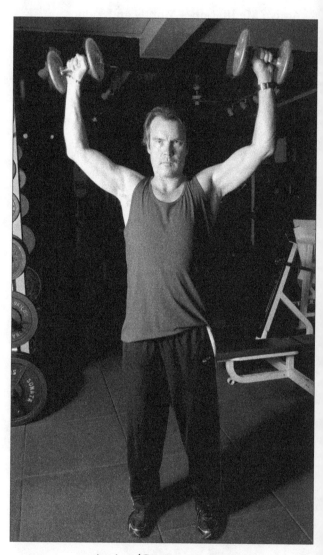

Action/Counter-action

Counter-action:

- Inhale; Lengthen energy from posterior dan tien up through torso, neck, and head as well as down through lower back and posterior legs.

- Exhale: Ground through feet as arms extend overhead with the same degree of force. Feel energy travel from armpits out through widened elbows as if elbows were an extension of the back's width.
- Inhale: Staying connected to your abdominal support and maintaining elbow alignment under wrists, return arms to starting position. Repeat.
- Be mindful to balance the drop of your lower back with the upward expansion of the upper back.

Action:

- Inhale: Visualize energy traveling up through lower abdominals as well as down through upper abdominals to establish a stable core.
- Exhale: Push resistance overhead using lateral shoulders without locking elbows. While pushing the weight away, draw energy into your abdominal center to manage your balance.
- Inhale: Use lateral shoulders to carry resistance back to the starting position. Repeat.
- Concentrate on the abdominals' strength and energetic force, giving vertebrae enough support to stay elongated.

Energy Orbit:

- **Isolated Connection.** Visualize the counter-action before engaging in the action. Counter-action: Cycle energy up the upper back, posterior shoulders, and triceps. Action: Orbit energy in through the biceps and anterior shoulders, and down chest and upper abdominals.
- **Unified Connection:** Counter-action: Extend a symmetrical energy orbit down the lower back and posterior legs. Action: Orbit energy up anterior legs and lower abdominals. Energize all eight energy orbits of the pattern through the dan tien. This step adjoins active and counter-active energies associated with the whole body in support of a shoulder-isolated connection.

Active Meditation—Morals and Values:

- Notice how the tailbone can tuck under, involving the lower back when one is in a standing position. This illustrates a lack of confidence in your abdominal support, transforming your relaxed support into artillery overdrive. Allow the abdominals to support you as you connect to outside resistance. Feel inward support and outward connection simultaneously.
- Guided meditation: I connect with authentic authority to what is happening in each moment.

BodyLogos Psyche-Muscular Observations for Shoulder Muscles

Here are examples of how to interpret mind-body expressions.

Size: Due to the tremendous skeletal range of motion in the shoulder joints, it is critical to recognize the joints' muscular complexity and their various directions and functions to ensure a challenge is executed properly.

🛑 When your action pushes the outside resistance beyond the designated point of return, you are then popping the challenge out of the intended muscle into another muscle. This tendency to bring in more muscle artillery illustrates a need to prove your value or the feeling that you should be better than you actually are.

🌀 To control range of motion, you need to stay connected to the weaker aspects of the shoulder muscle group. As you begin to depend on the quiet reserve of the smaller, weaker muscles more—and the dominance in the larger stronger muscles less—you will begin to experience a sense of inherent value and an air of competence. As you harness your movement to stay within the designated range, meditate on the value of less. Valuing less as more enables you to recognize when you are reaching away from yourself for outside approval. At the heart of all shoulder movements is the want for personal integrity.

Posture: Maintaining a symmetrical stance that supports balanced muscular development ensures independent strength in each shoulder and recognizes the importance of balanced strength in yin (left) and yang (right) aspects of the self.

🛑 An imbalanced shoulder action will cause one shoulder to lift upward toward the ear while the other remains properly dropped downward through the shoulder blade. This condition signifies that the lifted side is trying to dominate the movement, while the dropped side is more relaxed with the movement. Dominating with the left side—yin—implies an inward, dark, passive principle is asserting itself, one that is more connected to your relationship with yourself. Dominating with the right side—yang—implies an outward, light, active principle is asserting itself, one that is more connected to your relationship with the outside world.

🌀 Stabilize using the mirror as a reference. Press slowly into your outside resistance with equal intensity from the right and left shoulders. Only go as high as your shoulders can stay square. While you balance the symmetry of your shoulders' stance, meditate on balancing the yin and yang principles within yourself and balance your attention between your inside world and outside world. And experience your shoulders' action being kept in check by way of their dualistic counter-action.

Ability: There are some muscles that seem like they don't exist. It's as if other muscles have done the work for so long that you don't recognize them anymore.

🛑 The trapezius muscle in the upper shoulders can be an over-controlling muscle. For some people, this problem is so severe that they don't experience their deltoid muscles—outer shoulders—any longer. If you experience the shoulders lifting upward at the start of every shoulder exercise, your trapezius muscle is initiating the movement rather than the desired deltoid muscles. The trapezius muscles are brought into action only after the movement extends the elbows above the chest's nipple line. When you are unable to experience the deltoid muscles, this indicates you are unable to experience your full width and worth.

🌀 Stabilize before starting a shoulder movement. Totally relax the weight of your arms and shoulder blades downward until you feel a slight stretch in the upper shoulders, the trapezius. Limit your arm's range of motion as you drag your elbows outward, never upward. Let the weight of your shoulder blades continue to drop your shoulders down as your arms travel through the exercise's range. Experience the weaker part of your shoulders. Meditate on giving the vulnerability of weakness a sense of belonging within you.

Meet the Models

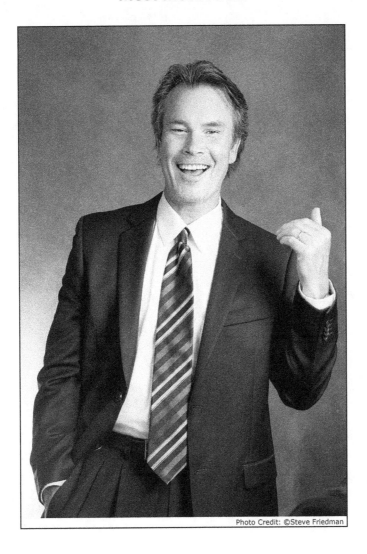

Photo Credit: ©Steve Friedman

Sean O'Connor

As a half-Irish, half-French boy, Sean started pumping iron in the fifth grade for two basic reasons. One was to defend himself against the New Jersey greasers, all Irish and Italian, who would cross his path on the way home from basketball practice and school dances. And two, he desired to knock long, glorious home runs out of his Little League ball park. He wasn't very successful at either, but strength training has remained a lifelong practice. Now, a fifty-eight-year-old award-winning and much-published playwright, screenwriter, and actor, Sean continues to use the gym to release troubling emotions and stay focused on his ambitions. In addition to sitting for two five-minute breathing meditations a day, Sean finds that "strength training is an active meditation that leaves [him] strong, vigorous, confident, and relaxed." And with his rather provocative grin, he adds, "It enlivens my cells."

Lesson 9

Determined Power Energy Pattern: Back, Triceps

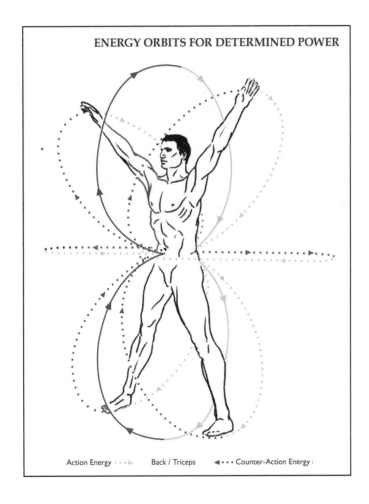

A downward force through the posterior body is what propels your body upward. Propelled from behind, like a bird springing into flight, this power is motivated by what feels like angel wings. This is the feeling of determined power.

Maintain essential alignment and direct the energy orbit of a breaststroke, and you will experience determined power. When you draw the shoulder blades downward and ground your lower back through your sitz bones and feet, you place your action behind you. This creates a clear path upward through the anterior body for focused attention on the task in front of you. Pulling your body's weight up off the floor or closing a jammed window employs this energy orbit, and it is how you remedy a forward shoulder slump.

Determined Power—Standing Ponder and Active Meditation
mindthebody.bodylogos.com/video12
(abbreviated description)

To get a feeling sense of determined power, stand with feet hips' width apart and knees slightly bent. Clasp hands together behind you with straight arms and locked elbows. This step will draw the shoulder blades together and drop them symmetrically down the back. Take a few deep breaths and allow the chest to rise. Experience your tension dropping behind you and your dan tien's life force effortlessly floating up in front of you. When your back muscles narrow, your chest muscles widen, supporting an expanded heart center. This broad, forward-opening stance enables you to distinguish the weight of your situation from a heartfelt perspective and discover your present viewpoint without distractions.

Back and triceps muscles use the determined power energy pattern. They both draw your posterior force down to the ground, then propel your anterior force up off the ground. This dynamic opposition between anterior and posterior planes bypasses the judgments held in the shoulders, freeing your heart energy and propelling it upward. Back exercises assume responsibility for keeping the heart uplifted, and triceps exercises push away what the heart deems insurmountable. This clears a path for you to connect sincerely as you move forward. As determined power descends energy down the entire posterior body and orbits it up the anterior body, you literally embody a smile. This gives rise to your chest, your smile of truth. This feeds your heart directly from your dan tien's central energy—spirit self—offering a poised grace as you connect with your life.

The Art of Strength

Practice Change

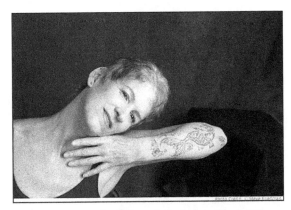

Henna tattoo of a fish swimming in fresh **Water**

Like **Water**,
Find power in flow.
When does a subtle flow
Give you the greatest support?
When does assertive force
Shape grace?

Determined Power
Is knowing when to assert yourself and
When to support yourself.
Be deliberate with your energy.
Preserve your life force.

Determined Power Energy Pattern as It Relates to the Back Muscles

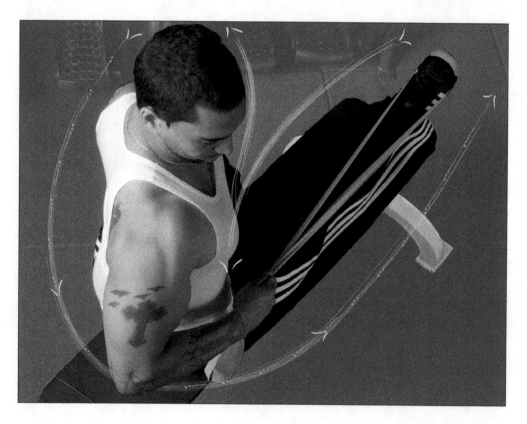

Visualize this energy pattern supporting all back isolations.

Introduction to Back Muscles

Theory of Yin and Yang

Yang: Active Muscle Group

Back Muscles:
- o Latissimus Dorsi
- o Teres Major
- o Rhomboids
- o Trapezius

Yin: Counter-active Muscle Group

Chest Muscles:
- o Pectoralis Major
- o Pectoralis Minor
- o Serratus Anterior

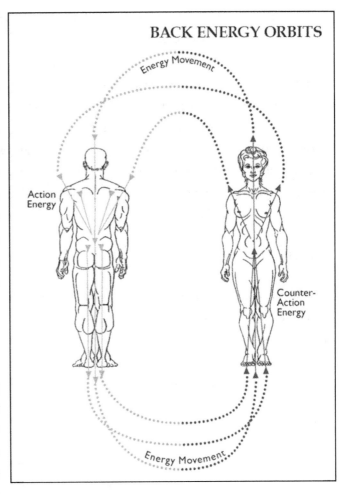

It can feel as if you're pulling your body out of the dregs of the earth to lift your body's weight up through gravity's force. A downward force through the back of the body elevates an equal upward force through the front of the body. An isolated pull from the back muscles (action), causes the chest muscles (counter-action) to lift toward the heavens. The back, it could be said, is working for the sake of the chest's lift and the heart center's openness. Commit to keeping the downward influence of the back's force connected to, and balanced with, the chest's ability to lift and open. Without this balance, the protective nature of the back becomes aggressive and disconnected from the heart.

Action: Protection

Your back muscles are like a shield protecting you from the aggressions of your inner or outer world. Your back's workout meditation can reconnect you with your courage and help you to face your fears or stand your ground. Explore what you need for a sense of safekeeping. Feel the strength and stature of your back's musculature. Experience it as both your ability to take care of yourself and to protect those you love. The degree to which you present your heart to the world is the degree in which you feel safe enough to do so. Notice the safe haven generated in heart by giving the back a deliberate course of action. When you feel safe within your self, you begin to experience greater freedom and safety in the world.

Counter-action: Smile of Truth

When contracting the back muscles, you can also meditate on expanding the counter-action of your chest muscles. Enjoy the opportunity to open your heart while in the care of your back's protection. Experience the delight of your heart's opening being as commanding as your back's protective eagerness. Notice the sense of devotion that swells up through the chest muscles in response to the back muscles' commitment to their needs, your needs. Feel your dreams emerging into the world and your happiness emerging into your dreams as a result of this cooperative, respectful, and loving internal relationship.

Five-Element Theory
Winter, Drilling Joints, Fear

Connection: Winter

The desire to hibernate in winter mimics the tendency your chest or heart has, which is to stay tucked in the safe shelter of the back's musculature. The back protects many vital organs byway of blocking the aggressions of the outside world, and the heart's well-being is its top priority. Feeling threatened causes an aggressive expansion in the back, not a contraction, showing off the back's muscular size rather than using its muscular strength—as in an animal's first line of defense in expanding its fur, gills, or quills. While this is initially useful for protection, the back's powerful command is lost when locked in an expansion that exceeds your true size. Without the powerful yang nature of the back muscles' freedom to fully contract, the chest muscles become cautious and hesitant to expand. Rather than the chest muscles and heart energy being free to stretch beyond their comfort zones and connect outwardly, they collapse inwardly and feel only the body's need to defend. When approaching a back exercise, concentrate on the internal relationship between the back and chest as the yang power that gives rise to your more vulnerable heartfelt yin nature.

Strength: Drilling Joints

The gliding nature of the shoulder blades is the primary bone mobility in any back exercise. When the back muscles lead in the dance with your chest, the shoulder blades glide together and apart. This motion causes the sternum to swell within the chest. The descending energy through the posterior body makes it possible for the chest to rise and move freely. Be resolved in employing the masculinity of the back without overshadowing your more feminine purpose of heart.

Meditation: Fear

Giving the back its full potential in range of motion and strength means giving the chest what it needs to feel empowered. If there is tension around the emotional vulnerability of the heart, this tension prevents the chest muscles from freely lifting, causing the back muscles to remain spread in a spastic-like defensive stance. At its worst, this renders the back muscles inoperative. It is imperative that the back and chest muscles operate as a team. This means the chest muscles realize the back muscles are right behind them as they courageously expand out of the safe but imprisoned security of the back cave. Only then can they connect to, and move with, outside resistance in a purposeful and commanding exploration. Be mindful of the dreams in your heart that ask the chest muscles to stretch and spur the back muscles to leap into purposeful action.

How to Isolate the Back Muscles

Feel It Contract

The back muscles need full articulation of the shoulder blades to properly isolate. The ability to glide the shoulder blades through a full range of motion, both inwardly and outwardly, prior to adding resistance gives you a reference point of the amount of range the muscle group has in the presence of a weighted challenge.

Shoulder Blade Grab Exercise

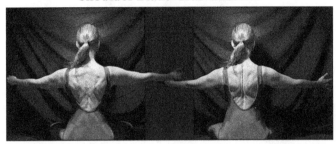

Exercise: Sit or stand with arms extended to the side. Pinch the shoulder blades together, keeping the arms relatively still. Then return to the expanded shoulder blade position. There is no need for the arms to travel backward or inward. Repeat this pattern until you feel clear about the range of motion and can successfully maintain symmetry between the right and left sides.

Feel It Release

Creating space between the shoulder blades releases residual tension that can collect in the middle back. Although most of us stand with a forward slouch (and overstretch the muscles between the shoulder blades), when you begin training and tightening up those foundational muscles, they can feel easily overtaxed and need a quick release.

Hollow Thigh Hug Stretch

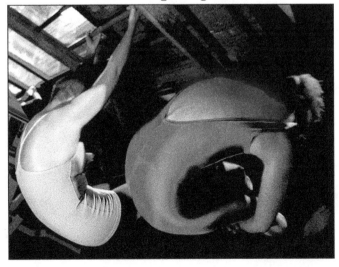

Exercise: Stand with feet shoulders' width apart, knees slightly bent, and body rolled forward over the waist. Hold hands behind the lower thigh or a stable bar in front of you. Contract the abdominal muscles, creating a

hollowed-out space between the thighs and abdomen. Expand the space between the shoulder blades as you exhale all tension out of the area. Explore changing the degree in which you bend the knees to find the back area that most needs the stretch. Hold it gently for five seconds or until you feel the muscles surrender. Repeat as needed.

Feel It Fatigue

The back muscles are very straightforward. They don't burn, scream, or holler when they are reaching muscle failure; they simply become unable to continue. At this point, it's more effective to rest and repeat the exercise. Don't transfer the challenge into your arms and shoulders.

Back Exercises

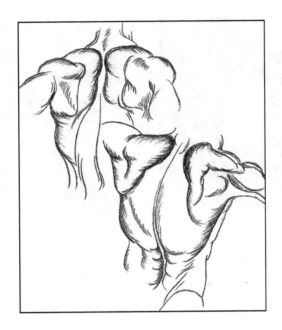

Back Muscles
Embody
Protection

Lat Pull Down

Pulley and Dyna-Band

Starting Position:

- Sit holding wide-grip handle of pulley or stand holding Dyna-Band overhead.
- Connect to dan tien and relax weight of skeleton through sitz bones and gushing spring points.
- Connect back muscles surrounding shoulder blades with outside resistance as you allow the back to fully expand outward.
- Commit to keeping upper back connected to the outside resistance while lower back remains quiet and grounded.

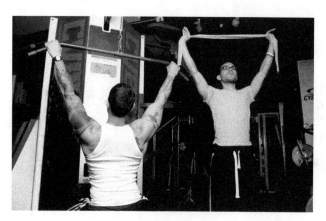

Starting Position

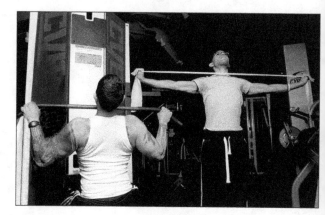

Action/Counter-action

Counter-action:

- Inhale: Visualize energy ascending from dan tien through abdominals and chest.
- Exhale: Lift sternum upward toward handle or Dyna-Band by allowing the head and neck to follow uplifting arch of upper spine.
- Inhale: Return chest and spine alignment to starting position. Repeat.
- Be mindful to keep your abdominals' upward force supporting your chest's expansion.

Action:

- Inhale: Connect back's width to outside resistance and relax shoulders.
- Exhale: Contract back muscles by drawing shoulder blades down and together, lowering handle or Dyna-Band toward chest. Visualize energy descending from shoulder blade channels through low back dimples and heel stirrups. (With a pulley handle, elbows will bend slightly to produce a full range of motion; with a Dyna-Band, elbows remain unchanged. Both approaches use shoulder blade movement to lead the range.)
- Inhale: Use the back muscles to carry outside resistance back to starting position by expanding the shoulder blades and elbows. Repeat.
- Concentrate on creating a curved coronal plane between back and chest muscles while maintaining a neutral spine through lower abdominals and lower back.

Energy Orbit:

- **Isolated Connection:** Visualize the counter-action before engaging in the action. Counter-action: Cycle energy up the chest from abdominal center. Action: Orbit energy down past the shoulders and shoulder blades to contract upper back.
- **Unified Connection:** Counter-action: Extend a corresponding energy orbit up the anterior legs and lower abdomen. Action: Orbit energy down the lower back and posterior legs. Energize all eight energy orbits of the pattern through the dan tien. This adjoins active and counter-active energies associated with the whole body in support of a back-isolated connection.

Active Meditation—Protection:

- Notice how passionately the chest rises when the protection of the back is present. Realize safe boundaries are a foundation for freedom. Explore freedom of heart through reverence of the self. Meet life rather than forcing it into being.
- Guided meditation: I am connected.

Seated Row

Machine and Dyna-Band

Starting Position:

- Sit aligned on million-dollar point, leg(s) extended forward with soft knees. Hold vertical handle of rowing machine or Dyna-Band ends with band's center stabilized under foot.
- Connect to dan tien and relax weight of skeleton through sitz bones.
- Connect back muscles surrounding shoulder blades with outside resistance as you allow the back to fully expand outward.
- Commit to keeping tops of shoulders relaxed down and away from ears.

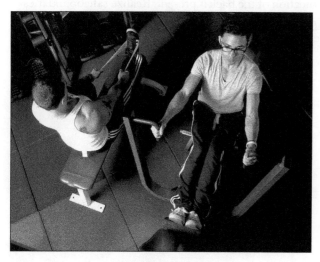
Starting Position

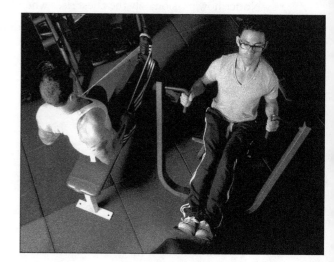
Action/Counter-action

Counter-action:

- Inhale: Visualize energy ascending from dan tien through abdominals and chest.
- Exhale: Open chest forward toward handle or Dyna-Band without rocking your weight off sitz bones by allowing shoulders to separate from chest. Keep elbows aligned behind wrists.
- Inhale: Return chest and shoulders to starting position. Repeat.
- Be mindful to keep heart open to the incoming resistance.

Action:

- Inhale: Connect back's width to outside resistance and relax shoulders.
- Exhale: Contract back muscles by drawing shoulder blades together. Visualize energy dropping from shoulder blade channels through low back dimples and sitz bones. Shoulder blades movement is initially met with straight arms, then elbows bend to permit full range of shoulder blades. Line up handle or Dyna-Band with solar plexus.

- Inhale: Use the back muscles to carry outside resistance back to starting position by expanding the shoulder blades. Repeat.
- Concentrate on preserving the connection between your upper back and outside resistance by using the biceps muscles sparingly when bending elbows.

Energy Orbit:

- **Isolated Connection:** Visualize the counter-action before engaging in the action. Counter-action: Cycle energy up the chest from abdominal center. Action: Orbit energy down past the shoulders to contract upper back.
- **Unified Connection:** Counter-action: Extend a corresponding energy orbit up the anterior legs and lower abdomen. Action: Orbit energy down the lower back and posterior legs. Energize all eight energy orbits of the pattern through the dan tien. This step adjoins active and counter-active energies associated with the whole body in support of a back-isolated connection.

Active Meditation—Protection:

- Notice how easily the smaller biceps muscles can interfere with the relationship between the larger back muscles and outside resistance. Acknowledge that the desire to get something (biceps) can obstruct you from protecting (back) a heartfelt connection. Appreciate who you are in relationship with over what you get from that relationship.
- Expression: I have all I need to succeed.

One-Arm Row

Dyna-Band

Starting Position:

- Sit aligned on million-dollar point with one foot extended forward and one foot on floor. Hold both Dyna-Band ends in one hand, with band's center stabilized under extended foot.
- Connect to dan tien and relax weight of skeleton through sitz bones.
- Allow shoulder blade holding Dyna-Band to spiral forward as you connect with back muscles.
- Commit to keeping your body weight equally distributed on both sitz bones.

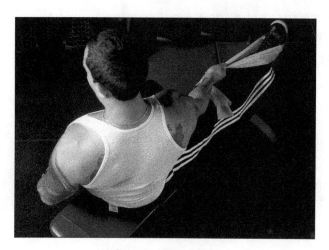

Starting Position

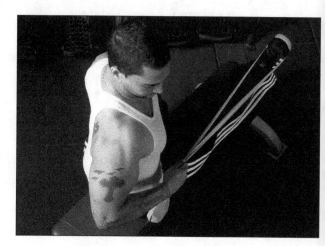

Action/Counter-action

Counter-action:

- Inhale: Visualize energy ascending from dan tien through abdominals and chest.
- Exhale: Allow torso to spiral at waistline by lifting sternum, opening chest, and spiraling up through crown of head. Keep elbow, wrist, and band aligned.
- Inhale: Torso unspirals and grounds through sitz bones as it is returned to starting position. Repeat.
- Be mindful to keep pelvis stable and essential alignment intact through spiral.

Action:

- Inhale: Connect back muscles to outside resistance and relax shoulders.
- Exhale: Contract only working side of back muscles by drawing shoulder blade inward toward median plane and spiraling waist. Visualize energy descending from both shoulder blade channels through sitz bones and expanding low back dimples. (Bend elbow only enough to permit full range of motion in shoulder blade. Keep Dyna-Band hand below solar plexus.)
- Inhale: Use back muscles to carry outside resistance back to starting position by expanding the shoulder blade and unspiraling waist. Repeat.
- Concentrate on maintaining the connection point with the upper back muscles rather than hanging from the various lower back joints involved in this complex spiral movement.

Energy Orbit:

- **Isolated Connection:** Visualize the counter-action before engaging in the action. Counter-action: Cycle energy up chest from abdominal center. Action: Orbit energy down past the shoulders to contract the upper back.
- **Unified Connection:** Counter-action: Extend a corresponding energy orbit up the anterior legs and abdomen. Action: Orbit energy down the lower back and posterior legs. Energize all eight energy orbits of the pattern through the dan tien. This adjoins active and counter-active energies associated with the whole body in support of a back-isolated connection.

Active Meditation—Protection:

- Notice how this complex movement can pull you out of your preferred abdominal support and into your lower back muscles. Use your abdominals' upward lift through the chest to stabilize your upper back's connection to both abdominals and the outside resistance, and to discern what range of movement is permissible. Pay close attention to and honor your stability first and foremost.
- Guided meditation: I empower my relationship with others by stabilizing my relationship with self.

Chin-Up

Chin-Up Bar

Starting Position:

- Hold chin-up bar with wide grip.
- Connect muscles surrounding shoulder blades with your body weight and allow your back muscles to expand outward. Do not hang from shoulder joints.
- Connect the dan tien to your lifting chest muscles and the pulling-back muscles to your body weight.
- Commit to keeping elbows under wrists and body positioned symmetrically between arms.

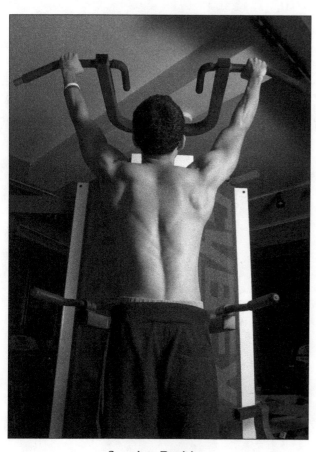
Starting Position

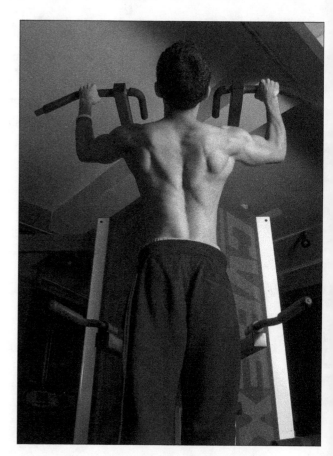
Action/Counter-action

Counter-action:

- Inhale: Visualize energy ascending from dan tien through abdominals and chest.
- Exhale: Open the chest to its widest possible position as the body is raised upward toward bar by lifting sternum and opening chest. Allow an arch in upper spine as chest rises.
- Inhale: Allow chest and sternum to return to starting position. Repeat.
- Be mindful that the chest is fully expanded at the height of the body's rise.

Action:

- Inhale: Connect back muscles to your body weight and relax shoulders.
- Exhale: Contract back muscles by drawing shoulder blades down and together. Visualize energy descending from shoulder blade channels through low back dimples and heel stirrups. Elbows align under wrists and bar as body rises.
- Inhale: Use the back muscles to carry your body weight back to starting position by expanding the shoulder blades. Repeat.
- Concentrate on the back muscles carrying your body's weight so your chest is free to rise above the challenge.

Energy Orbit:

- **Isolated Connection:** Visualize the counter-action before engaging in the action. Counter-action: Cycle energy up the chest from abdominal center. Action: Orbit energy down past the shoulders to contract the upper back.
- **Unified Connection:** Counter-action: Extend a corresponding energy orbit up the anterior legs and lower abdomen. Action: Orbit energy down the lower back and posterior legs. Energize all eight energy orbits of the pattern through the dan tien. This adjoins active and counter-active energies associated with the whole body in support of a back-isolated connection.

Active Meditation—Protection:

- Notice how you feel when your chest is free to expand at this elevated height. It is as if your heart were reaching for heaven. Appreciate every inch of movement the back muscles offer you with the knowledge that, as you gain strength, you will gain mastery in opening your heart.
- Guided meditation: I support my heart opening.

BodyLogos Psyche-Muscular Observations for Back Muscles

Here are examples of how to interpret mind-body expressions.

Size: The range of your back's motion won't allow the chin-up bar or Dyna-Band to touch the chest or the shoulder joints to lift toward the ears. This would extend the movement into the arms or shoulders. Allow the range of the shoulder blades to dictate the size of the movement.

🛑 A movement that bumps the bar or Dyna-Band into the chest indicates the need to forcefully pull things inward to feel safe or successful. The biceps have replaced the back muscles, pulling the elbows and wrists out of alignment. This points to a need to control your environment, and no doubt you will get the protective care you crave to feel safe.

🌀 Allow the movement of your body, the bar, or Dyna-Band to be dictated by the back's muscular strength and shoulder blades' range of motion. Recognize the truer, smaller range of motion in your back muscles as all you need for protection. Experience safekeeping when connected to your inner strength instead of an outer performance. As your movement remains limited to your back's capacity, feel safely cocooned in your own devoted guardianship.

🛑 Extending the back's upward momentum into the shoulder joints expands the movement beyond the range of your back muscles, lifting your shoulders toward your ears. This is a sign of not recognizing your own ability to protect yourself or defend your value.

🌀 Contain the expanding back muscles to the shoulder blades' range. As your back muscles experience a greater connection with outside resistance, experience a greater ability to stand up for yourself and say, "That's far enough!" Be your own sanctuary. As you protect your shoulders from overexertion, feel how you are protecting your value and loving yourself.

Posture: If the action and counter-action of a back movement aren't balanced, the weight of your body motivates the movement rather than your muscle strength.

🛑 When the action of the back muscles pull downward and the counter-action of the chest muscles fail to expand upward, these changes throw your weight back and collapse alignment, indicating a fear of showing your true self. This reflects that the heart is hiding in the back's strength.

The Art of Strength

Keep the descending direction of the shoulder blades connected to the outside resistance, equal with the ascending liberation of the sternum lifting away from your abdominal center. Feel the undercurrent of the chest or heart reaching up for personal freedom to encourage the back's strength. Experience openheartedness.

Ability: The inability to experience or discern back muscle isolations inhibits all movement in the upper torso.

When your shoulder blades offer very little range to initiate a back movement, kneading the surrounding muscles is helpful. The shoulder blade grab exercise (p. 193) will bring awareness to the muscles of the back. This frozen shoulder blade state indicates a freeze in your proclivity to protect yourself.

Once you get the shoulder blades familiar with the motion, introduce a light resistance and experience how the chest or heart opens when you pinch the muscles of the back. Experience the self-determination and pride that accompany acting on your own behalf. Protecting yourself is an act of love.

Meet the Models

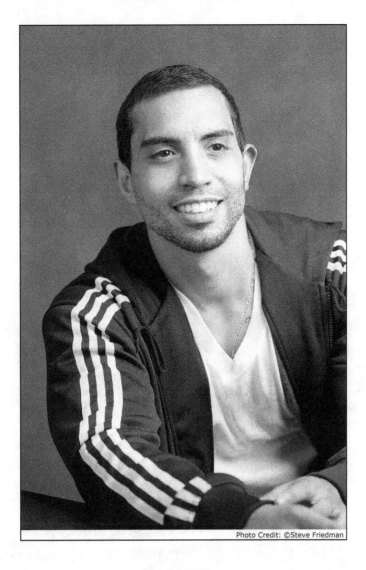

Tomas Milan

A New York City property manager of Cuban and Dominican descent, he says he feels like a superhero in his sculpted physique. Strength training has given him a platform where he realizes personal development and is motivated to live from his heart. He says, "When I graduate to a new level of resistance, I feel like I have accomplished something great!" Reaching "the zone" is his focus—a feeling of aligned energy, a meditative state that keeps him at ease and competent in his life.

Determined Power Energy Pattern as It Relates to the Triceps Muscles

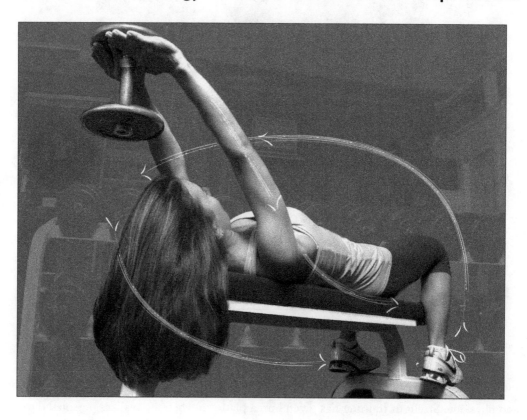

Visualize this energy pattern supporting all triceps isolations.

Introduction to Triceps Muscles

Theory of Yin and Yang

Yang: Active Muscle Group

Triceps Muscles:
- o Triceps Brachii
- o Anconeus

Yin: Counter-active Muscle Group

Biceps Muscles:
- o Biceps Brachii
- o Brachialis
- o Brachioradialis
- o Pronator Teres

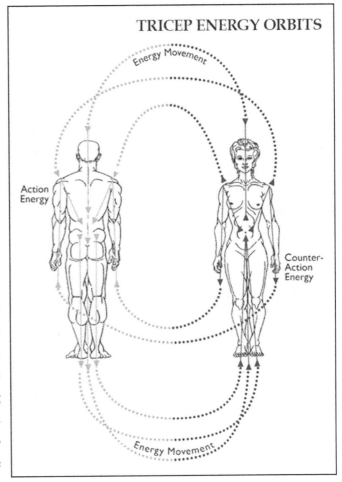

The experience of isolating the triceps muscles is one of distancing your chest or heart away from an outside resistance. Imagine extending an arm out in front of you, palm open as if to stop traffic. As the triceps (action) contracts up the back of the arm, the biceps (counter-action) extend down the front of the arm. This assertion energetically grounds you through the posterior body and lifts your anterior body through the chest. The body's energy orbit is committed to keeping your chest's position lifted above the assertion, to pushing away an outside resistance.

Action: Pushing Undesirables Outward

Here is an opportunity to empower your ability to say and mean, "No, thank you." To create positive change in your life, you first clear out the influences, external or internal, that aren't supporting where you are now and where you want to go. Connecting these influences to a muscular challenge enables you to gather your will, strength, and determination to deliberately and graciously let go of what was and make room for what is to come.

There are those overwhelming times, however, when it's hard to be clear on what it is you need to let go of. If everything feels equally important, meditate on creating space. Notice how giving the mind-body connection a direction to feel in, rather than to think in, will reveal what is important to you. By simply relaxing into your intuitive and instinctual natures with the intent to create space, the aspects of your life that are stifling you become clear. The answers are within you and will inform you when you direct your attention and movement deliberately.

Counter-action: Pulling Desirables Inward

When contracting the triceps muscles, you can also meditate on the expanding counter-action of your biceps muscles. Once you have cleared space in your environment, adjusted your physical standpoint, and transformed your mental viewpoint, you are able to direct your attention toward what you want to create next in your life. Your expanding biceps muscles—the muscles that pull desirables inward—are no longer recreating the past and are now available to consider fresh connections. Experience the space and freedom you have created for positive change to unfold and ponder what you are desiring in your new relations moving forward.

Five-Element Theory
Spring, Crushing Joints, Anger

Connection: Spring

When planting a spring garden, you have the added exuberance of longer days and warmer temperatures; your added vitality asserts your best efforts to learn from last year's garden experience before diving in. The sole purpose of the triceps muscles is to push away things that aren't in your best interest. Realizing what isn't working—be they physical objects or mental habits, goals or dreams—means rejecting choices you once made. As you change your priorities in life, it's imperative that you make room for the new. Letting go of the old, however, can feel uncertain. Take advantage of the energetic orbit descending through the lower back and let go of your anxiety about change, the unfamiliar, and the unknown. When approaching a triceps exercise, release the limitation of moving forward with your past. Concentrate on where you are going, free of where you have been. What is no longer true for you now will then be allowed to fall away.

Strength: Crushing Joints

The hinge joint of the elbow splits the action (triceps) and counter-action (biceps) as it pushes objects away from you. Once the biceps' energetic counter-action releases away from the shoulder and chest muscles, the triceps' strength can connect cleanly with the outside resistance. This connection creates an orbit of movement that coincides with the same opposition between the chest and back muscles and can then unlock and channel out any mind-body conflict barring your ability to let go of what is blocking your heart from being open. To push away a block is to recognize the viewpoint that created the block and then decide differently. Be resolved in taking responsibility for creating or perpetuating your internal conflicts; only then can you eliminate what is blocking your heart.

Meditation: Anger

Pushing away undesirables is a death of something in your life that, if you don't look beneath the surface, can keep you in a state of bitterness or resentment. You may feel slighted by the void created from the loss, but it's also a new beginning. Just as water naturally fills an unoccupied space, so will new life. The energetic expansion of the biceps muscles, as you contract the triceps, can feel like a rainbow of future possibilities before you. Be mindful of your biceps' speed of expansion matching the triceps' speed of contraction. Over-asserting your biceps could shadow the need to resolve your feelings of loss. This distracts you from fully dissolving your initial reaction while also causing the shoulder muscles to get needlessly involved, spewing expectations as to what should be rather than what is.

How to Isolate the Triceps Muscles

Feel It Contract

The significant range of motion that both wrists and shoulders bring to movement can obscure the simple extension of the elbow joints in a triceps exercise. To experience an isolated elbow extension, stabilize these surrounding joints. This will give you the reference point needed to recognize the triceps muscles and enable you to place greater responsibility in their isolated muscular strength.

Supine Elbow Lift with Pressed Fingertips

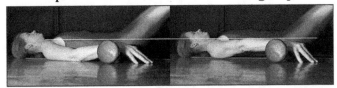

Exercise: Lie supine with knees bent and feet flat on the floor. Rest the front of one wrist over a large dumbbell (eight to ten pounds), placing your fingertips gently on the floor. Allow the shoulders to relax and the weight of your shoulder blades to surrender into the floor. Slowly lift your elbow off the floor as you gently press your fingertips into the floor. Maintain the relaxed and weighted placement of the wrists, shoulders, and shoulder blades. Your triceps can now be the sole initiator of the elbows' lift. Repeat until you can cleanly isolate the triceps muscles.

Feel It Release

To successfully stretch the triceps muscles, it's necessary to first extend your shoulder joint to its full range and then continue into the triceps' range. You can use your opposite hand to stabilize the elbow in the shoulder stretch or lean against the wall to effortlessly maintain the shoulders' range so you can concentrate on the triceps muscles' stretch.

Overhead Shoulder Blade Touch Down Stretch

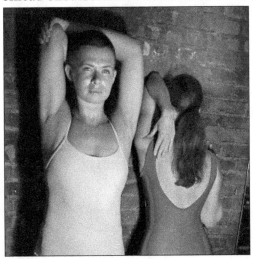

Exercise: Hold one elbow overhead as close to the ear as possible or stand facing a wall, approximately six inches away. Place one hand on wall at chest level to support your torso's weight and the other arm extending straight above your shoulder with the palm of the hand against the wall. Lean your body into the supporting

hand, directing the armpit of extended arm toward the wall until you feel the shoulder stretch. To continue into the triceps stretch, keep your shoulder blade dropped and bend the extended arm's elbow, touching the same shoulder or shoulder blade with fingertips. Relax the shoulder blade down as you continue to reach the elbow up. Breathe the stretch into the triceps muscle.

Feel It Fatigue

Triceps muscles are big talkers. They will cry mercy way before they are exhausted. Being unable to keep your chest lifted and shoulders dropped indicates that your triceps muscles are truly exhausted.

Triceps Exercises

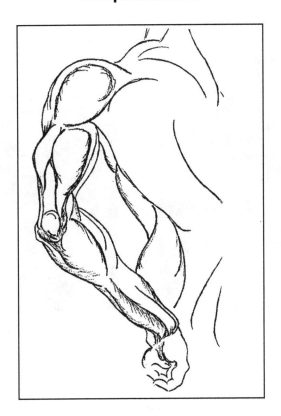

Triceps Muscles
Embody
Pushing Undesirables Away

Lying Overhead Triceps Extension

Dumbbell

Starting Position:

- Lie supine on bench, knees bent and feet flat on bench or bench legs.
- Hold one end of dumbbell with both palms up and keep bar in vertical direction.
- Position dumbbell over forehead, not over chest.
- Relax shoulders and drop shoulder blades' weight into bench.
- Connect to dan tien and preserve natural curves of the spine.
- Commit to using abdominal muscles to keep sacrum on the bench and lower back quiet in its natural arch throughout the movement.

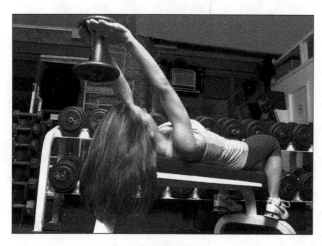
Starting Position

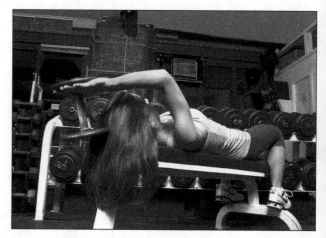
Action/Counter-action

Counter-action:

- Inhale: Visualize energy lifting from dan tien through chest, anterior shoulders, and biceps as elbows bend and dumbbell lowers above crown of head.
- Exhale: Lengthen biceps as arms extend while maintaining shoulder and elbow positions.
- Inhale: Keep dumbbell handle vertical as you return to starting position and use your abdominal muscles to leverage the destabilizing weight distribution of overhead movement. Repeat.
- Be mindful that elbows remain stable in their position as forearms travel with the outside resistance.

Action:

- Inhale: Carry outside resistance to crown of head by bending elbows to approximately a 90-degree angle.
- Exhale: Extend arms, flexing wrists at the top so dumbbell bar remains vertical, and visualize the triceps' downward force connecting to the shoulder blades.
- Inhale: Triceps return arms to the starting position and maintain a relaxed and neutral lower back. Repeat.
- Concentrate on keeping the arms at a slight backward angle between elbows and shoulders constant.

Energy Orbit:

- **Isolated Connection:** Visualize the counter-action before engaging in the action. Counter-action: Cycle energy up the chest, anterior shoulders, and biceps from abdominal center. Action: Orbit energy down the triceps, posterior shoulders, and upper back.
- **Unified Connection:** Counter-action: Extend a corresponding energy orbit up the anterior legs and lower abdomen. Action: Orbit energy down the lower back and posterior legs. Energize all eight energy orbits of the pattern through the dan tien. This adjoins active and counter-active energies associated with the whole body in support of a triceps-isolated connection.

Active Meditation—Pushing Undesirables Away:

- If you're not connected to your abdominal center, notice that the lower back will arch beyond its natural curve when bringing resistance overhead. This animates how the fear of pushing something away can overshadow genuine care of self. When doing this exercise, imagine standing up for yourself and connect to the quiet certitude of your spirit self residing in your dan tien. A relaxed commitment around self-care will permeate your abdominal support.
- Guided meditation: I create the environment I live in.

Kickback

Dumbbells

Starting Position:

- Stand with feet hips' width apart, knees slightly bent, and dumbbells in hand.
- Bend at hips with a natural spine, aligning neck and head with spine.
- Fold elbows, positioning them behind rib cage near the body, with palms in.
- Relax shoulder blades down the back, keeping chest forward and shoulders wide.
- Connect to dan tien, lengthening spine back through sitz bones and forward through crown center.
- Commit to keeping abdominal muscles lifted to meet weight of spine and outside resistance.

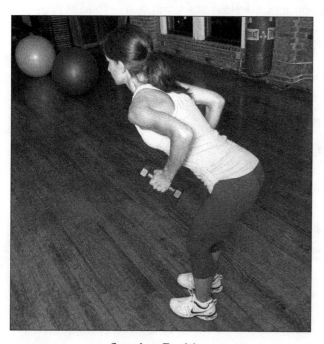

Starting Position

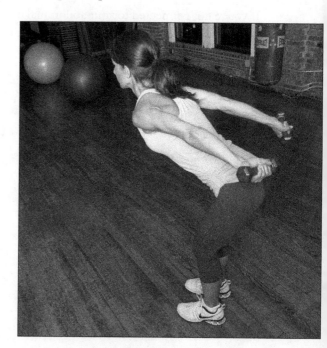

Action/Counter-action

Counter-action:

- Inhale: Visualize energy lifting from dan tien up through heart and crown centers.
- Exhale: Lengthen biceps as forearms extend. Open and lift chest to counter the backward extension of arms with outside resistance.
- Inhale: Neutralize the chest's forward lift as you return arms to starting position. Repeat.
- Be mindful to keep body weight stable on feet's gushing spring points. No rocking from heels to balls of feet.

Action:

- Inhale: Connect triceps muscles to outside resistance.

- Exhale: Extend forearms behind body by visualizing the triceps' force being grounded by the shoulder blades' drop. Support body position by balancing the downward length through the lower back with the upward lift through the chest.
- Inhale: Carry resistance with triceps back to starting position and maintain elbows position. Repeat.
- Concentrate on maintaining a clean forward bend in hip joints. Do not round torso at waist.

Energy Orbit:

- **Isolated Connection:** Visualize the counter-action before engaging in the action. Counter-action: Cycle energy up the chest, anterior shoulders, and biceps from abdominal center. Action: Orbit energy down the triceps, posterior shoulders, and upper back.
- **Unified Connection:** Counter-action: Extend a corresponding energy orbit up the anterior legs and low abdomen. Action: Orbit energy down the lower back and posterior legs. Energize all eight energy orbits of the pattern through the dan tien. This step adjoins active and counter-active energies associated with the whole body in support of a triceps-isolated connection.

Active Meditation—Pushing Undesirables Away:

- Notice how fervently the torso can throw itself forward, pitching your weight back and forth on your feet to overthrow the resistance. Meet the resistance with your triceps and experience their true capacity. Exert only the force needed to connect with the outside resistance and choose a weight where you are able to stay grounded through your alignment and open across your chest. There is no need to prove yourself—simply choose a resistance with which you can connect.
- Guided meditation: I allow for difference in strength and sensibilities.

Standing Overhead Triceps Extension

Dumbbell and Dyna-Band

Starting Position:

- Stand with feet hips' width apart and knees slightly bent.
- Hold dumbbell palms up overhead, bar in a vertical position. Or hold one end of Dyna-Band overhead and hang opposite end behind body. Bend both arms and grab Dyna-Band behind you at waist. Extend both arms (up and down), bracing back arm against body.
- Connect to dan tien and relax both shoulder blades downward.
- Commit to straightening arms as fully as a dropped shoulder blade position will allow.

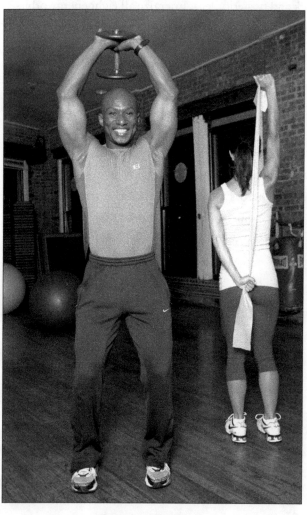

Starting Position

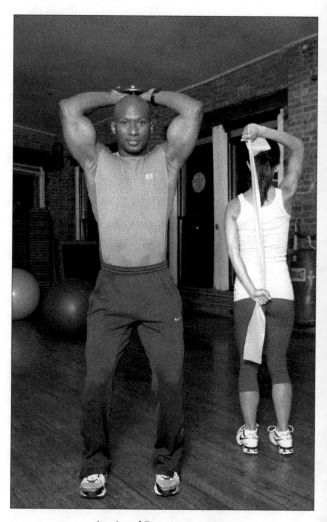

Action/Counter-action

Counter-action:

- Inhale: Visualize energy lifting from dan tien through chest, anterior shoulders, and biceps as overhead elbow(s) bends to a 90-degree angle.

- Exhale: Lengthen bicep(s) as you extend back to starting position. Keep chest lifted and maintain shoulder and elbow placement. Repeat.
- Inhale: Maintain biceps' reach upward and elbow placement as elbow(s) rebends. Change sides when using a Dyna-Band.
- Be mindful that the biceps energy is what reaches up through elbow joint(s).

Action:

- Inhale: Connect triceps muscles to outside resistance as elbow(s) bend 90 degrees.
- Exhale: Triceps extend arms back to starting position, flexing wrists so dumbbell handle remains vertical. Visualize the triceps' force grounding with the shoulder blades. Repeat.
- Inhale: Triceps muscles carry resistance back to bent arm position. Change sides when using a Dyna-Band. Do not flex wrist when using Dyna-Band.
- Concentrate on keeping the elbows as close to your ears as possible; elbow position must consider a comfortable shoulder rotation for easy completion of the exercise's entire range of motion.

Energy Orbit:

- **Isolated Connection:** Visualize the counter-action before engaging in the action. Counter-action: Cycle energy up the chest, anterior shoulders, and biceps from abdominal center. Action: Orbit energy down the triceps, posterior shoulders, and upper back.
- **Unified Connection:** Counter-action: Extend a corresponding energy orbit up the anterior legs and lower abdomen. Action: Orbit energy down the lower back and posterior legs. Energize all eight energy orbits of the pattern through the dan tien. This step adjoins active and counter-active energies associated with the whole body in support of a triceps-isolated connection.

Active Meditation—Pushing Undesirables Away:

- Notice the elbow placement that makes your shoulders most comfortable and recognize it as your personal reference point or need. Maintaining this shoulder position is valuing your needs in the face of challenge or adversity.
- Guided meditation: I honor and value my needs.

One-Arm Triceps Push Down

Pulley and Dyna-Band

Starting Position:

- Stand with feet hips' width apart and knees slightly bent.
- Face pulley and hold single-grip handle. Or hold one end of Dyna-Band in front of body with a bent arm while opposite end is hung over shoulder, supported by extended arm behind the body.
- Keep palm down when holding pulley handle and palm in when holding Dyna-Band.
- Place front bent elbow forward of coronal plane and connect to abdominal support.
- Commit to keeping shoulders symmetrical through this asymmetrical workload.

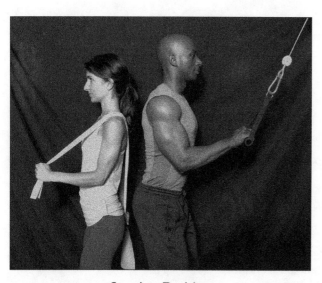

Starting Position

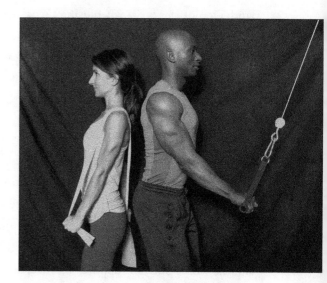

Action/Counter-action

Counter-action:

- Inhale: Visualize energy lifting from dan tien through chest, anterior shoulders, and biceps.
- Exhale: While biceps muscles lengthen, keep elbow placement stable and maintain width of chest and shoulders.
- Inhale: As arm is folded back to starting position, adjust lift of chest to counter the reduced force with outside resistance. Repeat and change sides.
- Be mindful that the ebb and flow of movement is vertical. Between the lifting chest and triceps extension, refrain from any horizontal swinging of elbow.

Action:

- Inhale: Connect triceps muscles to resistance.
- Exhale: Triceps extend arm as you ground downward through shoulder blades. Do not transfer work to forearm or hand.

- Inhale: Use triceps to carry resistance back to starting position. Repeat and change sides.
- Concentrate on maintaining the grounding influence of your shoulder blades to keep triceps connected.

Energy Orbit:

- **Isolated Connection:** Visualize the counter-action before engaging in the action. Counter-action: Cycle energy up the chest, anterior shoulders, and biceps from abdominal center. Action: Orbit energy through the triceps, posterior shoulders, and upper back.
- **Unified Connection:** Counter-action: Extend a corresponding energy orbit up the anterior legs and low abdomen. Action: Orbit energy down the posterior legs and lower back. Energize all eight energy orbits of the pattern through the dan tien. This adjoins active and counter-active energies associated with the whole body in support of a triceps-isolated connection.

Active Meditation—Pushing Undesirables Away:

- Notice how lifting the chest opens your heart center. Feel clear about your choice to clear away an undesirable influence. Experience "no" as taking responsibility for yourself.
- Guided meditation: I decide.

BodyLogos Psyche-Muscular Observations for Triceps Muscles

Here are examples of how to interpret mind-body expressions.

Posture: When one muscle group oversteps the domain of another, it disrupts postural alignment and interferes with the balance of muscular development. This situation reveals what specific muscles you overexert or underutilize.

STOP When the shoulders overpower the triceps, this situation pushes the chest down, rocks the elbows back, and replaces much of the triceps' contribution to the exercise. As a mind-body connection to morals and values, overbearing shoulders reflect your need to defend your value or integrity when pushing something away. This shoulder domination collapses your heart or chest, making it difficult to motivate your will. Pushing something away in this fashion begins to feel hopeless.

The anguish of pushing something away can bring up feelings of unworthiness or doubt. Misaligned or indoctrinated values can be experienced as personal judgments, condemning yourself or others, and results in keeping your heart energy in a state of perpetual immobilization. Give your triceps the opportunity to lead and allow yourself to explore inwardly what keeps your heart center truly smiling.

Coordination: Some exercises feel awkward and/or complicated. Keeping the elbows placed, the lower back long, the shoulders wide, and the chest up, in addition to doing the triceps exercise, can be more than you can manage. Sometimes an exercise can just feel too complicated.

STOP You need a strong, stable center to keep your elbow placed and your torso quiet in a triceps exercise. Stop if your torso is moving about as your forearm travels up and down. Pull in your lower abdominals and relax your lower back, ground through your feet, and lift through your chest. These two oppositions balance your energy orbits for postural alignment and connection with your dan tien. Maintaining this connected alignment is more important than the exercise itself, since it is prioritizing physical integrity over physical performance.

Approach the movement slowly and mindfully. Let your new alignment focus your intention to gain a sense of placement and belonging in the world. Through your meditation, push away or let go of all that is distracting you from maintaining personal stability.

Ability: The balance of strength between biceps and triceps indicates the balance of strength between pushing things away versus pulling thing inward.

> 🛑 If your triceps are substantially weaker than your biceps, feel into their trepidation and incite the triceps exercises with purpose. This imbalance indicates you are uncomfortable when pushing life away or uncomfortable when choosing yourself over another.

> 🌀 Create a meditation in regard to saying no that excites you and motivates your triceps. Inspire the ability to push undesirables away and realize doing so is your responsibility.

> 🛑 If your triceps are substantially stronger than your biceps, explore the nature of your triceps' strength. This imbalance shows your comfort in pushing life away and choosing yourself over another.

> 🌀 Meditate on the nature of pushing things away and notice whether it creates true happiness for you; or adversely, whether you are creating defenses that feed a hyper-protective reaction to living.

Meet the Models

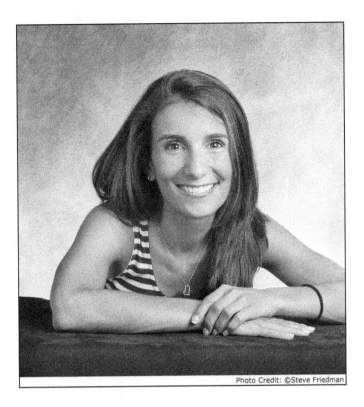

Kristen Delle Donne

This twenty-five-year-old Italian beauty has a passion for family, cooking, travel, entertaining, and of course, fitness. She was motivated to start strength training to become an accomplished softball pitcher, and though she was a committed athlete, Kristen chose teaching in the sciences as a career. She believes strength training keeps her body strong and her mind focused. She shares, "The focus, concentration, and motivation required in strength training provide mental and physical results in my life." In addition to the inward attention to herself at the gym, Kristen takes a little time each day to quietly reflect on the outward gifts surrounding her in life. Her attractiveness is surely attributed to recognizing and soaking up the beauty she experiences in her life.

Lesson 10
Creating Forward Energy Pattern: Chest, Quadriceps

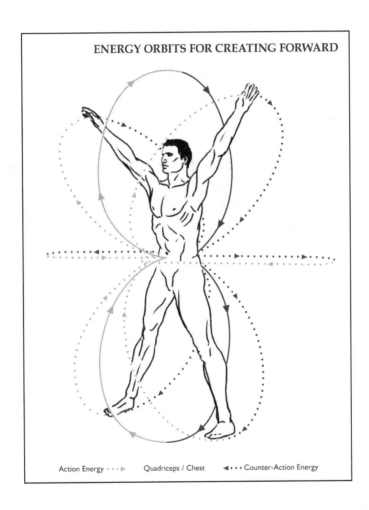

That satisfied feeling that wells up in your heart when you lean back in your desk chair and review the work you just produced is the feeling of "creating forward." You are committed to accomplishing a task and completely involved in its doing. Your body, mind, and heart are all immersed in creating your vision.

This is an energy pattern that elevates and unites your three primary power centers: jing, chi, shen. Refining your dan tien energy—shen—is experienced as a motivation to act on your spirit's behalf—jing. Chi is the communication between body and spirit. Creating forward energy offers you a readiness for action, an urgent excitement about what is ahead, and a vital sense of knowing everything will be okay. It not only inspires you to walk, jog, and run—this energy inspires speaking, problem solving, and brainstorming.

Creating Forward—T-Shirt Strip and Active Meditation
mindthebody.bodylogos.com/video13
(abbreviated description)

The sensation of creating forward energy is experienced when you take off a T-shirt. Stand with your feet hips' width apart and knees slightly bent. Cross arms in front of you as if grabbing the bottom edges of an imaginary T-shirt. Lift T-shirt off overhead as if turning shirt inside out. In doing so, become aware of the dynamic upward lift through the anterior legs and torso while simultaneously there is a gentle descent through the posterior torso and legs. This forward lift excites forward propulsion. Feel how that forward propulsion is present in mind and body.

Chest and quadriceps exercises utilize the creating forward energy pattern. They both quickly connect you to what is right in front of you, aligning your life force with what the universe has presented to you. Chest exercises move you forward by incorporating the desire for happiness. Quadriceps exercises move you forward by incorporating the desire to thrive. Both muscle groups provoke social scrutiny—stepping into the world to be seen and judged.

Orbiting energy upward from the quadriceps (movement forward) to the chest (smile of truth) and relaxing it downward to surrender the shoulders (moral values) help to relieve judgments regarding past heartfelt choices that hasten your forward progress. This prepares you for truthful reflection to guide future choices and propel forward movement, while simultaneously relieving tense shoulders that accompany the uncertainty of new frontiers. With your shoulders and their trepidations settled down, you are available to connect forward with clear vision and an open heart.

The Art of Strength

Practice Change

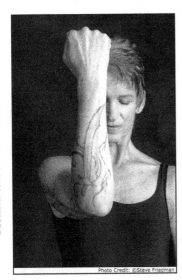

Henna tattoo of a **Metal** sword

Like **Metal**,
Sharpen your senses into life-sculpting tools.
Recognize your aptitude
to successfully cut through disorientation.
Recognize the ways your attitude
Can senselessly perpetuate disorientation.

Creating Forward
Is knowing the value of stepping into life
With authenticity and self-love.
Be you.
Live you.

Creating Forward Energy Pattern as It Relates to the Chest Muscles

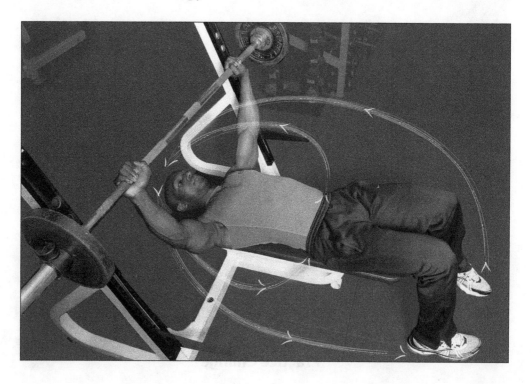

Visualize this energy pattern supporting all chest isolations.

Introduction to Chest Muscles

Theory of Yin and Yang

Yang: Active Muscle Group

Chest Muscles:
- o Pectoralis Major
- o Pectoralis Minor
- o Serratus Anterior

Yin: Counter-active Muscle Group

Mid- and Lower-Back Muscles:
- o Latissimus Dorsi
- o Teres Major
- o Rhomboids
- o Trapezius

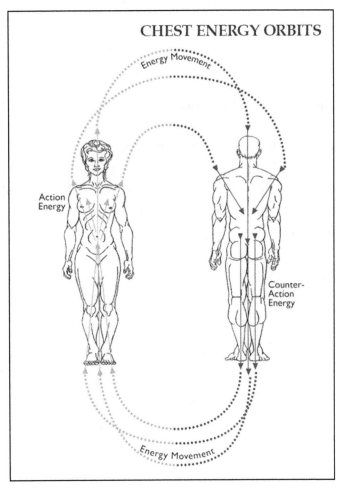

As if the sun were rising through your chest (action) and the moon were setting through your back (counter-action), engaging the chest muscles feels like an emergence. These opposing energies create an energetic orbit that circles the entire body, uplifting the anterior body through the brow while grounding the posterior body through the heel stirrups of the feet. Feel the heart center shift forward while the shoulders relax back. Commit to matching the inspired lift in the chest with a downward surrender in the upper-middle back.

Action: Smile of Truth

As an external sheath for the emotional seat of your existence (your heart center), chest muscles can teach you about your capacity to feel and about the true nature of happiness. To feel happiness is to be aware of, and in pursuit of, your aspirations and dreams. As you work the chest muscles, let your heart center experience the fruit of your dreams. Literally feel your chest smile as you offer it to the world through your active connection with your dreams. Notice how this smile of truth, expressed through the chest's radiance, projects your inner beauty outwardly into the world.

Counter-action: Protection

When contracting the chest muscles, you can also meditate on the expanding counter-action of the back muscles. The best support the back muscles can offer the chest's effort is to yield to the chest's more yin expression. As you work the chest muscles, ease the defensive and protective qualities that live in the back muscles. Notice how supple the back muscles can be as the movement in your chest progressively swells. Boldness is needed to surrender the back's protection just as it is needed to believe in the chest's dreams. As you deliberately release the back muscles, feel a newfound boldness clearing the way for your heart's vision.

Five-Element Theory
Autumn, Splitting Joints, Sorrow

Connection: Autumn

Autumn's gradual unveiling brings forth the nakedness your heart center feels when it connects to life. Pay particular attention to your dan tien feeding the chest's lift, like the tree's trunk supporting its bare and vulnerable branches. With a heightened awareness in the chest, you become better connected to the joy that lives in your heart center. With your abdominals' support, you are connected to the spirit of your heart's aspirations and dreams. When setting up for chest exercises, concentrate on uniting the smile that lives in your heart center with the life force that fuels your dreams.

Strength: Splitting Joints

The discs between vertebral bodies of the spine and the splitting connective tissue between the three aspects of the sternum are what allow the chest muscles to swell. Leading from the chest muscles feels subtle because cartilaginous connective tissue provides only partial mobility. You are looking more for a greater internal sensation than an external chest movement. The deeper you connect in the chest muscles, the more supple the surrounding cartilaginous tissues become, offering a yielding environment for the heart and lungs. Together, the emotions of the heart (which carry your joys) and lungs (which carry your sorrows) help you decide what you truly want for yourself and your life. Be resolved in fully connecting the chest muscles with the outside resistance before you move and continue to expand the muscles throughout your movement.

Meditation: Sorrow

In the quest to become successful in life, you can easily insist on forward propulsion. Eagerness turned to impatience becomes disappointment. The lungs (sorrow) and heart (joy) are nestled between the back and chest muscles. Together, they show you the full rainbow of emotions you contain. Haste can cause you to pinch the back muscles to quickly lift the chest, substituting the chest's more subtle connection. This doesn't strengthen heartfelt connections. It feigns a smile of truth and connects instead with the back's protectiveness. Eagerness turns to sorrowful discouragement. Patience in finding your chest muscles is found by slowing down the need to move. Feel the weight of the shoulder blades and back muscles settle downward as the chest muscles lift upward, giving your actions confidence and clear connection. Be mindful of the back muscles as a partner who supports the grace within the chest rather than as an overpowering protector replacing the chest.

How to Isolate the Chest Muscles

Feel It Contract

Traditionally, praying hands connect you to your heart center. This rendition creates an isometric resistance that awakens the musculature of the chest so you can present your heart outwardly to the world.

Praying Hands Exercise

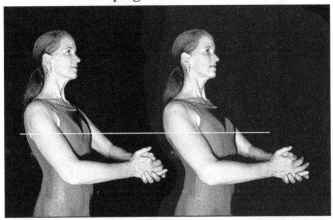

Exercise: Sit, stand, or lie supine with palms together and elbows wide. Direct an upward swell through your zhong heart center. Engage the chest muscles to lift your breast rather than aiming to move your bones. Feel the chest's gentle strength pass through the arms unimpeded to produce an inward pressure between the hands. The forward swelling of the chest will subsequently drag the associated ribs and vertebrae slightly forward, creating a subtle and relaxed arch in the upper back. This spinal arch is a natural consequence of the chest's upward swell and the isolated connection between the chest and back in this energy pattern. If this arch is prohibited or exaggerated, your shoulders will take over as the active muscle group. Release the isometric pressure between the hands and allow your alignment to return to neutral. Repeat until you can successfully isolate the chest muscles independently of the back and shoulder muscles.

Feel It Release

This chest opener separates the breasts at the heart center and elongates the sternum. If you have trouble experiencing the chest muscles in a contraction, exploring this stretch may bring about a greater understanding of what lifted chest muscles feel like.

Dyna-Band Circle Stretch

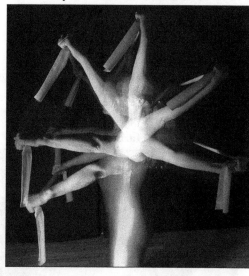

Exercise: With feet hips' width apart, knees slightly bent, and abdominal muscles gently engaged, hold Dyna-Band with a wide grip. Circle straight arms forward, then up overhead, and back behind the shoulder blades. Progressively separate the breasts so the shoulders can rotate back with straight arms. Reverse the circle up overhead, forward, and down in front. Slowly repeat the circle three to six times, pausing at the tightest aspect of the circle, just behind the head, to relax the shoulders and soften the chest muscles. You are looking for a chest stretch. If you encounter shoulder pain, widen your grip on the Dyna-Band.

Feel It Fatigue

When the muscles of the chest start fatiguing, they quietly retreat, and the shoulder muscles will take over. Be strict with your form. Practice keeping the chest muscles (smile of truth) connected to your action rather than your shoulder muscles' (moral values) judgments. When the chest muscles can no longer connect and transfer the challenge over to the shoulders, conclude the exercise. As the chest muscles develop, they will become more and more able to stay connected. Be patient and wait for the chest's connection to motivate you into greater challenges. Until then, let the chest muscles teach you the subtleties of heartfelt connection.

Chest Exercises

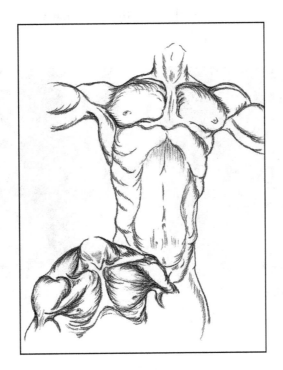

Chest Muscles
Embody
Smile of Truth

Lying Chest Press

Barbell

Starting Position:

- Lie supine on flat bench, knees bent, and feet grounded on floor or bench.
- Hold barbell slightly outside shoulders' width and connect to dan tien. Elevate bar off rack over chest or nipple line with straight arms.
- Experience the resistance and weight of arms and shoulders as one weight; channel this weight into the bench through dropped shoulder blades.
- Commit to connecting the chest muscles directly with resistance using arms and shoulders only to balance weight.

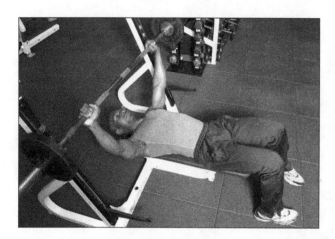

Starting Position

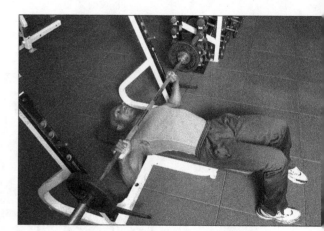

Action/Counter-action

Counter-action:

- Inhale: Bend elbows directly under bar. Feel elbows as an extension of the back's width by visualizing energy descending from the back of the head to the heels.
- Exhale: Relax the weight of shoulders downward through shoulder blades as the resistance is pushed upward with arms extended. Allow the upper back to follow the lift of the chest.
- Inhale: Keep shoulder blades and elbows heavy under the bar as arms rebend. Repeat.
- Be mindful that the upper back arch follows the chest's lift with the same degree of movement the chest offers.

Action:

- Inhale: Connect chest muscles to resistance and bend elbows to lower weight to chest.
- Exhale: Contract the chest to extend arms maintaining bar placement over nipple line. Visualize ascending energy rising from abdominal support. Chest will be highest when the arms reach their full extension. Do not lock elbows.

- Inhale: Use chest muscles to carry weight back to bent-arm position. Repeat.
- Concentrate on the chest muscles staying connected to the resistance throughout entire range of arm movement.

Energy Orbit:

- **Isolated Connection:** Visualize the counter-action before engaging in the action. Counter-action: Cycle energy down the triceps, posterior shoulders, and upper back. Action: Orbit energy up through the abdominals, anterior shoulders, chest, and biceps.
- **Unified Connection:** Counter-action: Extend a corresponding energy orbit down the lower back and posterior legs. Action: Orbit energy up the anterior legs and lower abdomen. Energize all eight energy orbits of the pattern through the dan tien. This adjoins active and counter-active energies associated with the whole body in support of a chest-isolated connection.

Active Meditation—Smile of Truth:

- Notice how leading from the chest draws the heart center forward and invites you to feel from your emotional body. The sincerity of your heart center permeates your effort and leads you toward what is most heartfelt and genuine. Experience the love that sits quietly within you. Be a beacon of love.
- Guided meditation: I am love.

Seated Chest Press

Machine and Dyna-Band

Starting Position:

- Sit back into machine or bench, million-dollar point grounded into seat, gushing spring points grounded into floor.
- Hold machine handles or Dyna-Band, palms down at nipple line.
- Connect to your dan tien to support resistance with the chest, positioning hands slightly in front of the body with bent elbows behind straight wrists.
- Commit to grounding your body's weight through your sitz bones.

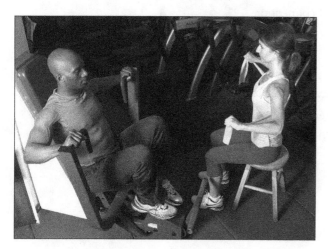
Starting Position

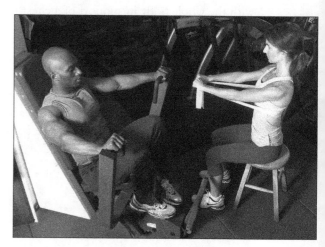
Action/Counter-action

Counter-action:

- Inhale: Visualize energy descending from occipital hollows through sitz bones and feel elbows' width as an extension of upper back's width.
- Exhale: Relax the weight of shoulders downward through shoulder blades as outside resistance is pushed forward with arms extended. Allow upper back to follow chest's lift.
- Inhale: Keep shoulder blades, elbows, and wrists at nipple line as you return to starting position. Repeat.
- Be mindful of your shoulders' weight resting through dropped shoulder blades.

Action:

- Inhale: Connect chest muscles to resistance as abdominals connect to chest muscles.
- Exhale: Contract chest to extend arms. Visualize energy ascending from abdominal support. Chest will be highest when arms reach their full extension; and hands will come together in front of nipple line when using a Dyna-Band.

- Inhale: Use chest muscles to carry arms back to starting position. Repeat.
- Concentrate on the chest muscles rising up from your anterior dan tien with the same intensity you are grounding down from your posterior dan tien.

Energy Orbit:

- **Isolated Connection:** Visualize the counter-action before engaging in the action. Counter-action: Cycle energy down the triceps, posterior shoulders, and upper back. Action: Orbit energy up through the abdominals, anterior shoulders, chest, and biceps.
- **Unified Connection:** Counter-action: Extend a corresponding energy orbit down the lower back and posterior legs. Action: Orbit energy up the anterior legs and lower abdomen. Energize all eight energy orbits of the pattern through the dan tien. This step adjoins active and counter-active energies associated with the whole body in support of a chest-isolated connection.

Active Meditation—Smile of Truth:

- In this grounded state, notice how grateful you are of the vulnerability in your heart center. As you relax your physical weight through your million-dollar point, experience the weightlessness of your heart center opening without judgments. Experience your tenderness as beauty. Be beautiful.
- Guided meditation: My vulnerability is beautiful.

Seated Chest Fly

Machine and Dyna-Band

Starting Position:

- Sit back into machine or bench with million-dollar point grounded into seat and gushing spring points grounded into floor.
- Hold machine handles or Dyna-Band with hammerhead grip (palms forward) and arms extended sideways at nipple line and slightly in front of coronal plane with soft elbows.
- Connect to dan tien to support chest muscles with resistance.
- Commit to maintaining the width of your back through your arms' reach.

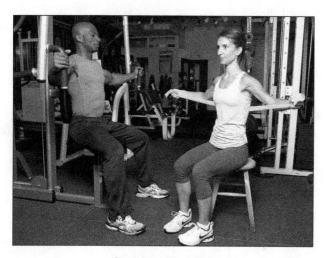

Starting Position

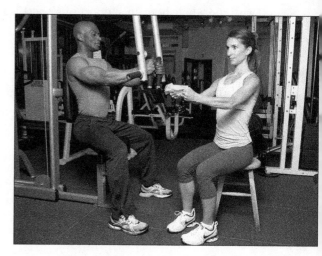

Action/Counter-action

Counter-action:

- Inhale: Feel arm span as an extension of back's width and visualize energy descending from occipital hollows through shoulder blade channels and sitz bones.
- Exhale: Relax the weight of shoulders downward through shoulder blades as outside resistance is pushed forward, creating a circular pattern with arms. Allow upper back to follow chest's lift as hands come together at nipple line.
- Inhale: Keep elbows soft and arms long as you are returned to starting position. Repeat.
- Be mindful that your elbows remain unaffected throughout your arms' motion.

Action:

- Inhale: Connect chest muscles to resistance as abdominals connect to chest muscles.
- Exhale: Chest muscles contract as arms circle forward. Visualize energy rising up from abdominals to chest. Chest will be highest when hands come together in front of body at nipple line.

- Inhale: Use chest muscles to carry arms back to starting position. Repeat.
- Concentrate on the chest muscles staying engaged with the outside resistance through the most lateral to the most medial aspects of the movement.

Energy Orbit:

- **Isolated Connection:** Visualize the counter-action before engaging in the action. Counter-action: Cycle energy down the triceps, posterior shoulders, and upper back. Action: Orbit energy up through the abdominals, anterior shoulders, chest, and biceps.
- **Unified Connection:** Counter-action: Extend a corresponding energy orbit down the lower back and posterior legs. Action: Orbit energy up the anterior legs and lower abdomen. Energize all eight energy orbits of the pattern through the dan tien. This step adjoins active and counter-active energies associated with the whole body in support of a chest-isolated connection.

Active Meditation—Smile of Truth:

- Notice how the chest can so easily rely on the back's greater strength and stature to initiate an outward connection. Recognize this internal dependency of the heart center leaning on the back's protection as a mirror of your external relationship dependencies. Experience dependence as permission to consider and accept yourself and then share yourself with others. Step into personal dependence and experience your courage to divulge its truths. Deliberately uncover what feels vulnerable with profound caring. Enjoy the depth of trust.
- Guided meditation: I trust myself and enjoy others.

Standing Chest Fly

Pulley

Starting Position:

- Stand between two pulleys. Hold handles with palms forward and arms outstretched sideways and slightly in front of coronal plane. Lunge one leg forward.
- Rock onto back leg as you bend elbows into waistline; then, staying connected to your dan tien, transfer onto front leg, extend arms forward, and press palms together at nipple line.
- Lean torso's weight onto abdominal center, support resistance with chest muscles, and maintain soft elbows and straight wrists.
- Commit to balancing a downward force through posterior body and an upward force through anterior body.

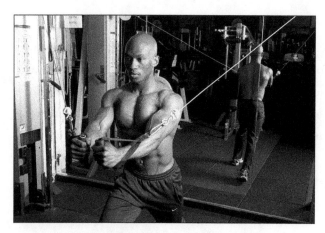
Starting Position

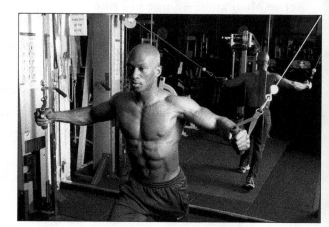
Action/Counter-action

Counter-action:

- Inhale: Open arms as an extension of back's width and visualize energy descending from occipital hollows through shoulder blade channels and down through heel stirrups.
- Exhale: Relax the weight of shoulders downward through shoulder blades as outside resistance is pushed forward, creating a circular arm pattern. As hands come together in front of nipple line, allow upper back to follow chest's lift.
- Inhale: Keep elbows soft and arms long as you return to starting position with a neutral spine. Repeat.
- Be mindful to keep movement's range in front of body within your peripheral span of sight.

Action:

- Inhale: Connect chest muscles to resistance and open arms side. Arms don't pass behind coronal plane.
- Exhale: Contract chest muscles and circle arm's forward. Visualize energy rising up from abdominals. Chest will be highest when hands touch in front of nipple line.

- Inhale: Use chest muscles to carry arms back to starting position and lean torso's weight onto abdominal center. Repeat.
- Concentrate on asserting from your chest muscles and allowing the subtle arch of your back muscles to move with them. Let the spine move freely between the chest and back muscle groups.

Energy Orbit:

- **Isolated Connection:** Visualize the counter-action before engaging in the action. Counter-action: Cycle energy down the triceps, posterior shoulders, and upper back. Action: Orbit energy up through the abdominals, anterior shoulders, chest, and biceps.
- **Unified Connection:** Counter-action: Extend a corresponding energy orbit down the lower back and posterior legs. Action: Orbit energy up the anterior legs and lower abdomen. Energize all eight energy orbits of the pattern through the dan tien. This step adjoins active and counter-active energies associated with the whole body in support of a chest-isolated connection.

Active Meditation—Smile of Truth:

- Notice how the constant outward pull of the outside resistance insists that you depend on your abdominal center. Experience your willingness to simultaneously assert your strength and expose your heart. Experience strength as opening your heart. Enjoy the growing tenacity of your heart center connecting.
- Guided meditation: I am available.

BodyLogos Psyche-Muscular Observations for Chest Muscles

Here are examples of how to interpret mind-body expressions.

Size: When opening the arms to the sides, as in a chest fly, keep the movement in your peripheral view. If the arms open so far that they travel outside your peripheral view, your shoulder blades pinch together. That places the resistance in the range of the back muscles, and the shoulders will need to assist in bringing the movement back into the range of the chest muscles.

🛑 Large movements that extend beyond your chest's limitations indicate moving forward with no awareness of, or respect for, your personal limits. This may be experienced as the tendency to propel yourself into things with an open heart but end up losing yourself in the process.

🌀 Contain your range of movement. Keep the motion in front of you and keep your back wide. With each repetition, allow the chest muscles to rise and arch the upper spine with your movement's forward push, and return the spine to its neutral starting position with each retreat. Experience the continuous ebb and flow of your heart energy connecting with an outside resistance. Experience the chest's push as your voice and the chest carrying the resistance on the retreat as your ability to listen. Be willing to experience what your heart is quietly reflecting without concern about proving your strength, success, or happiness.

Posture: The sensation of engaging the chest muscles is like feeling the ocean swell under your breast. It is subtle and composed yet commanding. If you're expecting a more explosive sensation from the chest, you will likely employ your shoulders to get it.

🛑 Rotating the shoulder blades off the bench or seat back means your shoulders have become part of the work force. Rather than playing a secondary role to balance the movement, they are dominating the softer voice of the chest. Your heart energy, then, doesn't get the opportunity to connect fully. Ideally, the shoulder blades remain relaxed back against the bench or seat back in a chest exercise. Your shoulders reflect your sense of value; leading with the shoulders rather than your chest suggests a need to prove your value or feeling that whatever your heart deems important isn't actually important. Using the shoulders in this way is a more superficial and defensive connection with outside resistance, and it's at the loss of the more subtle deep connection with your heart energy.

🌀 Before you engage the chest, relax the shoulder blades down the back and continue to relax them throughout the set. Be curious about new sensations in the chest as the shoulders retreat from their safeguarding. Literally, feel as though your heart energy is moving forward in your chest cavity with each repetition. It's possible that connecting with your chest or heart feels subtler and more "supernatural" than you imagined. To find this connection, you may initially need to lessen the weight of resistance.

Coordination: Collapsing in any aspect of the body, muscular or skeletal, leads to a less effective exercise and a disconnection between your body and the resistance.

Using your elbows to control a chest exercise weakens their function to keep your back wide. Back width, moreover, is crucial for giving the chest the support it needs to connect with and lift the outside resistance. Elbow collapse is when they fold inward toward the back rather than being an extension of the back's width, and it diminishes the connection between the chest and resistance. Your triceps are then manipulating the weight before the chest can get there. This triceps manipulation implies the need to push the outside resistance away before it touches your chest or heart.

Slow down and don't extend your arms. Allow the chest muscles to connect with the resistance at a slower speed and let the arms also be pushed forward from the chest. Take the time to truly feel the chest muscles connect before you begin moving. Explore what a heart connection is. As you relinquish the triceps' tendency to keep things at arms' length, recognize you are leaving room for something else to be offered.

Meet the Models

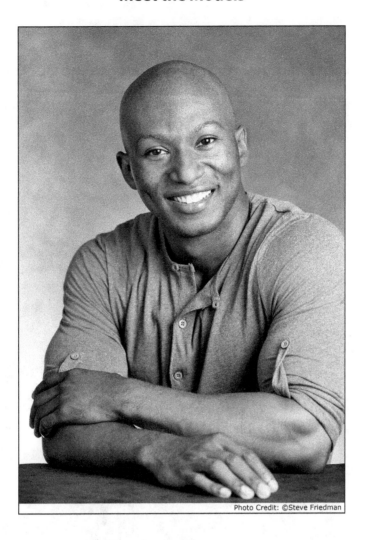

Mark Plaisir

As a singer or songwriter, Mark frequently gets lost in his music. Exercise provides the same oasis, whereby his focus is entirely on his connection to his body in motion. As a skinny grade-school boy back in Haiti, Mark got picked on. Now his physique wins him much praise and adoration. He says with a bright smile and a chuckle, "Compliments are a lot of fun!" Strength training has put him back in the control seat of his life so he can retain the vulnerable side of his nature for creating and performing his music.

Creating Forward Energy Pattern as It Relates to the Quadriceps Muscles

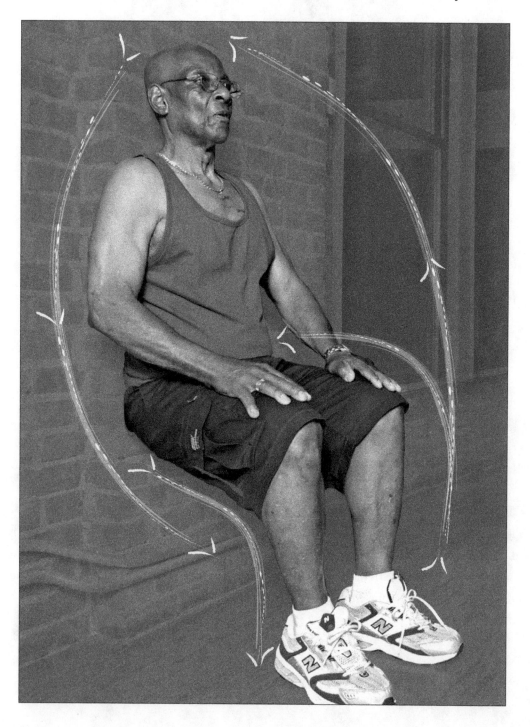

Visualize this energy pattern supporting all quadriceps isolations.

Introduction to Quadriceps Muscles

Theory of Yin and Yang

Yang: Active Muscle Group

Quadriceps Muscles:
- Rectus Femoris
- Vastus Lateralis
- Vastus Intermedius
- Vastus Medialis
- Sartorius

Yin: Counter-active Muscle Group

Hamstring Muscles:
- Semimembranosus
- Semitendinosus
- Biceps Femoris

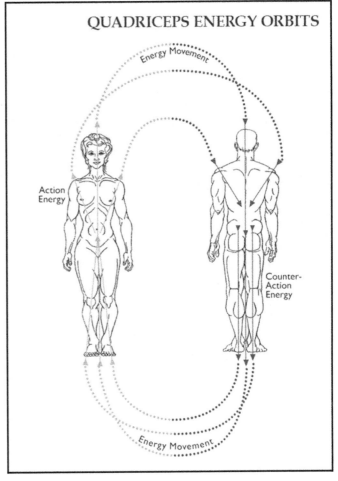

The feeling of driving down the highway in a convertible car, wind blowing your hair back and body pressed against the seat back, orients you in a quadriceps exercise. As the quadriceps muscles contract (action), they create an upward force through the entire anterior side of the body like the wind. The hamstring muscles (counter-action) oppose the wind, grounding downward through the entire posterior side of the body. When working the quadriceps muscles, commit to grounding through the shoulder blades, tailbone, and heel stirrups while lifting the abdominal muscles and chest, supporting the natural curves of the spine.

Action: Movement Forward

Moving forward is among the greatest challenges you face in life, since it requires the greatest amount of physical energy and mental determination to carry out. When you use the muscular thrust of the quadriceps muscles as a time to tap into your vision for yourself in the world, you deliberately channel their tremendous energy output toward your dreams. Whether you have a specific goal in mind or feel empowered in knowing that you can create your life forward deliberately, this mind-body connection empowers your sense of self in the world. Notice your excitement when driven toward a dream. Let the power of the quadriceps muscles remind you of this drive when entering uncharted territories of your life.

Counter-action: Movement Backward

When contracting the quadriceps muscles, you can also meditate on the expanding counter-action of the hamstring muscles. As the muscles that move you backward in space, the hamstrings release to extend under your quadriceps actions to move forward. Feel how your past has prepared you for where you are now going and release the need to micromanage your every move. Or experience how past perceptions or indoctrinations may no longer serve you, and as you release the hamstring muscles, also loosen your grip on keeping them in tow. Trust yourself to move forward intuitively.

Five-Element Theory
Spring, Crushing Joints, Anger

Connection: Spring

A spring planting brings forth precious bounty. Creativity and reflection as well as foresight and strategy are needed to set up and ensure this bounty. There are infinite ways to move ahead. Your choices are what define your individuality and the way in which you touch life and are touched by life. Quadriceps muscles move you forward in space to direct you toward your life's dreams. The uplifting anterior force in a quadriceps exercise rises up through your body, heart, and mind, inspiring new directions and possibilities. The grounding posterior force releases fear stagnating in the lower back that can block your strength and destabilize your alignment. Concentrate on organizing the energy orbits of your entire body before connecting the quadriceps muscles with an outside resistance. In this way, your whole being will be brought forward as an aligned and cohesive source of creative power.

Strength: Crushing Joints

The quadriceps muscles are responsible for the forward extension of the leg from the knee joints and assist in lifting the thigh upward from the hip joints. The quadriceps muscles' tremendous execution of force can overload the knee joints if the relationship between the action and counter-action isn't first in place. Balanced attention between energy forces sets up a safe and strong alignment that grants safety and freedom of movement. Be resolved in connecting to the resistance from the belly of your quadriceps muscles before you begin movement. This resolve ensures that you are in the muscles rather than in the joints and enables your quadriceps' force to freely support the energetic stretch of your energy centers.

Meditation: Anger

Moving ahead in life requires a series of decisions. Decisions can be judged as right or wrong, good or bad, acceptable or unacceptable. The dread of judgment or the anger accompanying a mistake can cause you to be tentative in your forward movement, yet without forward movement your commitment to life is undermined, distorted, or paralyzed. The commitment to a vision or to moving forward with a dream asks for an organized and balanced mind and body. Enduring the journey's distance to your dream's fruition also asks that you embrace a decisive direction in a relaxed manner. Decisiveness grants you clear intent, focuses your attention, and connects you to your intuition—spirit self. Be mindful of the need to relax in your journey forward, to balance clear intention with genuine connection. Recognize tentative moments as the need to balance decision-making with relaxation, ensuring that your direction forward is connected to your dream's purpose and its destination.

How to Isolate the Quadriceps Muscles

Feel It Contract

It's common to use the lower back muscles when asserting the quadriceps muscles. This could be attributed to the fear of moving forward—hence, tucking your tail under. To avoid this misalignment, it's helpful to experience quadriceps' isolation with your back fully supported. This reference point will help establish the relaxed back of essential alignment at the start of any quadriceps exercise and sets you up to easily recognize when the back muscles engage involuntarily.

Lying Leg Extension Exercise

Exercise: Lie supine, one knee bent with foot flat on the floor and the other leg extended with a soft knee over a tube. Notice the natural curve of the lower back, the degree of space between your waistline and the floor, and where your sacrum bears down into the floor. As you straighten the knee of the extended leg, maintain this lower back curve and weight distribution. With the lower back muscles relaxed and the spine's neutral position implemented, you will feel the weight that was once in the heels' connection to the floor clearly transfer into the quadriceps muscles' isolation.

Feel It Release

The most pertinent aspect of stretching the quadriceps muscle is to keep the legs parallel. Keep the inner thighs against your vertical plumb line or median plane so the knee joints stay aligned and protected. The quadriceps muscles can then release their customary safeguarding of the knees.

Standing Foothold Stretch

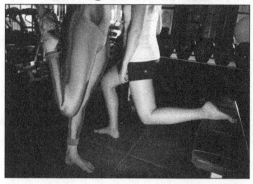

Exercise: Stand with abdominal muscles lifted and inner thighs together. Bend one knee and hold foot in hand or bend the knee and place the foot on a bench behind you. If you are holding the foot in hand, pull the foot up toward your buttock as you lengthen the quadriceps down toward the floor. If you have placed your foot on a bench, bend your supporting knee. Be sure your supporting foot is forward enough so the knee doesn't bend in front of the toes. In either case, you can use a pole or wall to support your balance.

Feel It Fatigue

Quadriceps muscles, due to their unparalleled size, use a lot of energy to motivate. When you exert them, you can quickly feel exhausted. Similarly, when you begin a new project, you can feel overwhelmed by the energy it will take to move it forward and can quickly feel exhausted. This start-up feeling of being overwhelmed isn't due to muscle exhaustion. It's more like beckoning a massive organism into action. Acclimate your quadriceps workout with a light, high repetition set or cardio warm-up. Once the quadriceps muscles are aroused, they can perform with much less defiance. Expect their willingness to ebb and flow with your level of available energy. The moment you feel discomfort with a lack of vitality creeping into your knees or lower back, rest before continuing. This is an indicator that your energy reserve or the quadriceps muscles themselves are too exhausted to continue with integrity. Discomfort with sufficient vitality indicates the need to realign your posture or lessen the outside resistance.

Quadriceps Exercises

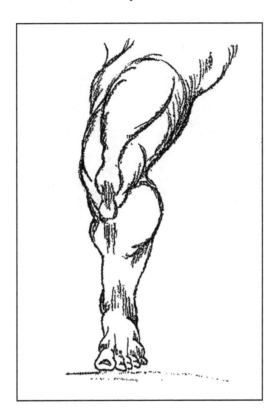

Quadriceps Muscles
Embody
Movement Forward

Seated Straight-Leg Raise

Stool or Floor

Starting Position:

- Sit with supporting knee bent and gushing spring points weighted on floor. Extend working leg in front of you with a soft knee.
- Sit directly on million-dollar point with your body weight on sitz bones.
- Use hands, if needed, to support alignment.
- Lengthen hamstring muscles downward and lift abdominal muscles upward to keep hip flexors soft.
- Commit to maintaining a long waistline.

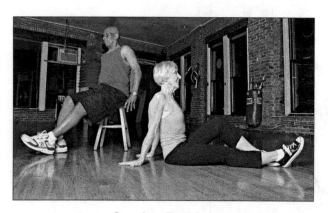

Starting Position

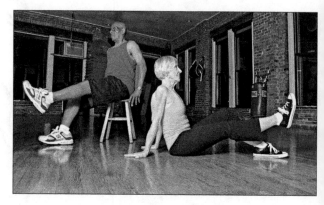

Action/Counter-action

Counter-action:

- Inhale: Hamstring energy elongates under both bent and extended legs. Visualize energy grounding down posterior torso, releasing shoulder blade channels and low back dimples.
- Exhale: Elongate hamstrings' energy beyond foot as leg lifts one to six inches off floor. Keep weight on sitz bones to avoid rolling back onto tailbone.
- Inhale: Keep knee lengthened as leg is returned to starting position. Repeat.
- Be mindful to keep leg reaching forward through a long yet soft knee joint.

Action:

- Inhale: Energy travels up the front of both bent and extended legs, and it lifts anterior torso from abdominals through chest.
- Exhale: Contract quadriceps muscles to lift leg one to six inches off floor. Experience the energy orbit in the legs separate from the energy orbit in the torso, aligning upper and lower bodies independently and permitting the 90-degree fold in the hip joints.
- Inhale: Carry leg back to starting position using quadriceps muscles. Repeat.
- Concentrate on the hip flexors, surrendering into the hip joint so the quadriceps energy can freely cycle around them into the hamstring's counter-active release. Work the belly of the quadriceps muscles as

far forward and away from the hip flexors as possible, keeping the femur bone articulation spacious in the hip joint.

Energy Orbit:

- **Isolated Connection:** Visualize the counter-action before engaging in the action. Counter-action: Cycle energy down the lower back and posterior legs. Action: Orbit energy up through the anterior legs and lower abdomen.
- **Unified Connection:** Counter-action: Extend a corresponding energy orbit down the posterior shoulders and upper back. Action: Orbit energy up abdominals, chest, and anterior shoulders. Energize all eight energy orbits of the pattern through the dan tien. This adjoins active and counter-active energies associated with the whole body in support of a quadriceps-isolated connection.

Active Meditation—Movement Forward:

- Notice how separating the energy orbit into torso and leg halves enables you to relax the hip flexors. Splitting the energy orbit offers added space where they adjoin. The hip flexors' hasty tendency to control needs this added space to thwart their controlling propensity, so the release coming from the hamstring's counter-action can support the quadriceps action instead. Value non-doing, release, and space.
- Guided meditation: Less is more.

Leg Extension

Machine or Dyna-Band

Starting Position:

- Sit in machine with ankles behind crossbar and knees aligned with crossbar's hinge. For a single leg extension with Dyna-Band, sit with supporting foot flat on floor. Tie Dyna-Band into loop, cross-wrap it around foot, and attach it to leg of stool.
- Weight drops through sitz bones. If using machine, relax back into seat back, maintaining natural curve in waistline.
- Commit to keeping crown as lifted as the million-dollar point is grounded.

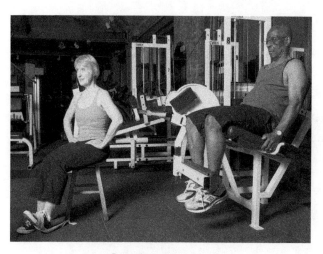

Starting Position

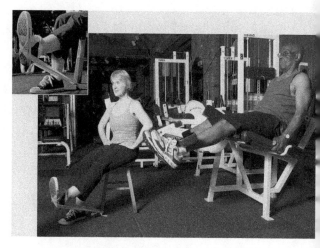

Action/Counter-action

Counter-action:

- Inhale: Elongate energy through posterior leg(s) and under resistance, and visualize energy grounding down posterior torso, releasing shoulder blade channels and low back dimples.
- Exhale: Elongate hamstring energy beyond foot to include resistance as leg(s) extends and sitz bones stay grounded in seat. Feel back of leg pressed into seat with the same degree of force as the ankles are pressed into crossbar. When working with the Dyna-Band, experience the inner thighs connecting on the median plane.
- Inhale: Keep lengthening under resistance as leg(s) is returned to starting position. Repeat.
- Be mindful to stay grounded through sitz bones to avoid tucking at waistline.

Action:

- Inhale: Energy travels up the front of both legs and lifts through anterior torso from abdominals.
- Exhale: Contract quadriceps muscles and extend to a straight leg(s). Experience energy passing through the knee(s) so as not to muscle the joint(s).

- Inhale: Carry resistance back to starting position using quadriceps muscles. Do not rest weight down between repetitions. Repeat.
- Concentrate on keeping quadriceps muscle connected to the resistance throughout the extension, knee bend, and the turnaround points.

Energy Orbit:

- **Isolated Connection:** Visualize the counter-action before engaging in the action. Counter-action: Cycle energy down the lower back and posterior legs. Action: Orbit energy up through the anterior legs and lower abdomen.
- **Unified Connection:** Counter-action: Extend a corresponding energy orbit down the posterior shoulders and upper back. Action: Orbit energy up the abdominals, chest, and anterior shoulders. Energize all eight energy orbits of the pattern through the dan tien. This step adjoins active and counter-active energies associated with the whole body in support of a quadriceps-isolated connection.

Active Meditation—Movement Forward:

- Notice how maintaining a neutral spine and staying weighted on your sitz bones improve your connection with the quadriceps muscles and your ability to determine boundaries that safeguard the knees and lower back. Appreciate your boundaries as a way of knowing yourself.
- Guided meditation: I am relaxed with who I am.

Leg Press

Machine

Starting Position:

- Lie on sled of machine with parallel feet placed on upper portion of foot platform. Keep feet hips' width apart and gushing spring points weighted.
- Hold handgrips, relax head on rest, and keep elbows inside pads.
- Extend legs to a soft knee position and maintain a neutral spine.
- Commit to spine's natural curve at waistline; do not press lower back into sled.

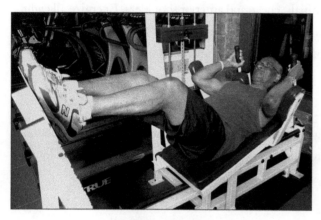
Starting Position

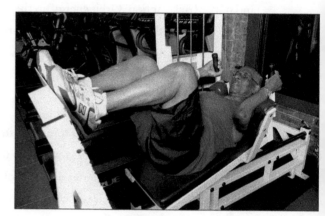
Action/Counter-action

Counter-action:

- Inhale: Relax weight through gushing spring points and push heels gently as knees bend to 90 degrees. Visualize energy grounding down posterior torso, releasing shoulder blade channels and low back dimples.
- Exhale: Continue grounding through posterior torso as your heels press and legs extend to a soft knee. Keep shoulder blades and sacrum equally weighted on sled.
- Inhale: Repeat knee bend. Bend only as far as you can keep sacrum properly weighted on sled. Do not tuck pelvis.
- Be mindful to surrender your torso's bones into the sled. Allow the combined weight of the sled and your body to be carried by the quadriceps and buttocks in this compound exercise.

Action:

- Inhale: Carry the combined weight of body and sled into a 90-degree knee bend and lift energy through anterior torso from abdominals.
- Exhale: Contract quadriceps and buttock muscles to extend legs back to starting position. Keep weight on gushing spring points as you push through heel stirrups.

- Inhale: Use quadriceps muscles to repeat knee bend. Allow a deep fold in hips throughout knee bend by keeping sacrum weighted on sled.
- Concentrate on keeping the hip flexors relaxed and waistline quiet in its natural curve.

Energy Orbit:

- **Isolated Connection:** Visualize the counter-action before engaging in the action. Counter-action: Cycle energy down the lower back and posterior legs. Action: Orbit energy up through the anterior legs and lower abdomen.
- **Unified Connection:** Counter-action: Extend a corresponding energy orbit down the posterior shoulders and upper back. Action: Orbit energy up the abdominals, chest, and anterior shoulders. Energize all eight energy orbits of the pattern through the dan tien. This step adjoins active and counter-active energies associated with the whole body in support of a quadriceps-isolated connection.

Active Meditation—Movement Forward:

- Notice whether the lower back muscles (fear) habitually jump into action the moment there is a significant challenge in the quadriceps muscles (movement forward). Explore your fears and switch off its automatic trigger to the challenges of forward growth.
- Guided meditation: I experience what I fear with curiosity, understanding, and resolve.

Parallel Squat

Wall or Free Standing

Starting Position:

- Stand with back against wall, feet parallel and hips' width apart, weight on gushing spring points, and arms relaxed. Freestanding is done without wall support.
- Keep hips and shoulder blades against wall and position feet forward enough to maintain a 90-degree fold at hip and knee joints. Freestanding will allow hips to travel back to the same degree that the chest travels forward in the knee bends. Keep knees behind toes at all times in both wall and freestanding options.
- Be mindful that waistline position stays neutral in both static and moving squats.

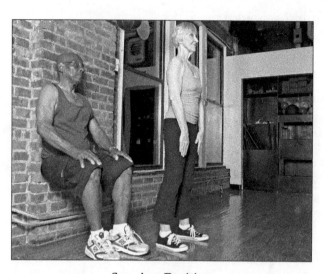

Starting Position

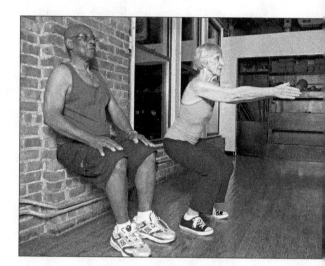

Action/Counter-action

Counter-action:

- Inhale: Lower million-dollar point toward the floor as you bend knees; visualize energy releasing through shoulder blade channels, low back dimples and heel stirrups.
- Exhale: Hold static wall squat for thirty seconds, breathing naturally and keeping spine neutral, then return to starting position. Keep spine relaxed through freestanding squat repetitions; inhale as you bend and exhale as you extend returning million-dollar point between anklebones.
- Inhale: In freestanding option, hips and knees are repeatedly bent; hips travel back while million-dollar point stays directed toward the floor behind feet.
- Commit to million-dollar point facing downward in wall and freestanding options.

Action:

- Inhale: Carry your body down to a 90-degree bend in hips and knees, and lift energy through anterior torso from abdominals.
- Exhale: Maintain a constant contraction up through quadriceps muscles and down through buttock muscles to carry out thirty-second hold or repetitions.

- Inhale: In freestanding option, repeat knee bend, keeping abdominals lifting torso weight out of hips to avoid misusing the hip flexors.
- Concentrate on lifting through the pubic bone and dropping through the tailbone to keep million-dollar point properly aligned with floor.

Energy Orbit:

- **Isolated Connection:** Visualize the counter-action before engaging in the action. *Counter-action:* Cycle energy down the lower back and posterior legs. *Action:* Orbit energy up through the anterior legs and lower abdomen.
- **Unified Connection:** *Counter-action:* Extend a corresponding energy orbit down the posterior shoulders and upper back. *Action:* Orbit energy up the abdominals, chest, and anterior shoulders. Energize all eight energy orbits of the pattern through the dan tien. This step adjoins active and counter-active energies associated with the whole body in support of a quadriceps-isolated connection.

Active Meditation—Movement Forward:

- Notice how lifting from your abdominal muscles (spirit self) connects you to your vitality, while a lack of abdominal lift ties you to the energy expenditure being used up in your leg's effort. Experience the vitality of moving ahead in life from your spirit self.
- Guided meditation: I choose vitality.

BodyLogos Psyche-Muscular Observations for Quadriceps Muscles

Here are examples of how to interpret mind-body expressions.

Posture: Although the quadriceps muscles are extraordinarily powerful, out of habit or urgency other muscles groups can come in to assist.

🛑 Tucking the buttocks under. This takes the abdominal support (spirit self) out of the exercise and gives the lower back (fear) the supporting role.

🌀 This employment of the lower back suggests a fear of moving forward in life. When extending the legs, be attentive that the waistline doesn't move when the knees bend. Experience the sitz bones being grounded and the million-dollar point facing downward into the seat or floor as you bend and straighten your knees. Experience a sense of relaxed self-assurance as your lower back releases into its natural arch and your abdominal muscles are reignited. As you surrender the fear of moving ahead and connect to what inspires you, you are actively manifesting your dreams. Envision your future.

Size: The large muscles of the quadriceps can overexert themselves, creating a movement of momentum rather than a deliberate action.

🛑 Controlling movement from your knees leads to joint breakdown. To maintain control, move slowly. Experience the hamstring muscle's energetic scoop under the outside resistance and its weight in the quadriceps muscles before you start moving, and continue to carry the resistance from this established connection point throughout the set. Overexerting the movement places a great deal of pressure on your knees and signifies an urgency to get somewhere other than where you are.

🌀 You can be taken aback when experiencing the significant resistance the quadriceps can handle and the effort needed to move the resistance. You can become unwilling to experience the hard work and instead throw the weight around. Rather than avoiding an experience of hard work, relax into it and feel it build a sense of personal empowerment and self-possession. Meditate on what you want to do with this personal power.

Ability: Sometimes sensitivity in the surrounding joints of a muscle prevents you from performing an exercise.

When knee pain cries out, stop moving forward in an exercise. Muscular tension, when in excess, will adversely affect the sinews (ligaments and tendons within joints). The knees, in particular, are irritated by the fear that lives in the lower back because your pelvis alignment is tested when challenging the legs. When up against this kind of habitual holding pattern, be very gentle with yourself. You are experiencing a deep-seated uncertainty. Internal tension causing chronic pain is a congestion of your own life force, a powerful opponent indeed.

Keep weight light or work without any resistance, move slowly, and listen to your knees' relationship with forward movement. Work within a pain-free range and meditate on a pain-free life. Send love and appreciation to your quadriceps for all the ways they have moved you forward successfully. Visualize a life you're not afraid of, enjoy the feeling of belonging, and feel nurtured by being curious about your body's cry. Notice what you are contemplating when the pain subsides and work to create that feeling in your life.

Meet the Models

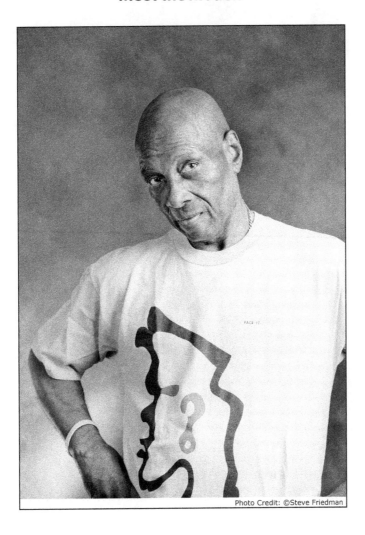

Clinton Alexander

After retiring as a dental technician at the young age of seventy-five, Clinton decided to come indoors from those seasonal pickup basketball games in the park to start a year-round strength-training program. "I'm from the Caribbean and have always preferred warm weather, so exercising inside during the winter months suited me well." Clinton started out playing soccer as a boy in Grenada and evolved into a basketball player who now plays for the New York City Old-Timers League. "Besides keeping my body operating at its highest level, strength training has brought an interesting focus into my life." Personal exercise for the well-being of his body versus athletic exercise for the well-being of his team has developed an integrated and meditative experience. As a young man, Clinton learned the importance of exercising to keep the body in shape; as a well-seasoned man, his workouts remind him that the mind and body are always operating as one.

Lesson 11
Suspending Judgment Energy Pattern: Hamstrings

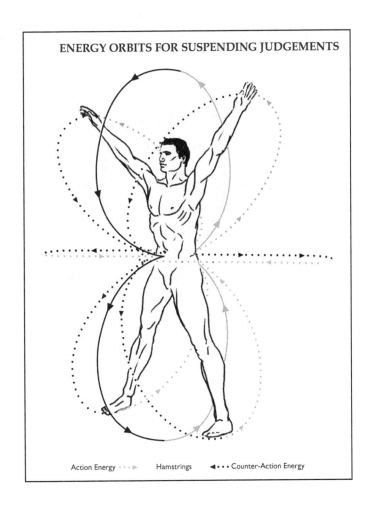

Leaning across the dinner table to clear the last plate gives you the feeling of the "suspending judgment" energy pattern. Your posterior body is stretching upward following your arm's forward reach, leaning your body's weight downward onto your abdominal center. It can feel as if you're falling forward onto the table if not for your abdominal strength catching your body's forward incline.

This downward force through the abdomen is atypical to its customary upward lift, giving your abdominal muscles (spirit self) a chance to connect to the earth rather than to the sky. This movement propels you forward from behind, suspending forward thinking and placing you in a state of presence for reflection and contemplation. Suspending judgment energy will hurl your weight forward for running fast or walking uphill since it provokes your body to fall forward. When maintaining essential alignment, however, the forward propulsion plunges straight down through the anterior body like a dropped object. This grounded halt places you in this very moment and is useful for writing and meditation practice.

Suspending Judgment—Standing Prayer and Active Meditation
mindthebody.bodylogos.com/video14
(abbreviated description)

To get the sensation of suspending judgment, stand with your feet hips' width apart in neutral alignment; start with your weight on your heels. Clasp hands in front of pelvis and bow your head forward. Experience the forward weight of your head pulling your neck up and out of the spinal column as you would imagine an arch of water spouting from a fountain. Take a few deep breaths in this position and relax your head weight. Feel how your mind and body slow down and a reverence for the present moment unfolds. Now, rock your weight forward onto the gushing spring points. You can imagine the weight adjustment feeling like a ski jumper leaning over his or her ski tips. Your need to move ahead is replaced with a need to lean into your center while experiencing the upward rush that is behind you. Allow this reverence to expand into gratitude for where you now stand.

Hamstring exercises are the only suspending judgment isolation of the body. They are the only muscle group that moves you upward and backward in space by shooting your energy up the back of the body and actively decompressing the fear and protection held in your lower and upper back muscles. With fearful protection diminished, the energy that orbits down the front of the body softly connects to your abdominal energy center (spirit self) and opens your hip flexors (control), allowing new reference points and conclusions to unfold from your past experiences.

Practice Change

Henna tattoo of the **Wood** of a cherry blossom branch

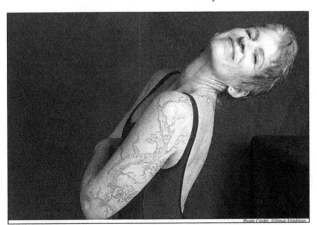

Like **Wood**,
Grow to express your beauty into being.
How do you share your spirit
In nondoing ways?
How do you infuse your essence
Into the things you do?

Suspending Judgment
Is knowing you are learning about your self
And your relationship with life;
Beauty is realized into being.

Suspending Judgment Energy Pattern as It Relates to the Hamstring Muscles

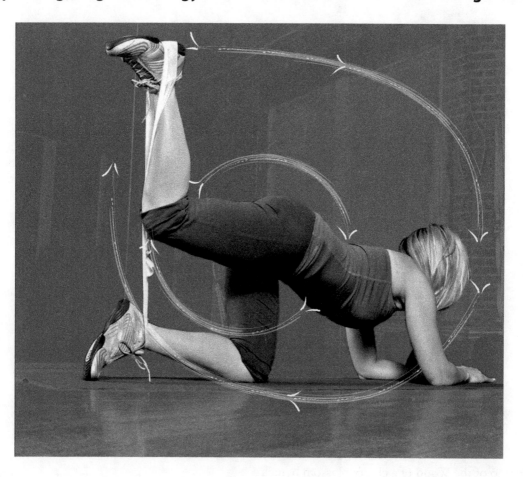

Visualize this energy pattern supporting all hamstring isolations.

Introduction to Hamstring Muscles

Theory of Yin and Yang

Yang: Active Muscle Group

Hamstring Muscles:
- o   Semimembranosus
- o   Semitendinosus
- o   Biceps Femoris

Yin: Counter-active Muscle Group

Quadriceps Muscles:
- o   Rectus Femoris
- o   Vastus Lateralis
- o   Vastus Intermedius
- o   Vastus Medialis
- o   Sartorius

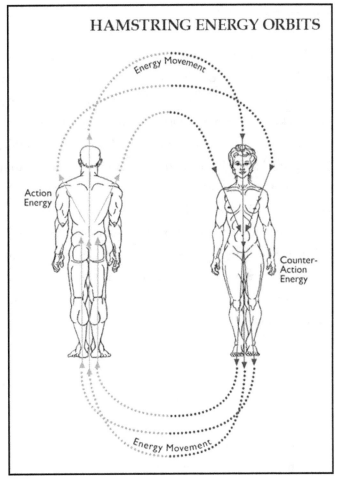

Imagine being a ski jumper. You can actually see the ski jumper leaning forward onto his or her abdominal strength and overriding his or her anterior leg support while simultaneously aligning his or her—spinal column, neck, and head—propelling the posterior body like a shooting arrow. The forward lean of the anterior body sends energy downward, while the energy of the posterior body is shooting upward, accelerating the ski jumper aerodynamically through the air. Contracting the hamstring muscles (action) instigates this same forward lean and propulsion, causing the quadriceps muscles (counter-action) to elongate. Commit to keeping energy centers aligned, maintaining an elongated spine and neck, and staying connected to the abdominals' stability as you release the grab of your iliopsoas muscles while in this energy orbit.

Action: Movement Backward

As you sculpt your hamstring muscles, you can consciously use their backward movement to sculpt personal integrity into your present and future actions. Reflect objectively on your past. Recognize behaviors and thoughts based on mindfulness versus behaviors and thoughts based on reactions. Contemplate your own truth as well as the truths of others. Notice how your beliefs have contributed to the outcome of your experiences. Feel empowered by the influence you have on the direction of your life, whether learned through positive or negative outcomes. Use your reflection to see who you have been, the way you have influenced others, and when you have felt most authentic.

Counter-action: Movement Forward

When contracting the hamstring muscles, you can also meditate on the expanding counter-action of the quadriceps muscles. Quadriceps muscles are highly used but not necessarily highly managed. Aligning the forward enthusiasm of your quadriceps muscles with your hamstrings' reflective nature helps clarify your next focus of attention. Knowing where you want to go in your future motivates your will to integrate and make peace with the aspects of your past that keep you from getting there. Rather than continuing to resent your bygone stories, you become curious about how your history can and has prepared you for your next journey.

Five-Element Theory
Spring, Crushing Joints, Anger

Connection: Spring

Turning over and irrigating spring soil reminds you of how the nutrients from last year's plantings lay the foundation for this year's planting. Returning to your roots regenerates, informs, and adjusts your future; these backward steps can create dynamic change in your forward steps. Hamstring muscles are responsible for moving you backward in space, a metaphor for moving backward in time. Reflecting back on the past can give you reference points to measure growth, assemble learned information, and review the beliefs forming your present perspectives about living. Reflection can also cause you to reignite and transform the regret from transgressions of the past. To support the open-minded outlook needed to reassess past actions, your movement needs to be connected to the essential intelligence of your dan tien. To allow a different response to the same mundane stimuli requires deliberate support from the abdominals (spirit self) and release of the fear, which is easily provoked by a leg challenge, living in the lower back muscles. Rather than attacking movement backward, as can happen when affronted with the past, concentrate on slowly connecting the hamstring muscles to the outside resistance with a quiet spine (central nervous system) and awakened abdominal center (spirit self). Create the change you want to see in your life first in your body.

Strength: Crushing Joints

The hamstring muscles' crushing qualities are fully responsible for flexing the knee joints and partially responsible for directing the legs backward from the hip joints. Setting the energy orbit into motion before the hamstring muscles connect to resistance keeps your experience out of the knee joints and in the belly of the hamstring muscles. Hamstring muscles stop the forward propulsion of life, giving you pause to connect in real time. The past becomes a compendium of lived experiences that have developed you toward personal responsibility or blame. Where the former supports growth, the latter contests it. When working the hamstring muscles, be resolved in appreciating each experience before moving on. This step will lead to appreciating the reality of life.

Meditation: Anger

Moving backward can feel irritating. It can spur on the concern of being left behind or having taken the wrong step forward. To neutralize these responses, be aware of your quadriceps muscles releasing as your hamstring muscles contract, reversing your energy's often-automatic forward drive. This energy shift releases expectations about the future so you can first find peace with the past and present moments. Be mindful of the quadriceps muscles' submission and let time stand still for the present moment to unfold. Recognize how the past has prepared you for this moment in time and realize the purpose of its unfolding. Embody the past and the future as a metaphysical tale teaching you about the richness of presence. Explore the universal purposefulness that has formed your life.

How to Isolate the Hamstring Muscles

Feel It Contract

Left to their own devices, the hamstring muscles will often bring the lower back (fear) and iliopsoas (control) in to help them when challenged. This tendency for the hamstrings to share responsibility or split off from their reflective nature is parallel with the challenge to stay connected within yourself when revisiting past hardships. Therefore, it's important to have a clear reference of what the hamstring muscles feel like as an isolation. You can then practice staying connected inwardly with the hamstrings (meditating on movement backward), while they stay connected with the outside resistance—the life challenge being reflected on.

Prone Knee Bend with Tube Exercise

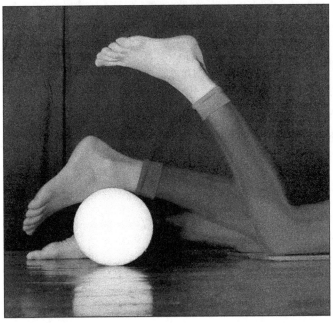

Exercise: Lie prone with one ankle resting over a tube. Notice the length in your lower back and openness in the front bend of your hip joints (iliopsoas). Relax the weight of your hip bones and knees equally into the floor. Slowly fold the bent knee further by asking the bottom of the foot to press toward the sky. As your hamstring muscle leads your movement, become aware of the tendency to engage the iliopsoas and lower back muscles, causing the knee to press into the floor and hip bones to release away from the floor. Encourage the hamstrings to stay connected by keeping the hip bones and knees connected to the floor. Return the leg to its starting position. Repeat until there is no extraneous involvement.

Feel It Release

Depending on the flexibility of your tendons versus your muscles, you could experience a hamstring stretch in the knee or hip joints rather than in the belly of the hamstring muscles. This misplaced stretch creates overly stretched joints and a decrease of flexibility and muscular strength. When a stretch is unable to penetrate a muscle, it limits the degree of accessible strength in that muscle.

Single-Leg Hamstring Stretch with Flexed Foot

Exercise: Sit tall on million-dollar point, extending one leg forward with a flexed foot. Place the center of a Dyna-Band at the ball of your foot, holding the Dyna-Band ends tight enough to enforce a relaxed flexion in the ankle. Keeping your extended leg straight, pull the Dyna-Band toward your belly button while drawing the belly button toward the Dyna-Band. This step elongates the spine, allowing the crown center and the million-dollar point to reach apart. It's often necessary to stretch through the upper calves' tightness before you can penetrate the belly of the hamstring muscles. Hold for fifteen to thirty seconds. Release and repeat several times. This can also be done while standing without a Dyna-Band.

Feel It Fatigue

Because hamstring muscles don't like to work alone, it's advisable to start slow and with moderate or light weight to develop their independence. Hamstring muscles are sensitive yet tenacious in nature. As they fatigue, they cry out; but with a gentle approach, they are given what they need to stay engaged for longer and longer intervals.

Hamstring Exercises

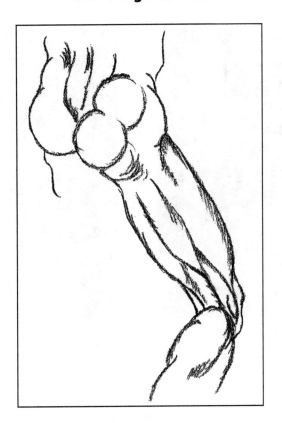

Hamstring Muscles
Embody
Movement Backward

Seated Leg Curl

Machine

Starting Position:

- Sit on machine with knees aligned at crossbar axis and ankles placed on crossbar. Slide leg brace down tightly over thighs.
- Hold handgrips and lean back into seat back, maintaining the natural arch of the waistline.
- Commit to relaxing body weight down through million-dollar point.

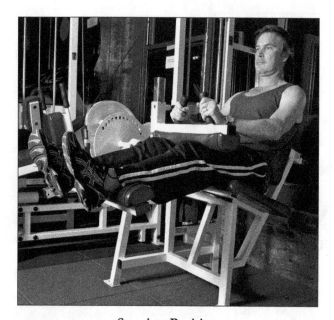
Starting Position

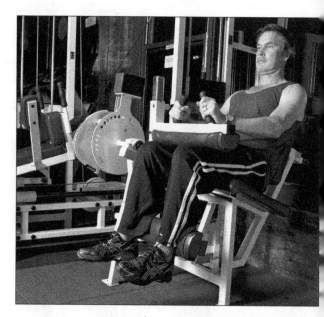
Action/Counter-action

Counter-action:

- Inhale: Lengthen energy away from seat through quadriceps and relax energy downward toward seat through chest and upper abdominals.
- Exhale: As knees are folded into a 90-degree flexion, direct your anterior leg energy outward. Secure your weight in the seat through the anterior torso's descending energy. Notice how separating the energy orbit into upper and lower body divisions gives you more stability.
- Inhale: Keep quadriceps' energy lengthening away from iliopsoas as legs are extended back to starting position. Repeat.
- Be mindful to ground your body's weight through your anterior torso's descending force.

Action:

- Inhale: Visualize energy lifting up posterior legs toward sitz bones while simultaneously elongating upper back up through occipital hollows.
- Exhale: Contract hamstring muscles to bend knees into a 90-degree flexion. Maintain natural curve of lower back. No tucking under or tipping back of tailbone.

- Inhale: Carry resistance back to starting position using hamstring muscles. Don't rest weight down between repetitions. Repeat.
- Concentrate on keeping iliopsoas relaxed in their folded position.

Energy Orbit:

- **Isolated Connection:** Visualize the counter-action before engaging in the action. Counter-action: Cycle energy down the low abdomen, iliopsoas, and anterior legs. Action: Orbit energy up the posterior legs and lower back.
- **Unified Connection:** Counter-action: Extend a corresponding energy orbit down the anterior shoulders, chest, and upper abdominals. Action: Orbit energy up back and posterior shoulders. Energize all eight energy orbits of the pattern through the dan tien. This step adjoins active and counter-active energies associated with the whole body in support of a hamstring-isolated connection.

Active Meditation—Movement Back:

- Notice how much grounding is needed to isolate the hamstring muscles and absolve the lower back of any input. Explore what the hamstrings are capable of on their own so you can develop from there.
- Guided meditation: Past choices aren't to be judged right or wrong—they are to show what has formed you.

Hydrant Hamstring Curl

Dyna-Band

Starting Position:

- Tie Dyna-Band into a loop and wrap around supporting ankle and working heel with a light-to-moderate intensity.
- Align elbows with shoulders and supporting knee with hip joint. Maintain a neutral spine by relaxing the heart downward between shoulders and lifting the abdominals upward to meet the coronal plane or spine.
- Lift extended working leg no higher than hip level.
- Commit to chosen height of working knee throughout exercise.

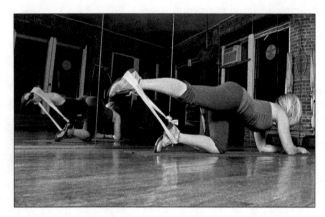
Starting Position

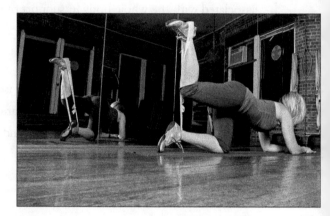
Action/Counter-action

Counter-action:

- Inhale: Lengthen energy through anterior torso and both legs. Energy will scoop under Dyna-Band attachment at working leg's heel.
- Exhale: The iliopsoas and quadriceps lengthen away from abdominals as the knee is folded to a 90-degree flexion.
- Inhale: Keep weight equally placed on elbows and knee as leg is returned to starting position. Repeat.
- Be mindful to connect your abdominal support to the weight of your torso, the working leg, and the outside resistance.

Action:

- Inhale: Energy travels up the back of both legs and continues through back, neck, and head.
- Exhale: Contract working leg's hamstrings and bend knee to a 90-degree flexion. Keep both inner thighs against body's medial plane to maintain a parallel position.
- Inhale: Control Dyna-Band with hamstrings and return to starting position. Repeat.
- Concentrate on connecting the belly of your hamstring muscles to the outside resistance rather than to the sinews of your knee joint.

Energy Orbit:

- **Isolated Connection:** Visualize the counter-action before engaging in the action. Counter-action: Cycle energy down the lower abdomen, iliopsoas, and anterior legs. Action: Orbit energy up the posterior legs and lower back.
- **Unified Connection:** Counter-action: Extend a corresponding energy orbit down the anterior shoulders, chest, and upper abdominals. Action: Orbit energy up back and posterior shoulders. Energize all eight energy orbits of the pattern through the dan tien. This step adjoins active and counter-active energies associated with the whole body in support of a hamstring-isolated connection.

Active Meditation—Movement Back:

- Notice how your attention can flip from supporting your alignment's integrity to connecting with an outside resistance. Strive to draw the outside resistance into your alignment integrity.
- Guided meditation: Connecting with another's integrity enables me to reevaluate my integrity.

Standing Hamstring Curl

Dyna-Band

Starting Position:

- Hook ankle of working leg through a tied Dyna-Band loop and stand on loose end of Dyna-Band with supporting leg. Create a light-to-moderate intensity. No band use is also an option, allowing you to focus intently on pelvis placement.
- Squeeze inner thighs to keep knees together and slightly bent. Place foot of working leg behind you.
- Position hips and shoulders square to the wall in front of you.
- Commit to keeping working foot behind the body throughout the exercise repetitions.

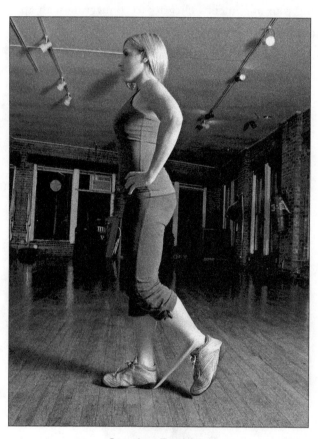

Starting Position

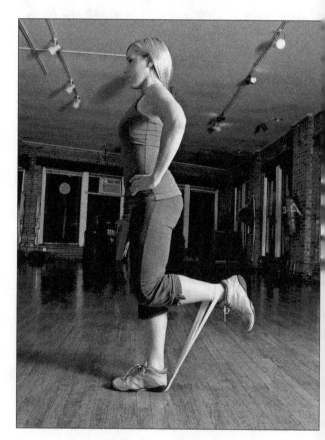

Action/Counter-action

Counter-action:

- Inhale: Lengthen energy down anterior torso, iliopsoas, and anterior legs. Feel as if you are scooping under Dyna-Band attachment at working ankle.
- Exhale: Lengthen quadriceps away from abdominals as knee is folded toward a 90-degree flexion. Keep body weight on gushing spring point with heel stirrup pressed, and don't bend at hips or waist.
- Inhale: As working leg is returned to starting position, keep gushing spring/heel stirrup marriage active on supporting side. Hold rail or bar if needed for balance. Repeat and change sides.
- Be mindful to keep sternum aligned above pubic bone on the anterior plane.

Action:

- Inhale: Energy travels up posterior legs and continues up back, neck, and head.
- Exhale: Contract working leg's hamstring and bend knee to a 90-degree flexion or less. Keep both inner thighs against body's medial plane to maintain a parallel position.
- Inhale: Control Dyna-Band using hamstring muscles and return to starting position. Repeat and change sides.
- Concentrate on keeping iliopsoas muscle elongated through hip joint and connecting the hamstrings' force with the outside resistance behind you on the posterior plane.

Energy Orbit:

- **Isolated Connection:** Visualize the counter-action before engaging in the action. Counter-action: Cycle energy down the lower abdomen, iliopsoas, and anterior legs. Action: Orbit energy up the posterior legs and lower back.
- **Unified Connection:** Counter-action: Extend a corresponding energy orbit down the anterior shoulders, chest, and upper abdominal. Action: Orbit energy up back and posterior shoulders. Energize all eight energy orbits of the pattern through the dan tien. This step adjoins active and counter-active energies associated with the whole body in support of a hamstring-isolated connection.

Active Meditation—Movement Back:

- Notice how grounding down through the abdominal muscles connects you inward while the upward extension of the spine propels you outward.
- Guided meditation: I am balanced.

Ball Squeeze

Gymnastic Ball

Starting Position:

- Lie supine with legs hips' width apart and resting on gymnastic ball. Choose a ball size that allows knee position to be at 90 degrees.
- Relax the body onto floor and ball with a neutral spine (natural arch at waist).
- Commit to shoulder blades and sacrum being connected to floor.

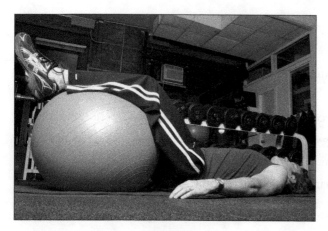

Starting Position

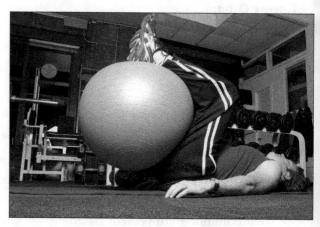

Action/Counter-action

Counter-action:

- Inhale: Lengthen energy down anterior torso, iliopsoas, and anterior legs.
- Exhale: As the ball is raised slightly off the floor, relax quadriceps and hip flexors downward. Hold ten to thirty seconds. Don't engage hip flexors.
- Inhale: Maintain ease in iliopsoas and quadriceps as the legs and ball return to starting position. Repeat.
- Be mindful to place axis of movement in hip joints without muscling from the hip joint.

Action:

- Inhale: Energy travels up posterior legs and continues up back, neck, and head.
- Exhale: Contract hamstrings to lift ball from the floor by directing heels through ball toward breasts, keeping hip joint spacious. Hold position for ten to thirty seconds.
- Inhale: Return ball to starting position. Repeat.
- Concentrate on pulling the outside resistance toward your heart center.

Energy Orbit:

- **Isolated Connection:** Visualize the counter-action before engaging in the action. Counter-action: Cycle energy down the low abdomen, iliopsoas, and anterior legs. Action: Orbit energy up the posterior legs and lower back.
- **Unified Connection:** Counter-action: Extend a corresponding energy orbit down the anterior shoulders, chest, and upper abdominal. Action: Orbit energy up back and posterior shoulders. Energize all eight energy orbits of the pattern through the dan tien. This action adjoins active and counter-active energies associated with the whole body in support of a hamstring-isolated connection.

Active Meditation—Movement Back:

- Notice that pulling resistance inward when abdominal energy is descending rather than ascending feels as if you're moving closer to the outside resistance rather than the resistance moving closer to you. Experience your hamstrings drawing your body's alignment into the outside resistance—drawing the higher vibration of your zhong heart center into your dan tien energy center (spirit self).
- Guided meditation: As I connect with life, I connect with heart.

BodyLogos Psyche-Muscular Observations for Hamstring Muscles

Here are examples of how to interpret mind-body expressions.

Coordination: Moving the legs backward is out of your range of vision, and you can become confused about where you are in space.

🛑 If you're more focused on your movement's destination than on the muscles getting you there, this focus causes you to grasp for whatever muscle or joints will get you "there" rather than being present in a deliberate journey of awakening. This shortcut shows a concern about appearing inept or weak. When you try to make a movement into a predetermined idea, you are creating an outcome rather than an actual arrival. Arriving involves exploring—a learning that unfolds. Know your intention and understand your range of motion; then let the combined arrival of you with the resistance be the exploration. Allow your movement to teach you.

Mind your alignment. A clean hamstring connection moves energy upward toward the buttock muscles, whose psyche-muscular comfort supports you in experiencing greater ease when asked to move backward in time and space. Reflecting through the uncertainties of your past can then offer a promising outcome. Meditate on actually creating connection and peace with your passing movement—each moment of movement as it passes. Experience appreciation where there was none, remorse where there needs some, and compassion for everyone. Feel how much more poise you have when you are consciously connected to your life and its movement.

Posture: When moving the legs backward, the tendency to overcompensate forward with your torso is high.

🛑 If you aren't stabilizing your torso's uprightness, stop and realign. A hamstring challenge descends energy through the anterior body, whereby the abdominals can inadvertently fall forward and cause skeletal alignment to collapse. Maintaining the ascending force through the posterior torso is what keeps the abdominals in their optimal placement to support the skeleton. The failure to stay uplifted through the back (fear and protection) suggests the inability to stay composed when reflecting on the past, since it awakens unresolved fears.

Keep your intention on maintaining essential alignment—your authenticity. Surrender all judgments until you feel connected to actual feelings as opposed to the resistance to feelings. As you move through the exercise, surrender all expectations in regard to your performance. Lower the weight and move smaller or slower. Appreciate how lifting out of fear-based judgments grants you an experience of personal fulfillment. Recognize what you have accomplished with a situation or your life so far.

Enjoyment: Left to your own devices, you wouldn't be choosing a hamstring exercise, but your trainer suggests it's good for you, and you agree, so you comply.

STOP Your hamstrings feel unenthusiastic. Something inside is screaming, "No." This signifies an abrupt refusal to reflect back on something currently unnerving you in life. Your past is actively being triggered and brought into light in the present.

Greet your hamstrings with the same care and concern you would like to be greeted with when visiting your past. Ask your hamstrings how much they are willing to get involved. Be respectful of their boundaries and appreciate any amount of connection they agree to give. In time, and with encouragement to work out in short easeful intervals, they will again become enthusiastic.

Meet the Models

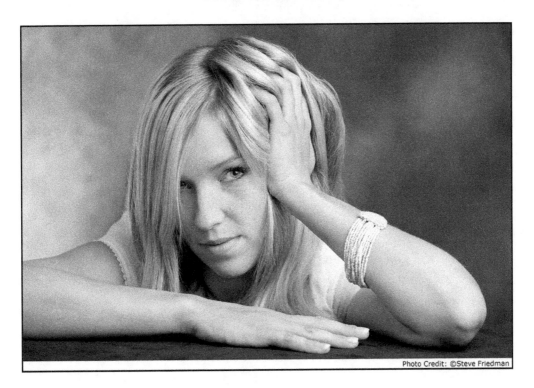

Hanne Torvinen

As a resident of Finland, Hanne's interest in different cultures, language, and travel has her here in the USA as a guest service agent with Hilton. She is a twenty-nine-year-old martial artist, who started strength training in high school to support her practice. She has been training ever since. She says, "I think the repetition of strength training is a great opportunity to be alone with my thoughts and set my mind free." Her stressful thoughts and worries are transformed into confidence. As her only meditation practice, besides chocolate and nature, strength training gives her greater strength and flexibility in mind and body.

Lesson 12

Universal Connection Energy Pattern: Buttocks, Inner Thighs, Calves

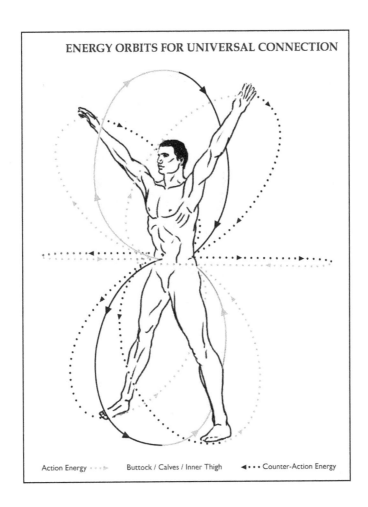

Visualizing the mathematicians' symbol for eternity—∞—as a vertical energy template for the human body conveys the experience of universal connection. This serpent-shaped energy pattern encourages the uncoiling of your essential alignment, making you a human antenna—creating a universal connection between earth and sky. This universal connection aligns your mind and body to create righteous and virtuous change in your life and in the world.

Universal connection energy joins the buttocks' unparalleled power and the inner thighs' connection with the central plumb line with the abdominals' centering strength, creating a core strength that lifts you up against gravity's mighty force. The opposing snakelike energy current of universal connection energy also positions you on your feet properly so your calves' upward rise can align and elongate your spinal column. Use this pattern to revitalize your energy when standing still or strolling, remedy hip discomfort, tackle static mental and physical conditions, organize thought and movement, and foster a sense of balance and well-being.

Universal Connection—Standing Corkscrew and Active Meditation
mindthebody.bodylogos.com/video15
(abbreviated description)

To familiarize you with the universal connection energy pattern, stand with your feet more than hips' width apart and legs turned out. Extend arms straight overhead. Position pelvis so far forward that it nearly lifts your heels off the floor and feel your buttocks engage under your abdominal center. Experience the weight of your shoulder blades snake down through the dan tien to the front of your hips, lengthening the iliopsoas muscles; experience your buttocks' force snake its newfound strength up through the dan tien to uplift your chest. Allow these opposing snakelike forces to reorganize your posture until you feel your neutral alignment unravel its tensions into essential alignment. Allow your attention to neutralize as the details of everyday living are replaced with a larger perspective. See your present life as a preparation for what is to come.

Buttock, calf, and inner-thigh exercises all use the universal connection energy pattern. Buttock exercises reinforce the central plumb line, calf exercises position the body's weight on your feet properly to align that central plumb line, and inner thigh exercises move you into the central plumb line. All three of these muscle isolations encourage your central plumb line to elongate vertically beyond the physical body to connect universally.

The Art of Strength

Practice Change

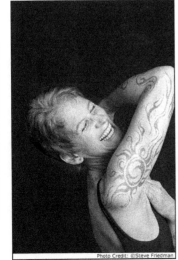

Henna tattoo of the sun's **Fire**

Like **Fire**,
Burn what is stagnant to make room for new life.
What is no longer relevant?
What have you outgrown?

Universal Connection
Is knowing your purpose
And feeling worthy of its fruition.
Success lives in you.

Universal Connection Energy Pattern as It Relates to the Buttock Muscles

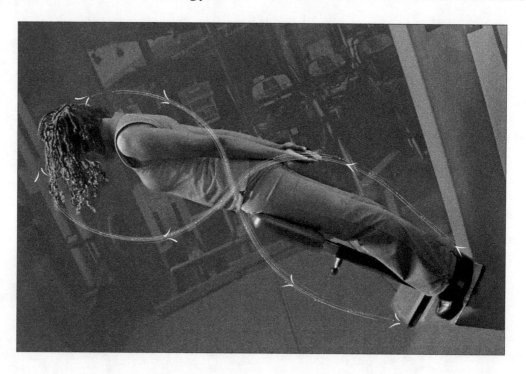

Visualize this energy pattern supporting all buttock isolations.

Introduction to Buttock Muscles

Theory of Yin and Yang

Yang: Active Muscle Group

Buttock Muscles:
- o   Gluteus Maximus
- o   Gluteus Medius
- o   Gluteus Minimus

Yin: Counter-active Muscle Group

Iliopsoas Muscle:
- o   Inferior Aspect or Hip Flexion
- o   Superior Aspect or Low Back

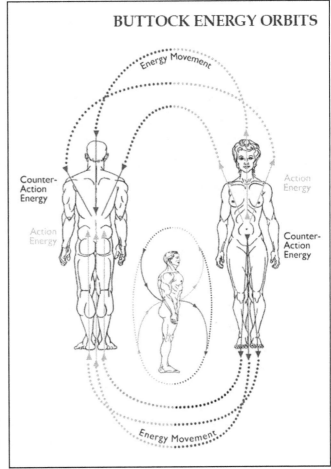

The unparalleled force of your buttock muscles powers your human eternity symbol. The buttock's energy snakes upward through your dan tien and connects to your upper abdominals' strength. This supports the upper back's energy to snake downward through your dan tien and connect to the iliopsoas muscles release. This intersection through your dan tien energy center is due to the snakelike iliopsoas muscles, whose origin connects to the lower vertebrae of the spine; after passing through your body's center, it attaches to the femur between the inner thigh and quadriceps muscles. The iliopsoas muscles, from lower back to hip flexor, releases as your buttock muscles engage. Your energy orbits are committed to preserving supple iliopsoas muscles so the buttock muscles' strength becomes accessible.

Action: Comfort

Padded strength is the offering of the buttock muscles, and with that we are able to find comfort in any life situation. Their unparalleled strength can both move you outward into the world in whichever direction you choose and pad a needed respite when you get there. The buttock muscles animate the seeking of both physical and psychological comfort.

Recognizing that you are intended to be comfortable gives you permission to be so. Discomfort, however, is a guide and motivator for spiritual development. It's the guide toward self-aligning comfort. Discomfort, though seemingly dark by nature, brings light to the ways you interfere with your own inner and outer contentment. Notice that the more involved the buttock muscles are in your workout, the more inwardly serene you become.

Counter-action: Control

When contracting the buttock muscles, you can also meditate on the releasing counter-action of the iliopsoas muscles. The iliopsoas muscle travels from the lower back through the pelvis and anterior hip, attaching at the inner thigh. The iliopsoas muscle ensures that you move ahead and stay upright, a parallel with social pressures to move ahead or outperform a competitor or your own previous performance. Controlling the outcome of your performance can become more important than being comfortable with your performance. The ability to lead from the buttocks allows the iliopsoas muscle to loosen its control, positioning the buttocks' strength in alignment with your abdominal center (your spirit self). Leading from the buttocks-abdominal duo ensures that the iliopsoas muscle can freely and simply align the torso and legs with the dexterous grace they were designed to implement rather than taxing their delicate agility with blind force.

Five-Element Theory
Summer, Pounding Joint, Joy

Connection: Summer

Summer days are the longest days of the year, offering added time and space for a more comfortable rhythm in life. The comfort offered by the buttock muscles has the same nature, offering added fat to rest on and exceptional strength to move from. Whether passive or active, the buttock muscles provide comfort. Without comforts in life, living becomes a task. Without addressing discomforts directly, life becomes a struggle. Just as a summer vacation rejuvenates your life force from a grueling work schedule, balancing your performance strengths with performance respites rejuvenates and restores your comfort in training and working hard. To initiate buttock exercises, concentrate on balancing passive and active aspects of your physical, mental, and emotional comforts.

Strength: Pounding Joints

Your hip joints offer a huge range of mobility, a range that can lead you out of the buttock muscles' domain. "Less is more" is a good motto to follow when challenging the buttocks. When initiating buttock movements, keep the buttocks' muscle belly carrying the challenge rather than stretching the buttock muscles into relinquishing their powerful influence. Be resolved in containing buttock exercises inside the range the buttock muscles can produce, with little to no stretch. In this way, you experience the comfort of self-assurance with every repetition. In contrast, slipping into the full range of motion your hip joints offer collapses you into the lower back and iliopsoas muscle. This outer edge of flexibility doesn't have the stability found in the belly of the buttock muscles. So suddenly fear and control are provoked due to muscle weakness and danger of injury.

Meditation: Joy

The basis of joy comes from living your truth. True joy requires little from the outside world. Well-being, purpose, gratitude, serenity, and peaceful actions account for joyful living. The psyche-muscular component of fear (lower back) and control (iliopsoas) adversely affects the comfort that lives in the buttock region. To keep the buttock muscles' strength (your comfort) leading a movement, maintain supple iliopsoas muscles. Some exercises require a quiet waistline, while others will require a tipped pelvis and rounded waistline. Either way, the iliopsoas muscles can remain pliant. Be mindful of the buttock muscles' core alignment strength; give the weaker lower back and iliopsoas muscles freedom from the unreasonable liability of supporting your alignment. Experience the joy of fearless presence. Support yourself from the buttocks' core strength rather than from the lower back or iliopsoas muscles' reactive tension.

How to Isolate the Buttock Muscles

Feel It Contract

To position the buttock muscles correctly in relationship with the abdominal muscles, you need to pitch the pelvis correctly under the rib cage. Because there is so much room for error at the waistline, a clear understanding of where the pelvis belongs is necessary. This alignment will release the excess tension held in the iliopsoas and lower back muscles, which return the responsibility of supporting your body's weight back to the buttock and abdominal strength.

Forward Body Rock Exercise

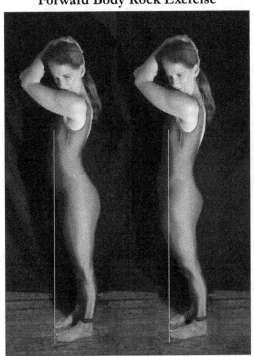

Exercise: Stand with parallel feet hips' width apart and legs straight. Rock your body's weight forward onto the gushing spring points of the feet; feel a downward surrendering of tension from the low back dimples through the heel stirrups and rotate the outer heels slightly inward without changing the feet to access the inner thighs. The lower back continues to lengthen downward without tucking the tailbone between the legs as the buttocks muscles engage under the weight of the torso. This pelvic position will place the million-dollar point directly between the ankle bones and elongate the iliopsoas muscles.

Feel It Release

The choice between operating from the fear in your lower back muscles or the comfort in your buttock muscles is a constant impasse, because they are in constant deliberation regarding your uprightness. Whenever stretching the buttock muscles, you will likely stretch the lower back muscles simultaneously, since they are in such close proximity to each other. The area in which you feel tightness or discomfort will tell you where your inflexibility is rooted and whether fear or comfort is eliciting the unwanted tension. Where too much tightness in either muscle group signifies overuse, lack of sensation would signify the absence of use.

Supine Buttock Release Stretch

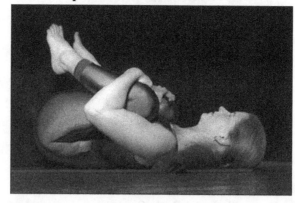

Exercise: Lie supine with knees folded into your chest. Hold at the knees or under the thighs so you can fully relax the hip flexors and thigh muscles. Take a deep breath. As you exhale, pull the knees toward your armpits, allowing the lower back to round into the floor and your tailbone to roll off the floor. Relax the buttock muscles, lower back, and hip flexors as you hold the position ten to thirty seconds. Repeat until your range of movement is easy. Be sure to keep knees separated so you don't squash your internal organs yet within your shoulders' width so you don't crush the hip flexors.

Feel It Fatigue

The buttock muscles with their superior strength don't scream when tired. They ache. As they begin to weaken, the tendency is to employ your lower back muscles for extra power. Rather than employing a fear-based weaker muscle or momentum, it's better to stop, recover, and return to the exercise with a clean connection.

How to Find the Iliopsoas Muscles

Feel It Contract

This is a muscle that generally needs no additional strength training; rather, it needs to surrender. Recognizing its presence is the first step in its retreat.

Iliopsoas Seated Knee Lift

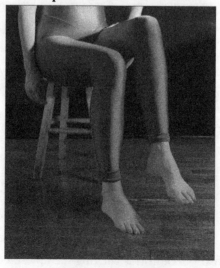

Exercise: Sit erect over million-dollar point and sitz bones with both feet flat on floor. Lift one leg two inches off the floor. Notice the rod-like muscle that flexes in the anterior hip joint. This is the inferior aspect of

the iliopsoas muscle. Notice the involvement in the lower back area. This is the superior aspect of the iliopsoas muscle. Repeat on the other side.

Feel It Release

Take time to expand through the more superficial thigh muscles (quadriceps) to then more gently stretch the internal pelvic muscles (iliopsoas).

Kneeling Butt Tuck Stretch

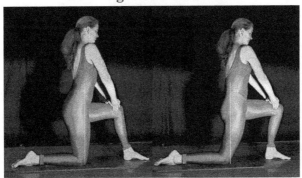

Exercise: Kneel with one knee on the floor under your torso and one foot on the floor in front of you. Rotate the kneeling foot slightly outward, rotating the quadriceps muscles slightly inward. First clench your buttock muscles; this will produce a slight tuck in the pelvis that stretches the more superficial quadriceps muscles and anterior hip flexors. For a deeper stretch that penetrates into the iliopsoas muscle, shift your weight slightly forward until a more penetrating stretch is felt. Hold the stretch until the quadriceps muscles relax and the iliopsoas muscle is fully extended. Release iliopsoas stretch after a few seconds since the muscles easily seize up. Repeat up to three times. Repeat on other side.

Feel It Fatigue

The iliopsoas muscles feel like a tightrope traveling vertically where the legs fold at the anterior hip. They will spasm or lock up when challenged to change, whether through a stretch or an exertion. Treat them gently. Never force an outcome. Rather, tap in with respect and curiosity. Use short stretch sequences.

Buttock Exercises

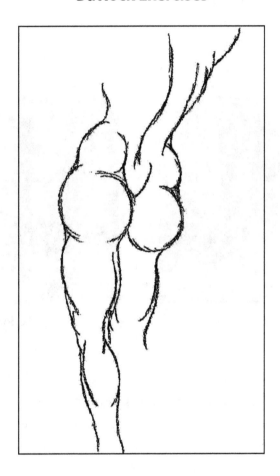

**Buttock Muscles
Embody
Comfort**

Hyperextension

Machine

Starting Position:

- Position feet on hyperextension foot platform hips' width apart. Fold body over pelvis brace so hip bones bypass the pelvis cushion. Relax and elongate into a long, neutral spine. Do not round back.
- Place hands together at lower back.
- Maintaining spinal alignment from million-dollar point to crown center. Gently compress abdominal and buttock muscles inward toward coronal plane.
- Commit to folding from the hips, not the waist.

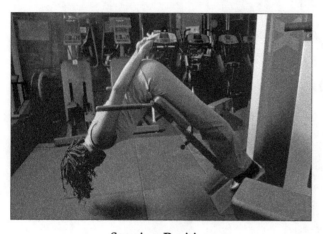

Starting Position

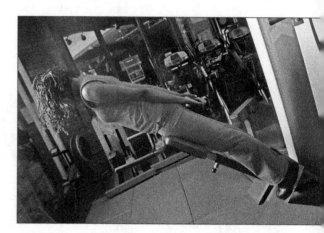

Action/Counter-action

Counter-action:

- Inhale: Visualize energy descending down back, snaking through the dan tien and down anterior legs.
- Exhale: Torso is extended forward and up to align spine on the same plane as legs' position as release of shoulder blades snakes through iliopsoas muscles to the quadriceps muscles.
- Inhale: Maintain length in spine as the hip joints are folded back to starting position. Repeat.
- Be mindful to keep lower back long and undisturbed through movement.

Action:

- Inhale: Connect buttock muscles with the resistance of your body's weight by pressing through your heels.
- Exhale: Contract buttock muscles to lift torso in alignment with legs. Visualize energy ascending up posterior legs and snaking through the dan tien to lift chest. Balance opposing forces to ensure the torso doesn't overextend into an excessive lower back arch.
- Inhale: Use buttock muscles to carry body weight back to starting position. Repeat.
- Concentrate on the buttock-abdominal relationship upholding neutral alignment so you can elongate farther and farther into essential alignment with each repetition.

Energy Orbit:

- **Isolated Connection:** Visualize the counter-action before engaging in the action. Counter-action: Drop energy down shoulder blades and snake it through dan tien and down iliopsoas muscles. Action: Orbit energy up contracted buttocks and snake it through dan tien and up upper abdominals.
- **Unified Connection:** Counter-action: Extend energy orbit down posterior torso, snaking through dan tien and down anterior legs. Action: Orbit energy up posterior legs and buttocks, snaking through dan tien and up anterior torso. Energize all eight energy orbits of the pattern through the dan tien. This adjoins active and counter-active energies associated with the whole body in support of a buttock-isolated connection.

Active Meditation—Comfort:

- Notice how eager the lower back is to replace the buttock muscles. This translates to your fear being quick to replace your comfort. Can comfort replace your fear? Experience comfort as a personal consideration and valid option rather than an extravagance.
- Guided meditation: Comfort is an expression of the self.

Dead Lift

Barbell and Dumbbell

Starting Position:

- Stand with feet hips' width apart, knees slightly bent, and weight on gushing spring points.
- Hold bar shoulder width apart with alternate hand grip—one palm forward and one palm back—or hold dumbbells with both palms back in front of thighs.
- Connect to abdominal center and elongate lower back muscles.
- Commit to hanging arms and resistance as one from the shoulder blades.

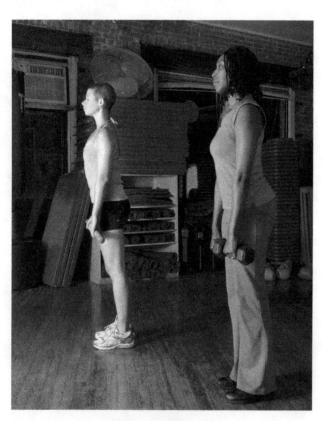

Starting Position

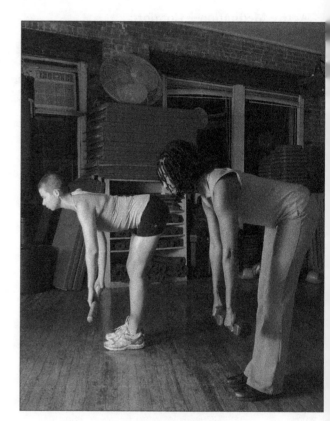

Action/Counter-action

Counter-action:

- Inhale: As hips fold, pubic bone reaches backward by visualizing energy descending down back and snaking through the dan tien and down anterior legs.
- Exhale: Realign pubic bone on anterior plane and lengthen iliopsoas muscles as torso is returned to starting position. Keep body weight on gushing spring points while releasing lower back tension through heel stirrups. Repeat.
- Inhale: Keep outside resistance hung from the shoulder blades in both bent-over and upright positions so you don't disturb shoulder placement.
- Be mindful to keep a long neutral spine from million-dollar point to crown center. Do not round back.

Action:

- Inhale: Fold at hip, creating no more than a 90-degree angle. Visualize energy ascending up backs of legs and buttocks, snaking through the dan tien and up chest.
- Exhale: Contract buttock muscles with the same amount of force that is grounding downward through heel stirrups. Return to starting position as the lower back's length elongates upward through the chest. Repeat.
- Inhale: Use buttock muscles to support body's weight and outside resistance as one.
- Concentrate on maintaining your shoulders' width as the arms' dead weight rotates in the shoulder sockets.

Energy Orbit:

- **Isolated Connection:** Visualize the counter-action before engaging in the action. Counter-action: Drop energy down shoulder blades and snake it through dan tien and down iliopsoas muscles. Action: Orbit energy up contracted buttocks and snake it through dan tien and up upper abdominals.
- **Unified Connection:** Counter-action: Extend energy orbit down posterior torso, snaking through dan tien and down anterior legs. Action: Orbit energy up posterior legs and buttocks, snaking through dan tien and up anterior torso. Energize all eight energy orbits of the pattern through the dan tien. This step adjoins active and counter-active energies associated with the whole body in support of a buttock-isolated connection.

Active Meditation—Comfort:

- Notice how the same uprising of energy that contracts the buttocks (comfort) also opens the chest (smile of truth). Attending to comfort aligns you with your heart. Experience the tenderness of self-love when comforting your own heart.
- Guided meditation: I am trustworthy to nurture my own heart.

Seated Abduction

Machine

Starting Position:

- Sit tall with machine's kneepads rotated outward. Position lateral side of legs against pads.
- Relax quadriceps muscles slightly inward to disengage iliopsoas muscles.
- Connect to abdominal center.
- Commit to keeping iliopsoas muscles relaxed.

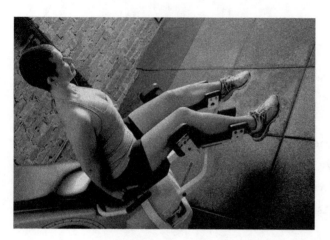

Starting Position

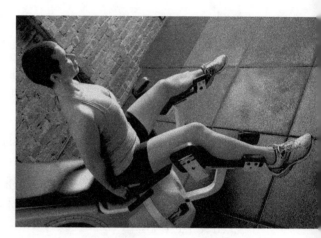

Action/Counter-action

Counter-action:

- Inhale: Visualize energy descending down back of torso, snaking through the dan tien, and continuing down the anterior legs.
- Exhale: Quadriceps lengthen away from iliopsoas as legs are separated, keeping quadriceps relaxed inwardly.
- Inhale: Stay grounded through sitz bones as legs are returned to starting position. Repeat.
- Be mindful to generate your force from the dan tien where the active and counter-active energies cross.

Action:

- Inhale: Visualize energy ascending up posterior legs and buttocks, snaking through the dan tien, and continuing up anterior torso.
- Exhale: Contract buttock muscles and direct heels outwardly to separate legs by directing the upward force of your buttock muscles through the upper abdominals and chest muscles. Don't press from the lateral knees.
- Inhale: Use buttocks to carry weight back to starting position. Repeat.
- Concentrate on keeping torso aligned over million-dollar point. No rocking your body.

Energy Orbit:

- **Isolated Connection:** Visualize the counter-action before engaging in the action. Counter-action: Drop energy down shoulder blades and snake it through dan tien and down iliopsoas muscles. Action: Orbit energy up contracted buttocks and snake it through dan tien and up upper abdominals.
- **Unified Connection:** Counter-action: Extend energy orbit down posterior torso, snaking through dan tien and down anterior legs. Action: Orbit energy up posterior legs and buttocks, snaking through dan tien and up anterior torso. Energize all eight energy orbits of the pattern through the dan tien. This step adjoins active and counter-active energies associated with the whole body in support of a buttock-isolated connection.

Active Meditation—Comfort:

- Notice how the iliopsoas muscles are quick to engage. To disengage them is to let go of control. Allow comfort to take on an unknown form. Explore the unforeseen comforts found in each moment. Expand beyond your expectations of a moment.
- Guided meditation: I am comfortable not knowing.

Sumo Squat

Dumbbell

Starting Position:

- Stand tall with legs rotated outward at hip joints, feet placed wider than hips, and weight on gushing spring points.
- Hold one dumbbell between legs on anterior plane using both hands. Hang arm and dumbbell predominantly from shoulder blades.
- Slightly bend knees to relax lower back and connect to abdominal support.
- Commit to lifting through abdominals and chest to oppose the downward weight of dumbbell through shoulder blades.

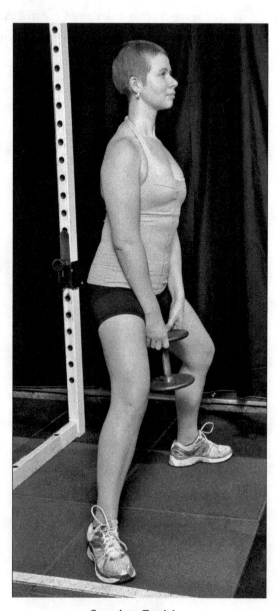

Starting Position

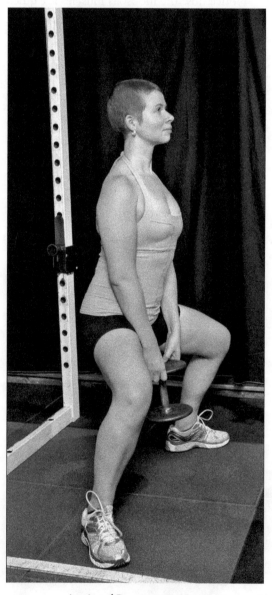

Action/Counter-action

Counter-action:

- Inhale: Visualize energy descending down the shoulder blades, snaking through the dan tien, and continuing down the iliopsoas and quadriceps. Align bending knees over, but not past, second and third toes until knees are approximately at a 90-degree flexion.
- Exhale: Feel the shoulder blades send energy down through the lengthening iliopsoas muscles as legs are extended back to starting position. Keep legs rotated outward at hips in sitting and standing portions of movement. Repeat.
- Inhale: Be sure body's weight drops behind kneecaps in knee bend and refrain from rotating knees forward of big toes. If knee pain occurs, keep range smaller.
- Be mindful to let arms and resistance hang from dropped shoulder blades.

Action:

- Inhale: Visualize energy ascending up posterior legs and buttocks, snaking through the dan tien, and continuing up chest. Lower hips into a turned-out squat, placing pelvis slightly behind coronal plane and chest slightly forward of coronal plane.
- Exhale: Contract buttock muscles to carry dumbbell and torso's united weight back to starting position by connecting the buttocks' upward energy to upper abdominal stability. Repeat.
- Inhale: Keep pelvis above knee level when in the deepest portion of squat and inner thighs always symmetrically relating to your median plane.
- Concentrate on uniting buttock and inner thigh strength with abdominal stability.

Energy Orbit:

- **Isolated Connection:** Visualize the counter-action before engaging in the action. Counter-action: Drop energy down shoulder blades, snaking it through dan tien and down iliopsoas muscles. Action: Orbit energy up contracted buttocks and snake it through dan tien and up upper abdominals.
- **Unified Connection:** Counter-action: Extend energy orbit down posterior torso, snaking through dan tien and down anterior legs. Action: Orbit energy up posterior legs and buttocks, snaking through dan tien and up anterior torso. Energize all eight energy orbits of the pattern through the dan tien. This step adjoins active and counter-active energies associated with the whole body in support of a buttock-isolated connection.

Active Meditation—Comfort:

- Notice how clearly you experience your core strength when you relax your body weight and the resistance into your core support—abdominals, buttocks, and inner thighs.
- Guided meditation: Strength is measured by my ability to relax.

BodyLogos Psyche-Muscular Observations for Buttock Muscles

Here are examples of how to interpret mind-body expressions.

Posture: When unable to maintain alignment through an isolated challenge, the workload is dispersed, and the intended muscle group's involvement is thwarted. This situation makes for a more superficial connection with the outside resistance.

STOP When the natural arch of your lower back is lost, you have lost essential alignment. If the alignment between the upward-reaching sternum and the downward-reaching pelvic bone isn't as dynamic as the resistance you're meeting, your spinal alignment will collapse or become rigid. This is an imbalanced relationship between the chest (smile of truth) and iliopsoas muscles (control). This also suggests a need to control your environment to be comfortable and a reluctance to trust your heart. The result of this mistrust is that the iliopsoas (control) and lower back muscles (fear) have to work harder to handle the challenge, and they consequently develop greater determination than the buttock muscles (comfort). This can be interpreted as "Fear is more revered or more comfortable than comfort itself."

Relaxing the lower back muscles before starting an exercise encourages the iliopsoas muscles to also relax throughout the exercise. Reach the sternum and pelvis bones vertically apart on the anterior plane as you feel your need to control your environment retreat. As your spine and central nervous system relax, your heart begins to lift freely once again. Enjoy the rising energy in your chest's expression as you simultaneously stand in the buttock muscles' unmatched strength. Experience freedom from fear (low back).

Size: The size of movement in an isolated muscle depends on its inherent flexibility and relative strength in relation to the resistance. If you don't connect the isolated muscle to the resistance before moving, you won't be exploring the muscles' flexibility; you will be exploring its associated joint's range of motion.

STOP When you lose the connection to your buttock muscles, pause from the exercise. Although buttock muscles support large, sweeping movements in the body, the core movement occurring in the pelvic area is quite small. When you thrust the pelvis, you are working the quadriceps or lower back or both. The comfort that could be found in the buttocks' strength is lost to an irritated low backache and fatiguing quadriceps.

Focus on the buttock muscles' constant connection to the movement. When you feel the movement shift out of the buttocks, you have gone too far. Limit your range of motion and focus your meditation on less being more. Experience how creating a smaller outer movement gives your inner movement greater command. Recognize comfort as an internal state rather than as an external show.

Enjoyment: If you find certain exercises a waste of time because you feel awkward or uncertain about their movement, you feel awkward or uncertain about the psyche-muscular component they carry.

🛑 Pause when your ability to lead an exercise from the buttock muscles feels inept. Often the relationship with the buttocks is one of apprehension. It may be the strongest muscle of the body, but your relationship with it can be vague.

Work smaller and slower, use lighter resistance, and be more curious about your buttocks' connection to resistance. Try new ways of relating to the buttock muscles through different exercises and approaches; value their quiet support until their strength is realized. When you begin to recognize the buttock muscles as the mega power they are, you can change your awkward uncertainty to purposeful resolve.

Meet the Models

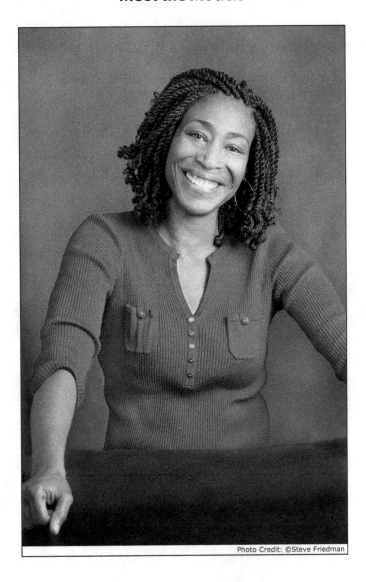

Vivianne Williams Kurutz

Vivianne is founding director of Harlem Center for Healthy Living (HCHL), a one-of-a-kind nonprofit, holistic living center in Harlem, New York. This forty-nine-year-old woman is passionate about being of service in the world and has chosen the devastating effects of lifestyle-related or preventable diseases as her mission. Fitness began so organically for Vivianne that she doesn't even remember its point of origin. Fitness has simply always been part of the flow of her life. She feels the practice of active meditation is an invitation to let go of unnecessary tension in the midst of effort. She says, "Meditation practice facilitates watching the ego and caring for myself in the process." Development of HCHL offers an education about what she inherently understood about health and wellness. Through HCHL classes in healthy cooking, mind-body movement, and ecological or community living, body therapy, individual health coaching, and wellness retreats, Vivianne shares her enthusiasm for living an active, athletic life. To keep her life's natural flow moving, Vivianne reads from the scripture and prays daily.

Universal Connection Energy Pattern as It Relates to the Inner-Thigh Muscles

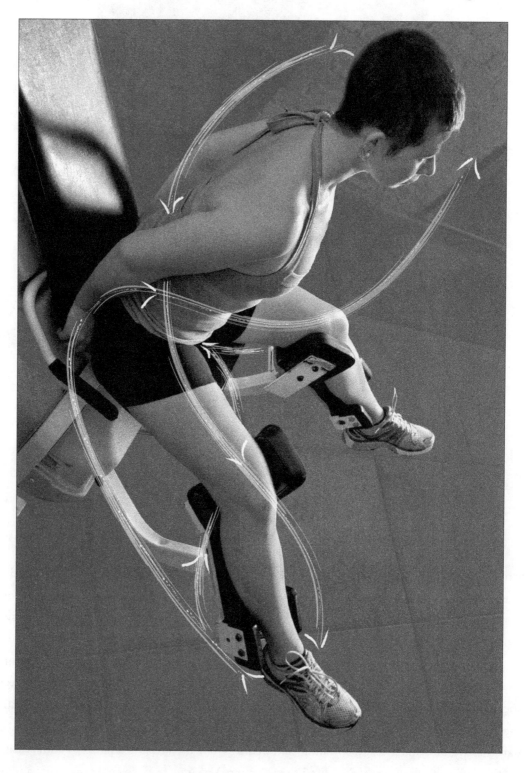

Visualize this energy pattern supporting all inner thigh isolations.

Introduction to Inner-Thigh Muscles

Theory of Yin and Yang

Yang: Active Muscle Group

Inner-Thigh Muscles:
- o Pectineus
- o Adductor Brevis
- o Adductor Longus
- o Adductor Magnus
- o Gracilis

Yin: Counter-active Muscle Group

Inner-Thigh Muscles:
- o Pectineus
- o Adductor Brevis
- o Adductor Longus
- o Adductor Magnus
- o Gracilis

This inward movement lives solely on the coronal plane; coupled with its upward active force, it gives the sensation of an outside resistance being sucked upward through your central plumb line. An inner-thigh contraction (action) provokes a symmetrical reaction from the other inner-thigh (counter-action) to uphold a square pelvis and healthy spine. This symmetrical attachment to the median plane generates an upward lift through the chest as well as a downward release in the lower back and iliopsoas. An action being channeled through your central plumb line, the most central aspect of your body, can feel frighteningly intimate. But releasing the fear-filled tension of the lower back flushes the trepidation around this intimacy away. Commit to flushing out any stagnation in active and counter-action forces before a movement begins for a clean connection with your plumb line, your essential alignment's foundation.

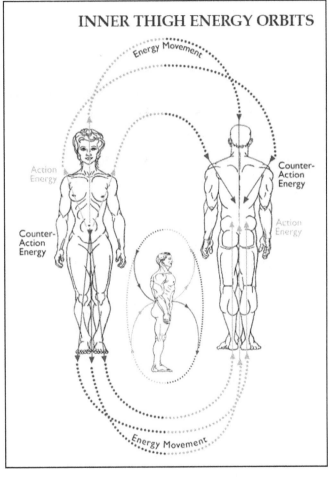

Action: Movement Inward

There is a quiet stillness that accompanies movement inward, a complete cognoscente that isn't associated with movement outward. Allow this quiet completeness to empower your sense of "now" and experience your ability to discern within each moment's "now" as it passes. Allow no need to move ahead of, or change anything about, anyone or anything. You are a witness to life's offerings and constantly deciding on what you would like to connect with—and to what degree. Notice when your inner thighs disconnect from a resistance and let another muscle group replace their connection. Is it the eagerness to move forward (quadriceps muscles), the need to control (iliopsoas muscles), or the fear of seeing yourself (lower back muscles)? Explore leading with the inner thighs and feel yourself being respected.

Counter-action: Movement Inward

When contracting the inner-thigh muscles, you can also meditate on the releasing counter-action of the inner-thigh muscles. That might sound confusing, but as the most medial muscles, the inner thighs are each other's opposing muscles. Their release is experienced as a lengthening, while their contraction is their connection with outside resistance. Their inward movement works closely with the abdominals (spirit self) to maintain both emotional balance and physical stability. As you move inward, appreciate what you have created in yourself. Feel the significance of who you are. Notice how relaxed you can be when considering your own competence and self-reliance. You're recognizing your own voice as the expert of your own experience. Acknowledge how exercising self-respect supports clear discernment inwardly and graceful communication outwardly.

Five-Element Theory
Summer, Pounding Joint, Joy

Connection: Summer

The long days of summer ask for an energized mind and body. The ample light and time to fully express yourself through vocation or recreation can leave you overwhelmed by personal choices or a lack thereof. This is seen in the body when the iliopsoas' and quadriceps' muscles' over-eagerness to control forward movement dominates the subtler sensation of the inner thighs' inward movement and "honor thyself" nature. Relaxing the iliopsoas and quadriceps muscles outwardly and gently rotating the inner thighs inwardly before you step forward connects you to your central plumb line and your sense of self. This alliance to your essential alignment energizes your creative life force. Concentrate on your inner-thigh muscles subduing the eager iliopsoas and quadriceps.

Strength: Pounding Joints

The inner thighs, iliopsoas, quadriceps, hamstrings, or buttock muscles can lead the ball socket joints of the hip and upper legs. The inner-thigh muscles generally have the quietest voice; hence, they require focused attention to be heard. Connecting the inner thighs with an outside resistance is like drawing the outside world into your center by way of the birth channel—pelvic floor. It's an intimate invitation whereby you feel yourself fully available and able to experience an outside resistance without interference of any kind. Be resolved in navigating through the more boisterous muscle groups of the hip and connecting with outside resistance through the inner thigh's soft-spoken yet keen-sighted nature.

Meditation: Joy

The central position of your inner-thigh muscles offers you poise. The more practiced you are in connecting your inner thighs (movement inward) with your abdominal center (spirit self), the more deliberate you can be with that poise. Once equipped inwardly with a strong sense of self, you can connect outwardly with joyful confidence and free expression. Poise is cultivated by drawing both strength (action) and ease (counter-action) equally from both inner thighs. This generates a downward calm through the lower abdominal and iliopsoas muscles, with an upward connection through the inner thighs and upper abdominal muscles. While lower abdominal muscles ground your stance, the upper abdominals lift your torso's weight out of your stance. The dan tien energy center's space is restored, and energy flow is reestablished. Be mindful of your creative life force flowing unimpeded, expanding your imagination to consider what was before unknown and unrecognizable.

How to Isolate the Inner-Thigh Muscles

Feel It Contract

Because the most superior inner thigh-muscles—your pectineus muscles—are also used in upward movement, it's easy to misidentify hip flexion as the entry into inward movement. An isometric (nonmoving) exercise helps to distinguish between these two actions of the inner-thigh muscles.

Seated Heel Kiss Exercise

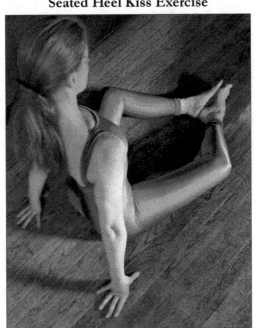

Exercise: Sit on the floor with the soles of the feet together in front of you and knees turned out. Place your feet in a comfortable distance in front of you. Maintain a grounded sit through the million-dollar point by using your hands behind you to assist in sitting upright. Without disturbing your knee position, gently press your heel stirrups together. As soon as you have a sensation of the inner-thigh muscles, recognized as a muscular connection to the sitz bones, release the pressure. Notice how exerting more force easily displaces your knee position, and you will then draw from the hip flexion for support. Repeat this gentle heel press without the hip flexion until you are clear about the degree of force your inner thighs can successfully isolate in an adduction movement.

Feel It Release

Although they are a fairly large muscle group, the inner thighs are delicate. Be sure to stretch them using only your body's weight and gravity—no bouncing or lunging your body's weight through them for a quicker result. Injury will most likely follow impatience and ultimately slow down your results.

Supine Frog Stretch

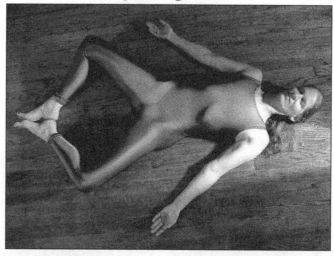

Exercise: Lie supine, soles of feet together, and knees turned out. Engage abdominal muscles gently to maintain neutral alignment. Do not push lower back into the floor. Place your feet a suitable distance away from the pelvis so a stretch is established in the inner thighs. Relax and allow gravity and the weight of your legs to increase the stretch. Extend the feet a little farther away from pelvis, relax, and use your legs' weight to stretch inner thighs again and again. Be sure to stretch the entire length of the inner-thigh muscles, from mid-thigh to pelvis, until legs are straight. Once they are fully straightened, rock the legs in and out to surrender any hip flexor resistance that may have collected while holding the stretch.

Feel It Fatigue

It's more important to build endurance in the inner thighs than brute strength. Stick to high repetition with moderate weight and range. When inner thighs begin to fail, lower back and hip flexor muscles will step in; stay vigilant to produce a clean adduction, even if an inward direction feels weak and powerless. As the inner-thigh muscles reach failure, a high-pitched tightness builds in the area. This is physically a delicate feeling; however, this delicate experience of self connects you to an inner strength and emotional sense of belonging. Be gentle and build slowly.

Inner-Thigh Exercises

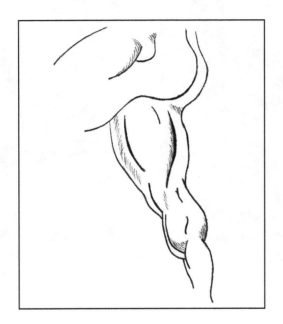

Inner-Thigh Muscles
Embody
Movement Inward

Seated Adduction

Machine

Starting Position:

- Sit in machine with leg pads rotated inward. Sit upright on million-dollar point with leg pads positioned at inner thighs and allow only a very light inner-thigh stretch.
- Rotate quadriceps outward and inner thighs inward.
- Use arms to support an upright torso position while dropping body weight through sitz bones.
- Commit to keeping hip flexors and quadriceps relaxed outwardly.

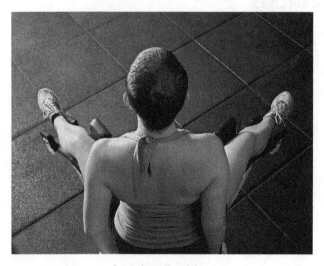

Starting Position

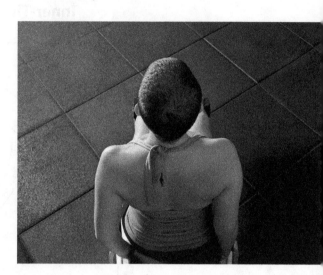

Action/Counter-action

Counter-action:

- Inhale: Visualize energy descending back of torso, snaking through the dan tien, and continuing down the hip flexors, anterior inner thighs, and quadriceps.
- Exhale: Relax your quadriceps outward to the same degree your inner thighs are motivated to move inward and keep energy orbiting down through pubic bone to the same degree energy orbits up through the sternum.
- Inhale: Keep legs turned out in the hips as they return to starting position. Repeat.
- Be mindful to lengthen the iliopsoas muscles away from the anterior dan tien to create space in hip joints and a constant connection with inner thighs.

Action:

- Inhale: Visualize energy ascending up posterior legs and inner thighs, snaking through the dan tien, and continuing up anterior torso.
- Exhale: Contract inner-thigh muscles, drawing legs to median plane. Experience the inner-thigh muscles leading the movement. Maintain your connection point using no momentum.

- Inhale: Use inner-thigh muscles to carry legs back to starting position. Repeat.
- Concentrate on drawing your inner thighs into your dan tien to stabilize your sitting position.

Energy Orbit:

- **Isolated Connection:** Visualize the counter-action before engaging in the action. Counter-action: Release energy down the middle back and snake it through dan tien and iliopsoas to continue down anterior inner thighs and quadriceps muscles. Action: Orbit energy up posterior inner thighs and snake it through dan tien and upper abdominals.
- **Unified Connection:** Counter-action: Extend energy orbit down the posterior torso, snaking through dan tien and down anterior legs and inner thighs. Action: Orbit energy up posterior legs and inner thighs, snaking through dan tien and up anterior torso. Energize all eight energy orbits of the pattern through the dan tien. This step adjoins active and counter-active energies associated with the whole body in support of an inner-thigh isolated connection.

Active Meditation—Movement Inward:

- Notice how the iliopsoas muscles are quick to grab hold of outside resistance, hindering the legs' freedom to rotate outward. Approach the resistance from the underbelly of the inner thighs to encourage the quadriceps and iliopsoas muscles to open away from pubic bone. Feel yourself open to a more intimate connection.
- Guided meditation: I open outward to connect with and share my inner beauty.

Lying Adduction

Floor

Starting Position:

- Lie supine in essential alignment with legs extended upward. Leg weight relaxes through sacrum, grounding pelvis into floor while maintaining natural lower back curve.
- Rotate legs outward with heels touching and toes directed outward.
- If iliopsoas or lower back grabs, support legs' weight with hands just above the knees.
- Commit to the natural curve of the lower back with legs positioned directly over pelvis.

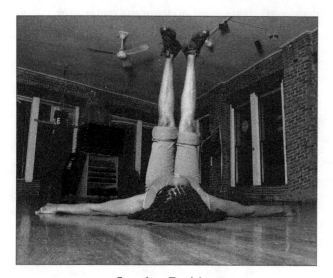

Starting Position

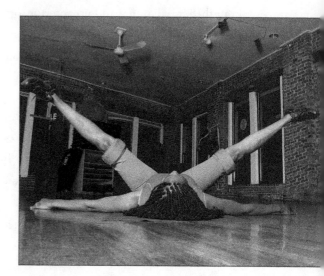

Action/Counter-action

Counter-action:

- Inhale: Visualize energy descending down back of torso, snaking through dan tien, and continuing down the quadriceps and anterior inner thighs as legs separate.
- Exhale: Anterior inner thighs follow quadriceps' relaxed outward rotation as legs return back to starting position. Avoid bouncing legs at outer stretch. Repeat.
- Inhale: Reopen legs to straddle position, being careful to maintain connection point and inner thigh involvement without overstretching inner thighs.
- Be mindful of grounding weight of legs through the sacrum to release iliopsoas muscles and minimize hip flexion.

Action:

- Inhale: Visualize energy ascending posterior legs and inner thighs, snaking through dan tien, and continuing up anterior torso as legs separate.
- Exhale: Motivate contraction through posterior inner-thigh muscles, drawing legs into median plane. Keep weight of sacrum and shoulder blades equally grounded into the floor. Repeat.

- Inhale: Use inner thighs to carry legs back to straddle position as you continue to rotate legs outward.
- Concentrate on your inner-thigh muscles controlling the movement by experiencing the weight of your bones, and stabilize your position through a balanced relationship with the median plane.

Energy Orbit:

- **Isolated Connection:** Visualize the counter-action before engaging in the action. Counter-action: Release energy down the middle back and snake it through dan tien and iliopsoas to continue down anterior inner thighs and quadriceps muscles. Action: Orbit energy up posterior inner thighs and snake it through dan tien and upper abdominals.
- **Unified Connection:** Counter-action: Extend energy orbit down the posterior torso, snaking through dan tien and down anterior legs and inner thighs. Action: Orbit energy up posterior legs and inner thighs, snaking through dan tien and up anterior torso. Energize all eight energy orbits of the pattern through the dan tien. This step adjoins active and counter-active energies associated with the whole body in support of an inner-thigh isolated connection.

Active Meditation—Movement Inward:

- Notice how the leg's position is determined by your flexibility. Recognize the leg's weight as your outside resistance and deliberately create a symmetrical inner-thigh stretch. The distance between legs is less important than your legs staying on their coronal plane. Support extreme flexibility with limited range and support lack of flexibility with additional stretching and by supporting the legs' weight with your hands. You are balancing the condition of your boundaries.
- Guided meditation: I challenge strength with flexibility and flexibility with boundaries.

Standing Straight-Leg Adduction

Pulley

Starting Position:

- Attach inside leg to pulley strap at ankle. Stand a distance away from pulley, which permits chosen weight to be lifted off stack with working leg extended sideways.
- Stand with legs parallel, hips and shoulders square to wall in front of you, and connect to abdominal center. Your essential alignment is in alliance with your standing leg. Outside arm may use a pole to stabilize position.
- Commit to keeping waistline still.

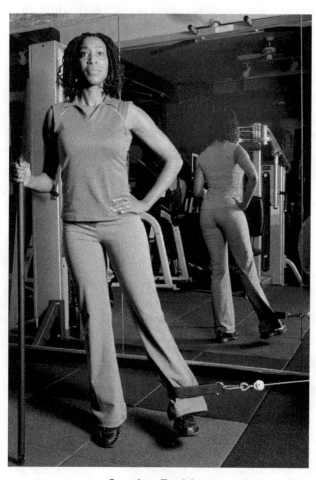

Starting Position

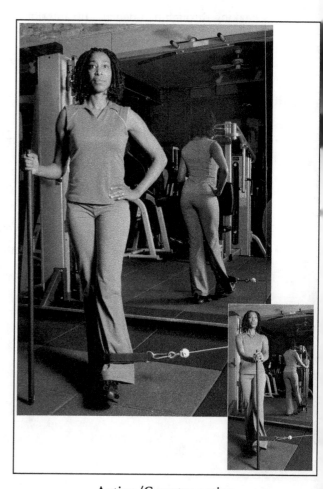

Action/Counter-action

Counter-action:

- Inhale: Visualize energy descending down back of torso, snaking through dan tien, and continuing down the anterior legs. Keep gushing spring/heel stirrup marriage active on standing leg.
- Exhale: Elongate both iliopsoas muscles to position inner thighs forward, as the working leg and resistance are dragged inward to median plane. Keep legs parallel and on coronal plane.

- Inhale: Elongate waist by lifting the upper abdominals upward away from grounded low abdominals as working leg is returned to starting position. Repeat.
- Keep your weight on gushing spring point while releasing energy through both heel stirrups.

Action:

- Inhale: Visualize energy ascending posterior legs and inner thighs, snaking through dan tien, and continuing up anterior torso.
- Exhale: Contract inner-thigh muscles, drawing working leg inward to meet supporting leg. Lift energy of both inner thighs upward toward dan tien. Notice how involved the buttock muscles are on your supporting side.
- Inhale: Use inner thighs to carry leg back to starting position. Repeat.
- Concentrate on supporting and working leg's continuous connection with the dan tien energy center.

Energy Orbit:

- **Isolated Connection:** Visualize the counter-action before engaging in the action. *Counter-action:* Release energy down the middle back and snake it through dan tien and iliopsoas to continue down anterior inner thighs and quadriceps muscles. *Action:* Orbit energy up posterior inner thighs and snake it through dan tien and upper abdominals.
- **Unified Connection:** *Counter-action:* Extend energy orbit down the posterior torso, snaking through dan tien and down anterior legs and inner thighs. *Action:* Orbit energy up posterior legs and inner thighs, snaking through dan tien and up anterior torso. Energize all eight energy orbits of the pattern through the dan tien. This step adjoins active and counter-active energies associated with the whole body in support of an inner-thigh isolated connection.

Active Meditation—Movement Inward:

- Keeping weight forward on the support leg's gushing spring point places the movement on the coronal plane, challenging your supporting buttock and abdominal muscles as well as the inner-thigh muscles. Buttocks, inner thighs, and abdominals are your core's stability.
- Guided meditation: I am stable in myself and need not control others.

BodyLogos Psyche-Muscular Observations for Inner-Thigh Muscles

Here are examples of how to interpret mind-body expressions.

Ability: When a domineering muscle group overrides a nearby submissive muscle group, the submissive muscle group needs to reclaim its position.

STOP If you are experiencing the quadriceps muscles during an inner thigh exercise, stop and realign. The quadriceps muscles (eagerness to move forward) are overriding the inner thighs (personal connection inward). This is often due to a lack of abdominal support (connection to self), causing the pelvis position to tuck or tip and your dan tien to lose its central placement. From this position, the quadriceps muscles are the only available muscles able to connect with the resistance.

In this case, lengthen your iliopsoas muscles while repositioning your million-dollar point under your dan tien. This shift will correctly place your pelvis under your rib cage and elongate the waistline. From this place, the inner thighs are in a leading position for the movement. As your inner-thigh muscles realign with your abdominal center, feel like you're coming home to yourself, readying yourself to connect with the world. Each inner-thigh squeeze brings a greater sense of inner strength, personal empowerment, and peace.

Coordination: If your inability to balance prevents you from attempting an inner thigh exercise, even with a brace to support the movement, you have lost the relaxed weight of your bones.

STOP If you are grasping for control or tensing to balance, realign, and begin again, using a pole to assist your balance when doing a standing exercise. This is a step toward balancing on your own, but only if you are still trying to balance by your own accord.

Use the pole to steady your balance, as opposed to leaning on it. The pole need not feel your body weight. Use your abdominal muscles—your connection to your spirit self—to initiate proper alignment. As you insist on your alignment and depend on your core's relaxed strength, you will find yourself much more capable and able to maintain your balance. With each successful movement, meditate on easefully taking personal responsibility for your own failures and successes. Experience an increase of personal accountability.

Enjoyment: If you enjoy inner thigh exercises, it would indicate that you enjoy personal growth and inward exploration. If you avoid inner thigh exercises, this would indicate that you'd rather not look inward too closely.

STOP Stop avoiding inner thigh exercises. Rather than doing none at all, do short sets in combination with other exercises until you begin to feel more successful or enthusiastic. Balance is what you are training for, so the ability to move both outward and inward is necessary for a healthy body and mind.

This avoidance indicates a compromise of self-acceptance. As you integrate inner thigh work into your regimen, experience it as your agreement time. You are checking in with yourself; you don't need anyone else's endorsement. Agreeing inwardly about something, whether you are happy or unhappy about it, motivates self-esteem and self-respect as clarity of thought replaces uncertainty. Enjoy being in the know about your own position in the world.

Meet the Models

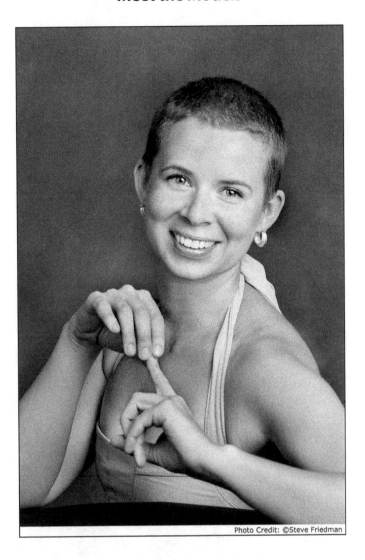

Photo Credit: ©Steve Friedman

Hiie Saumaa

Hiie Saumaa, PhD, teaches and writes about somatic practices and meditation. She offers classes and workshops in mind-body techniques: BodyLogos, Nia, and JourneyDance. She teaches literature and philosophy at Columbia University and writes on interconnections between somatic practices, the meditative mind-body, twentieth-century literature, and theories of movement and consciousness. Her focus is to inspire her students, inside and outside academia, to cultivate balanced strength and move through life with dancing joy. This very accomplished thirty-two-year-old Estonian intellectual says, "Meditation in strength training gives my movement purpose; it grounds, centers, and allows me to make discoveries about my holding patterns, habitual ways of thinking and acting, and creates positive change." Her interest in fitness started at the age of seventeen out of her love for health and healing. She feels, "The human body is infinitely fascinating and our greatest teacher!" After a day of active meditation activities—writing, dancing, music (choral singing and flute)—Hiie welcomes the ending of her days with prayer and yoga postures.

Universal Connection Energy Pattern as It Relates to the Calf Muscles

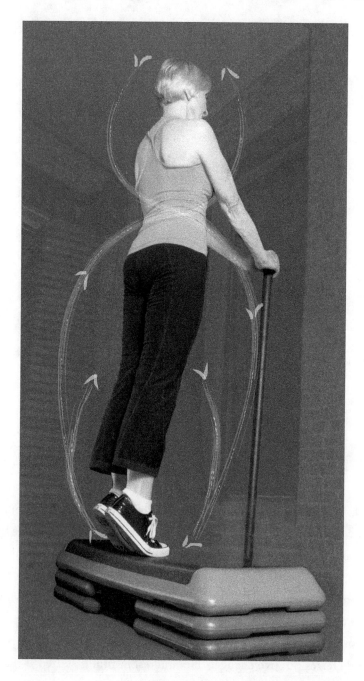

Visualize this energy pattern supporting all calf isolations.

Introduction to Calf Muscles

Theory of Yin and Yang

Yang: Active Muscle Group

Calf Muscles:
- Gastrocnemius
- Soleus
- Popliteus
- Flexor Hallucis Longus
- Flexor Digitorum Longus
- Tibialis Posterior

Yin: Counter-active Muscle Group

Shin Muscles:
- Tibialis Anterior
- Extensor Digitorum Longus
- Extensor Hallucis Longus
- Peroneus Tertius
- Peroneus Longus
- Peroneus Brevis

The stance of a gymnast about to spring across the mat embodies calf energy movement. The posterior legs lift up through the anterior torso (action), readying the calves to spring into action, while the posterior torso grounds through the anterior legs (counter-action), permitting the calves to land safely with the shins' support. Commit to maintaining the opposing snakelike forces through your body's length, especially through the dan tien, where these forces intersect.

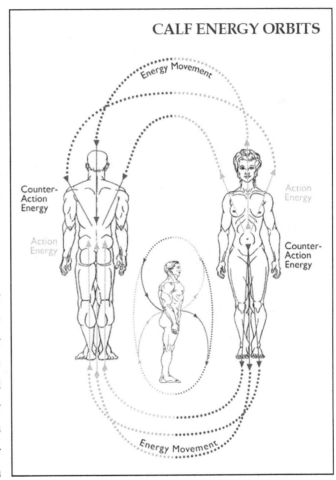

Action: Determination

Your calf muscles lift you up and out of your stillness. The determinations they carry lift you up and out of your burdens. Just as you can recover swiftly from life's occasional misfortunes, calves embody the ability to be inspired, strive ahead, and stay on a path of personal growth and self-discovery in daily life. The determination of your calves swiftly recovers from daily challenges. Notice how your determination becomes energized when you celebrate your growth and newfound wisdom rather than depending solely on what you are producing. Living a dream is built on learning your dream; enjoy every nuance and detail of your dreams through your calves' nature.

Counter-action: Grounded

When contracting the calf muscles, you can also meditate on the expanding counter-action of the shin muscles. The shin muscles balance and ground you together with the muscles of the feet. This sense of groundedness carries a relaxed strength, giving you confidence in your ability to maneuver with grace. Recognize the graceful support and acute sensitivity the shin muscles offer your calves' determination. Know your ability to rescue your balance due to the shin muscles' dexterity. Feel your resilience to navigate through challenges. Experience grounded determination. Experience the traction to go for your dreams.

Five-Element Theory
Spring, Crushing Joint, Anger

Connection: Spring

Spring glimpses of warmth ramp-up the calf muscles' willingness to perform, but be prudent. It is important that you keep them warm and dry as the weather fluctuates to support their enormous responsibility. Because of their small size and big assignment to support and mobilize your entire body's weight they are characterized by determination. Use this determination to maintain the subtle weight distribution needed for Essential Alignment rather than muscling yourself into action. Keep your body's weight forward on your Gushing Spring points and equally dropped through your Heel Stirrups. This not only keeps the calves energized, it employs the buttock muscles to help them support your body's weight.

Strength: Crushing Joints

The ankle joints, operated by the calf muscles, are less typical hinge joints, since they allow a slight degree of rotation or of side-to-side movement. This added mobility asks for greater due diligence in maintaining the precise alignment favored by hinge joints. Be watchful that you position your body's weight along the metatarsals of the second and third toes, rather than the big toe or little toe. This weight distribution will align the foot properly to develop the calf muscles evenly, medially and laterally. Be resolved in maintaining joint alignment through a full range of motion—heel raises and knee bends. Avoid sickling your ankles inwardly or winging them outwardly. Misalignment in ankle, knee, and hip joints weaken entire leg.

Meditation: Anger

The exhilaration of determination—the psyche-muscular component of the calf muscles—can overwhelm the mind and overburden the body. The momentum of elation can spin out of control and before long come to an abrupt stop. Suddenly, you are being dragged through life, and the spirited connection you once had has been lost. Your attention gravitates toward the twang of negative thinking and irate confusion that accompanies the loss of inspiration. A twang of an equally halting nature can suddenly stop your body in its tracks if you accelerate through the feet and ankles too abruptly. Recognize the calves' counter-action—the downward weight through the shins—giving your calves' determination a balanced and grounding force. This balance is found by connecting the bottom of your feet to the earth's universal energy. Combine the energetic lift of your calves, which passes through the buttocks and upper abdominals, with the energetic descent of your shoulder blades that passes through the iliopsoas and shins. Be mindful of your weight staying securely on your gushing spring points so the release of tension can navigate through your heel stirrups.

How to Isolate the Calf Muscles

Feel It Contract

Due to the complexity of the foot—each is operated by twelve muscles, twenty-six bones, and seven thousand nerve endings, all of which the calf muscles influence—it can be challenging to feel the relatively simple six-muscle calf grouping. The calf muscles are bigger and stronger than the muscles that articulate the feet, yet the nerve density of feet makes their articulations more sensitized. To separate the sensation of the calf from the articulation of the foot, focus on slowly pressing the body's weight up and down below the level of toe flexion.

Flat-Footed Calf Raise Exercise

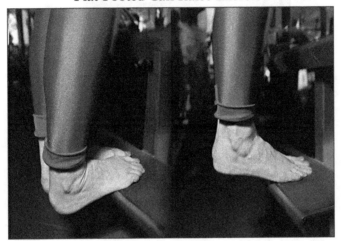

Exercise: Stand on a stair with heels dropped below the step and body weight on gushing spring points. Keep knees, ankles, and toes together; stabilize your balance by holding a railing. Feel your weight fully placed over the gushing spring points as you slowly relax down through your heel stirrups. Then contract the calves, raising the heels to the same level as the step but no higher. Do not press down through the balls of your feet; simply keep the weight placed on the gushing spring points. Return the heels to the starting position without rocking your weight back. Repeat until you feel the movement motivated by the calf muscles rather than shin or feet muscles.

Feel It Release

As an amazingly small muscle group for propelling your entire body's weight, the calf muscles need a lot of support-releasing tension. They walk, run, jump, and skip your weight all around town. To counter all this quick-twitch activity, stretch slowly.

Stair Heel Drop Stretch

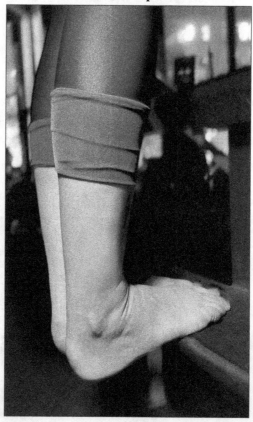

Exercise: With straight legs, stand on a stair with the gushing spring points supported on the step. Keep knees, ankles, and toes together. Relax heels down below step level. The weight of the body is aligned over the gushing spring points, while the heel stirrups release downward to stretch the calf muscles and exercise the ankles' full range of motion. Once you have reached a full stretch in the calves, gently step out of it. Do not linger or force this weight-bearing stretch. A weight-bearing stretch allows for greater range and sensation, but holding a weight-bearing stretch for too long in the calves can cause spasms or overstretching.

Feel It Fatigue

Calf muscles are tenacious but can also be a bit reckless. Their fatigue is felt as tightness. The rigidity of this fatigue asks for slow-to-moderate speed and range of motion as well as aligned movement. Failure to address their rigidity and accommodate their fatigue can result in abrupt pain or injury. They are mighty yet sensitive like the thin legs of a thoroughbred; work them and stretch them respectfully.

Calf Exercises

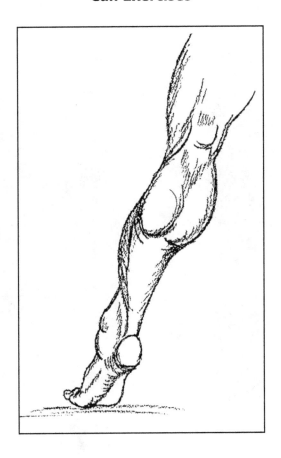

**Calf Muscles
Embody
Grounded Determination**

Hyperextended Calf Raise

Step

Starting Position:

- Stand with gushing spring points near the edge of step, position feet together, and drop heels below step. Single-leg calf raise is also an option.
- Support your balance with a bar or railing.
- Commit to keeping both big toes and both heels together throughout movement.

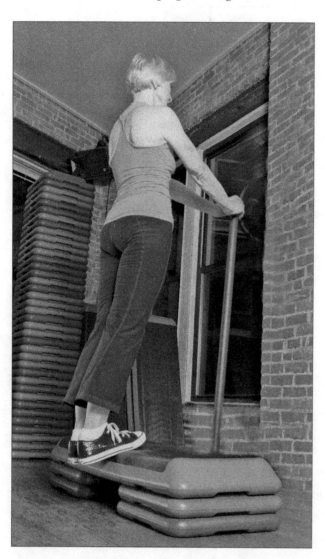

Starting Position

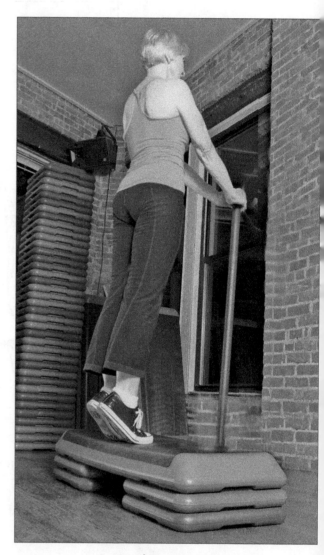

Action/Counter-action

Counter-action:

- Inhale: Visualize energy descending down back of torso, snaking through dan tien, and continuing down the anterior legs to gushing spring points.

- Exhale: Elongate muscles along front of shins and ankles as heels are raised. Recognize your elongated ankles aligning with your elongated iliopsoas muscles.
- Inhale: Relax front of ankles through gushing spring points as they are returned to starting position. Repeat.
- Be mindful to keep million-dollar point, dan tien, and zhong heart center aligned.

Action:

- Inhale: Visualize energy ascending through calves and posterior legs, snaking through dan tien, and continuing up the anterior torso.
- Exhale: Contract calf muscles to lift heels. Send energy up to the buttock muscles and inner thighs, then connect their strength with the upper abdominal lift.
- Inhale: Use calves to carry heels back to starting position. Repeat.
- Concentrate on connecting the ascending buttock and inner thigh energy up and under your upper abdominals and chest.

Energy Orbit:

- **Isolated Connection:** Visualize the counter-action before engaging in the action. Counter-action: Drop energy down the middle back and snake it through dan tien and iliopsoas, then down anterior legs to shin muscles. Action: Orbit energy up the calves to buttocks, snake it through dan tien, and continue to upper abdominals.
- **Unified Connection:** Counter-action: Extend an energy orbit down the posterior torso and snake it through dan tien and down anterior legs. Action: Orbit energy up the posterior legs and snake it through dan tien and up anterior torso. Energize all eight energy orbits of the pattern through the dan tien. This step adjoins active and counter-active energies associated with the whole body in support of a calf-isolated connection.

Active Meditation—Determination:

- It is important to cross the opposing S curves directly in your center of gravity—dan tien energy center. If too far forward, the upward S curve (action) will throw the anterior ribs forward; if too far back, the downward S curve (counter-action) will throw the posterior ribs back. Recognize front and back planes of the body; position the crossing of active and counter-active energies at absolute center.
- Guided meditation: I am centered.

Weighted Hyperextended Calf Raise

Machine

Starting Position:

- Lie supine on machine sled with gushing spring points positioned on lowest aspect of footplate. Keep feet together, legs straight, and drop through heel stirrups.
- Connect to abdominal support and maintain natural curve in lower back.
- Commit to keeping legs long, not locked, through the knee joints.

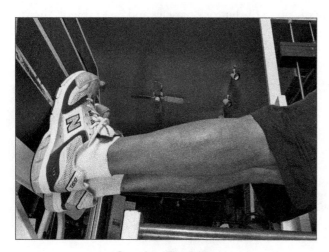

Starting Position

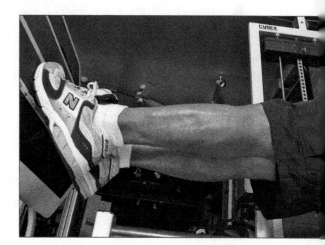

Action/Counter-action

Counter-action:

- Inhale: Visualize energy descending down back of torso, snaking through dan tien, and continuing down the quadriceps and shins to gushing spring points.
- Exhale: Elongate shin muscles as heels are raised. Recognize and honor the more limited range of motion in the ankle when heels are kept together and feet stay aligned between second and third metatarsals.
- Inhale: Relax front of ankles as heel stirrups are returned to starting position. Repeat.
- Be mindful to keep inner legs and ankles against median plane to stay connected to abdominal center.

Action:

- Inhale: Visualize energy ascending through calves and posterior legs, snaking through dan tien, and continuing up anterior torso.
- Exhale: Contract calf muscles to lift heels, using alignment of feet and ankles to connect your entire body with the median plane. Machine's sled and your body glide upward as one.
- Inhale: Use calf muscles to carry heel stirrups back to starting position. Repeat.
- Concentrate on legs' energy orbits to deliver power rather than depending solely on the brute force of your calf muscles for power.

Energy Orbit:

- **Isolated Connection:** Visualize the counter-action before engaging in the action. Counter-action: Drop energy down the middle back and snake it through dan tien and iliopsoas, then down anterior legs to shin muscles. Action: Orbit energy up the calves to buttocks, snake it through dan tien, and continue to upper abdominals.
- **Unified Connection:** Counter-action: Extend an energy orbit down the posterior torso and snake it through dan tien and down anterior legs. Action: Orbit energy up the posterior legs and snake it through dan tien and up anterior torso. Energize all eight energy orbits of the pattern through the dan tien. This step adjoins active and counter-active energies associated with the whole body in support of a calf-isolated connection.

Active Meditation—Determination:

- Notice how small the calves are in relation to the huge task of carrying your body's weight. Recognize the necessity to lift the burden of your weight out of the calves' responsibility so they can elevate you rather than relentlessly catch your fall. Utilize your energy alignment and core strength of buttocks, inner thighs, and abdominal muscles to lighten the load for the calf muscles.
- Guided meditation: I am aligned with my dreams and aspirations.

Calf Raise

Dumbbells or Eyes Closed

Starting Position:

- Stand with feet together, arms relaxed at sides; hold dumbbells and/or close eyes.
- Connect to abdominal support and activate the gushing spring/heel stirrup marriage.
- Hang your arms like dead weight from the shoulder blades. If holding resistance, commit to experiencing the outside resistance as an extension of your arm's weight.

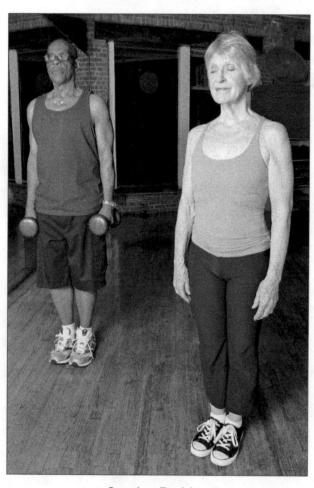

Starting Position

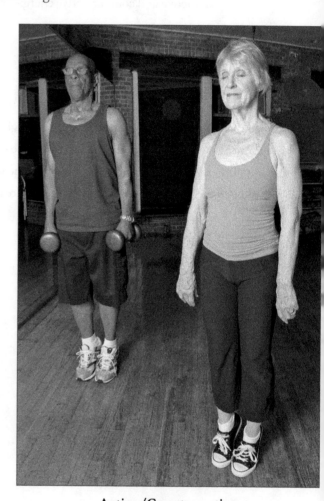

Action/Counter-action

Counter-action:

- Inhale: Visualize energy descending down back of torso, snaking through dan tien, and continuing down the quadriceps and shins to gushing spring points.
- Exhale: Elongate shin muscles as heel stirrups are raised. Feel the weight of your bones lightening through their precise alignment.

- Inhale: Relax front of ankles as heel stirrups are returned to starting position. Repeat.
- Be mindful to keep your shoulder blades heavy and shoulder blade channels committed to the heart center's upward rise through the crown center.

Action:

- Inhale: Visualize energy ascending through calves and posterior legs, snaking through dan tien, and continuing up anterior torso.
- Exhale: Contract calf muscles to raise heel stirrups up through open heart and crown centers, as if rising to the heavens. Use your core—buttocks, inner thighs, and abdominal muscles—to maintain alignment and assist calf muscles in lifting body weight upward.
- Inhale: Use calf muscles to carry heel stirrups back to starting position, maintaining your heart and crown centers' upward lift. Repeat.
- Concentrate on the support your alignment offers your overall muscular strength and ability as you experience both groundedness and weightlessness through your bones.

Energy Orbit:

- **Isolated Connection:** Visualize the counter-action before engaging in the action. Counter-action: Drop energy down the middle back and snake it through dan tien and iliopsoas, then down anterior legs to shin muscles. Action: Orbit energy up the calves to buttocks, snake it through dan tien, and continue to upper abdominals.
- **Unified Connection:** Counter-action: Extend an energy orbit down the posterior torso and snake it through dan tien and down anterior legs. Action: Orbit energy up the posterior legs and snake it through dan tien and up anterior torso. Energize all eight energy orbits of the pattern through the dan tien. This step adjoins active and counter-active energies associated with the whole body in support of a calf-isolated connection.

Active Meditation—Determination:

- Notice how uniting with an outside resistance attaches a layer of doubt to your ability. Experience your essential alignment extended toward both earth and sky. Trust this elongated alignment is connecting you to your universal parents—the greater knowing of earth and sky. Experience alignment as your spirit's safekeeping.
- Guided meditation: I stretch into the unknown so I can relax in my essence, where true safety lies.

Calf Raise Turned Out

Floor

Starting Position:

- Stand with heels together and legs gently turned out. Keep your hip bones forward and tailbone dropped so your million-dollar point stays aligned between anklebones when rotating legs.
- Rotate legs only to the degree in which you have rotation in hip joints; be sure knees bend over the second and third toes. Commit to supporting your turnout by keeping inner thighs relating to your median plane.

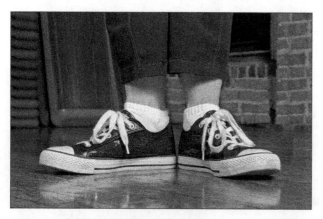

Starting Position

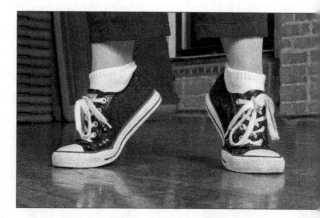

Action/Counter-action

Counter-action:

- Inhale: Visualize energy descending down back of torso, snaking through dan tien and iliopsoas, and continuing down anterior inner thighs, shins, and gushing spring points.
- Exhale: Elongate iliopsoas and shin muscles as heels are raised. Relax balls of feet and tops of feet so the gushing spring points spread out onto the ground.
- Inhale: Relax front of ankles as heels are returned to starting position. Repeat.
- Be mindful to keep iliopsoas muscles soft and elongated so your million-dollar point stays dropped between anklebones.

Action:

- Inhale: Visualize energy ascending through calves, posterior legs, and buttocks, snaking through dan tien, and continuing up anterior torso.
- Exhale: Contract calf muscles to raise heels and keep inner thighs rotating toward median plane.
- Inhale: Use calves to carry heels back to starting position. Repeat.
- Concentrate on the buttocks' support giving the hip flexors freedom to relax and rotate outward.

Energy Orbit:

- **Isolated Connection:** Visualize the counter-action before engaging in the action. Counter-action: Drop energy down the middle back and snake it through dan tien and iliopsoas, then down anterior legs to shin muscles. Action: Orbit energy up the calves to buttocks, snake it through dan tien, and continue to upper abdominals.
- **Unified Connection:** Counter-action: Extend an energy orbit down the posterior torso and snake it through dan tien and down anterior legs. Action: Orbit energy up the posterior legs and snake it through dan tien and up anterior torso. Energize all eight energy orbits of the pattern through the dan tien. This step adjoins active and counter-active energies associated with the whole body in support of a calf-isolated connection.

Active Meditation—Determination:

- Notice how the calves (determination), buttocks (comfort), and inner thighs (movement inward) come together to encourage your anterior pelvis to open freely. Allow yourself to feel comfortable with your innermost desires and sensuality; be determined to express what is real for you.
- Expression: I enjoy my body.

BodyLogos Psyche-Muscular Observations for Calf Muscles

Here are examples of how to interpret mind-body expressions.

Posture: Alignment is necessary to develop balanced strength in a muscle group. Without alignment, lopsided posture, injury, or accident will eventually follow.

STOP If the ankles splay at the top of a calf raise, this movement draws your attention away from the medial line of the body, disrupts essential alignment, and will only develop the lateral side of the calf muscles. Keep your ankles aligned, weight between second and third metatarsals in foot, throughout an exercise to develop both the medial and lateral sides of the calf muscles equally. This alignment connects you to your abdominal support, your primary balance muscle.

As you gently align your ankles, notice your inner thighs becoming involved. Experience your median plane connecting the low abdomen, inner thighs, and ankles like a mannequin's central beam of support. This medial line connects the grounded determination of the lower leg to your sense of self in the abdominals. As you perform a calf exercise, experience yourself as confident, determined, and tenacious.

Coordination: The ability to execute an exercise in such a way that it leads to improvement shows coordination. The inability to combine the requirements needed to repeat an exercise shows a lack of coordination, and repetition is needed to create change.

STOP The inability to balance makes you unable to continue an exercise. Either you have abandoned your abdominal center or tension has collected in your lower back muscles or both. This would indicate an abandonment of self and an attachment to fear. It is imperative that the energy lifting through your lower back muscles at the sacrum continue their upward sweep through the upper abdominal muscles, or you will have no abdominal support––your primary balance muscles.

Giving up the familiar fear-based holding pattern of the lower back––at the lumbar curve––can feel more frightening than the fear itself. As you allow the upward force traveling through the dan tien to connect the sacrum to the upper abdominals, you will find lumbar tension unnecessary. You may experience a sense of relief in not needing that tension to hold you up anymore. You are elevating your energy centers' alliance, readying yourself to create the life you want. Allow yourself to ease into this relaxed elevation with poise. As your relaxation allows you to balance, feel the words "Yes, I can." Be your potential.

Size: Recognizing a muscle's full range of motion is required for a stretch, but for strength, the range of motion is limited to the muscles' ability to stay connected. Staying connected with the calf muscles while executing their full range is the challenge.

STOP If your feet are tiring from a calf exercise rather than your calves, you are pressing the top of the foot through the balls of the feet rather than lifting the heels from the bottom of the foot. Pressing from the top of your foot's arch may be taking you out of the calf muscles and exhausting the foot muscles. The top of your movement needs to have the same command of balance as the bottom; you have simply arrived at an elevated platform. When you allow the metatarsals to expand as the heels rise, more ball of the foot stays on the ground, supporting your balance. A pop-up finishing point compresses the foot, indicating that the tenacious process of determination (calf muscles) has been replaced by a fleeting performance destination to feel emotionally grounded but physically compromised (shin muscles).

Connect to feeling grounded by separating it from feeling determined; recognize that determination is the journey to becoming grounded. Meditate on the sense of satisfaction gained when completing a task at your greatest potential. Appreciate the hard work and commitment—determination. Then feel the hard work done, a sense of arrival—groundedness. Love the process of growing as you love the destination of succeeding. Experience calf exercises as a series of determined accomplishments that generate a grounded sense of belonging in the world.

Part 3
Life Is Outside Resistance

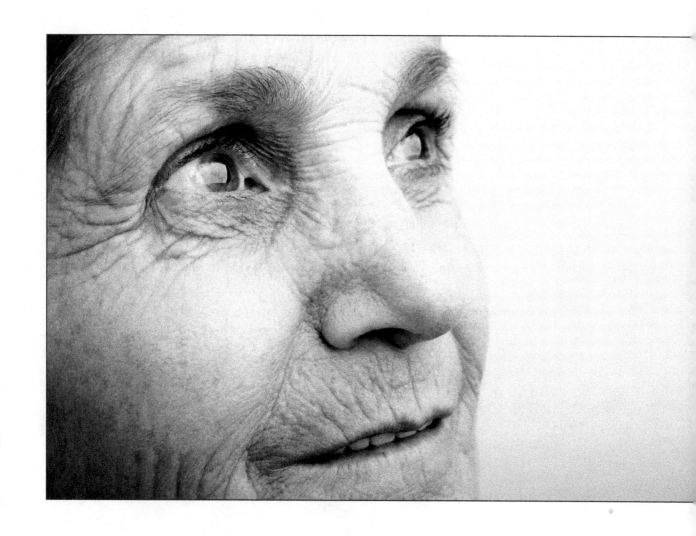

Overview

Lesson Chapters 13–15

> Liberate your potential,
> Strengthen your effectiveness,
> And you create a meaningful relationship with life.
>
> —Tammy Wise, BodyLogos

This final section will explain how to design workouts to liberate your strength to freely connect with your aspirations in life.

Part 3 shows you how to holistically appraise the condition of your strength, to consider your physical disturbances, emotional discontent, personality, lifestyle, and beliefs as contributing aspects of strength. Then use this appraisal to discern your condition's pattern.

Part 3 further develops the concept that, to liberate your highest self, you have to feel the weight of your movement rather than just go through the motions. And the most effective way to balance your attention between a "thinking mind" and "intending spirit" is through a "feeling body." You learn to witness this balance or lack thereof in your workout so you can recognize it in your daily posture.

Part 3 recognizes that what is true in one domain of strength applies to the others. This understanding develops perceptual strength—the ability to connect mind, body, and spirit—to become your highest self. This perceptual strength inspires the ability not only to change who you're being in life but also to create the life and environment that serve your highest self's purpose.

Part 3 makes Tao strength training a lifestyle discipline using the resistance found in life to distinguish between emotional fears and spiritual intuition, defusing reactions and restoring intention.

Part 3 acknowledges the larger picture of one's spiritual immortality and, in so doing, imparts an urgency to create meaningful connections in life by practicing active meditation, recognizing one's own inner alchemy, and developing as a psyche-muscular spiritual human being.

> When a person is alive, he is soft and supple.
> When a person dies, he becomes hard and rigid.
> When a plant is alive, it is pliant and tender.
> When a plant is dead, it becomes dry and brittle.
> Hence, the hard and rigid are companions of the dead.
> The soft and supple are companions of the living.
>
> —Lao Tzu, *Tao Te Ching*

Physical Transformation Chapter

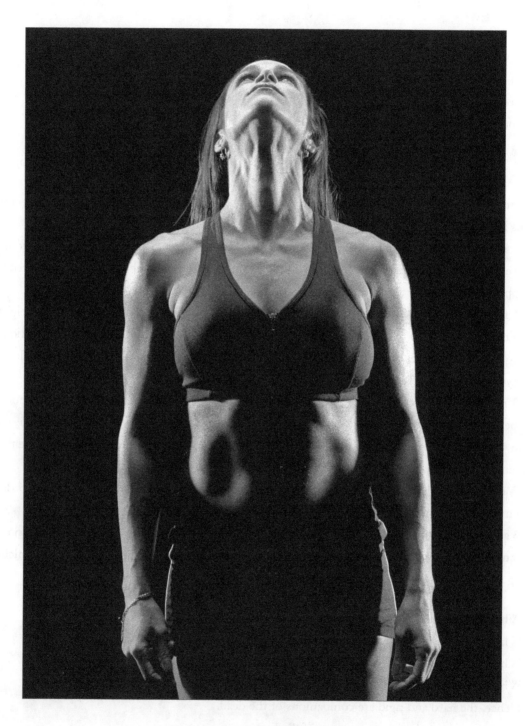

The yin and yang of physical grace
Lie in the collaborative relationship between
Alignment and stability.

Lesson 13
Sculpt the Body

The Master does his job and then stops.
He understands that the Universe is forever out of control
And that trying to dominate events goes against the current of the Tao.

—Lao Tzu, *Tao Te Ching*

Peace is found by balancing your life, not controlling life.

—Tammy Wise, *BodyLogos*

Attend to the Moment

Understanding theory and guidelines in energy alignment is a starting point. But by recognizing where we are in each moment, we can use energy alignment to support the fluctuation of workouts and everyday life. Movement integrity is based on balancing yin and yang muscular responsibilities within the constantly changing conditions of our minds and bodies. We are asked, therefore, to constantly discern where we are starting. The Taijitu symbol depicts balance not as a straight split but as a flow. To create balanced movement, our attention won't always require a fifty-fifty split between active and counter-active forces. Instead, balance asks us to flow between opposing forces as needed. Attending to the moment is the ability to adjust our movement's balance of forces while considering our posture's existing, tension-ridden imbalances.

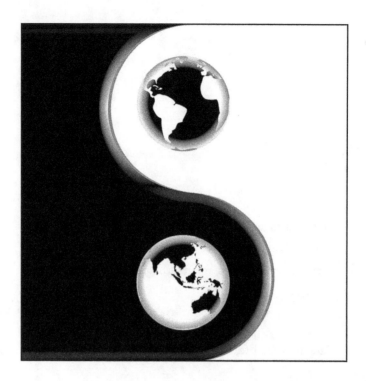

We are always transitioning from various demands, locations, or identities. A workout may fall between work life and home life. Maybe you are coming into your workout over-stimulated or fatigued. You may want to get pumped for the day's tasks, or maybe you need to lighten up for an evening date. Recognizing yin (counter-active) energy as calming and yang (active) energy as invigorating allows you to motivate the outcome you want.

By managing where your attention is, you adjust the subtle needs of each day's workout.

By establishing a clean relationship with the connection point—the place where counter-active energy transitions into active energy—we have freedom to place more or less focus on yin or yang influences as they relate to the outside resistance. With this variable, we are able to create a workout that is aligned with the ebb and flow of our energy level and the fluctuating conditions of our minds and bodies.

~ feel into this ~

Balance through Attention

Place greater attention on the yang aspect of your energy orbits—action—to create a more assertive, gregarious, and outwardly motivated workout.

Place greater attention on the yin aspect of your energy orbits—counter-action—to create a more peaceful, graceful, and introspective workout.

This is a subtle but effective variable that adds tremendous benefits to your overall experience. It offers you a workout choice. You can experience strength training as hard or soft, assertive or tranquil, outgoing or reflective. Their shared criterion, however, lies in keeping your connection point with the outside resistance precisely between the active and counter-active forces.

Be in the moment of a workout, look at your posture, experience your mood, and recognize whether you are stuck in your body or on a subject. What energy orbit and physical strength is needed to create balance in your posture's skeletal alignment? What meditative focus is needed to create physical, emotional, and mental alliance? Choose three to six muscle groups (including abdominals) that together support your intention. Decide on one to three exercises for each of those muscle groups that challenge the muscle from various angles. Connect to the resistance by first establishing essential alignment and visualizing the energy orbits. Then establish your connection point and balance the active and counter-active pathways of your movement. Place the psyche-muscular focus within the created energy pattern. As the energy pattern becomes balanced and you stretch your essential alignment, you are transforming the direction of your life. Value each exercise as a unifying tool for your mind, body, and spirit. Set up your workout for success in your inner and outer worlds.

- Observe your present condition and set an intention.
- Choose three to six muscle groups, including abdominals.
- Decide on one to three exercises for each muscle group.
- Establish essential alignment and visualize the energy orbit.
- Establish your connection point and balance active and counter-active pathways.
- Meditate on your isolated psyche-muscular component.
- Experience mind, body, and spirit as a unified team.

Holistic Self-Appraisal

To make positive change in your life, you first need to know where you are in relation to where you want to be. When it comes to sculpting the self, this means knowing who you are and how that "who" is affecting your overall strength. Well-being, as it pertains to the condition of your life force, is affected by the following:

- Physical disturbances—pain and tension, numbness, and weakness
- Emotional discontent—emotional avoidance and mental judgment
- Personality—coping mechanisms
- Lifestyle—organization of time between work, socializing, self-care, and hobbies
- Beliefs—underlying convictions

Before you can connect to the foundational strength you already have, you need to know where the tension and weakness lie that derail you from your strength. Ask yourself the following:

- Where am I concerned about my body?
- What subject triggers me into an emotional reaction? What subject turns me off?
- How do I manage my reactions?
- How do my reactions organize my priorities in life?
- What beliefs are causing me to steer my life in ineffective directions?

Discerning Your Condition

Once you recognize the ways you presently manage resistance through your body, mind, and lifestyle, you have a clear understanding of the areas where tension has sculpted your way of being. These are the areas in which you aren't standing in your strength. Physical disturbances clearly direct you toward the muscle group needing your focus, but mental discontent may ask you to refer to the psyche-muscular blueprint to direct your focus until the mind-body relationship becomes apparent. Lifestyle patterns are created by a cacophony of misdirected reactions that define your particular form of emotional chaos and direct your focus toward multiple psyche-muscular misalignments.

The root of your condition may be physical or mental; either way it affects your spirit's ability to shine through. No matter where your holding pattern is rooted, the expressions of misalignment create a consistent and recognizable pattern. By identifying your pattern's nature, you can establish a general framework to craft a mind-body strength-training workout. Your pattern is hyper, hypo, or hyper/hypo.

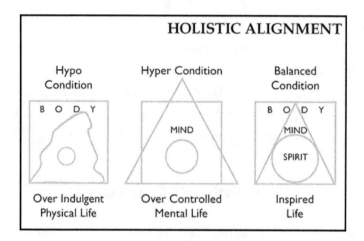

- Hypo-reaction conditions: These personalities want the world to take care of them and operate from a place of lack. They tend to focus on being liked or valued; have an eroded self-worth and confidence; and suffer from inflammation, over-extension, weak boundaries, and self-punishment. They are often defensive, self-critical, and over-indulgent; and they tend to distract themselves with entertainment, consumption or deprivation, contention, and sex—a victim posture.
- Hyper-reaction conditions: These personalities want to take care of the world and operate from a place of abundance. They are often rigid, hide their feelings, are over-controlling, and are rejecting of compromise. "Should be" and "must be" are guiding principles. They have tensed-up muscles, experience limited range of motion, are resistant to change, and tend to believe they can handle anything. They are thinkers who exercise their wills and have an ambivalent relationship with emotions—a survivor posture.
- Hyper/hypo-reaction conditions: They vacillate between hyper and hypo but don't quite find center; they stay frozen in uncertainty.

Take, for example, a thirty-two-year-old Broadway dancer who is riddled with injuries and has chronic inflammation body wide from years of dancing. She's currently teaching yoga and high-intensity cardio classes between gigs. To preserve her body, she recently tried to make the move from the chorus to leading lady but was told she was "sexy, not love-interest pretty." This feedback sent her into a spiral of emotional self-doubt and left her feeling intensely critical of her body, her purpose, and her talent. She continually blames her injuries for her circumstances and over-indulges in physical and emotional self-punishment. She's caught in a *hypo-reaction condition*, misled by an underlying belief that she must extend beyond her limits to be loved.

On the other hand, take a forty-seven-year-old IT director who suffers from intense shoulder and low-back pain. He is recovering from corrective surgery for a herniated disc. He prides himself on his ability to shoulder incredibly high levels of stress and trauma, but they take their toll on his body in the form of joint pain and high blood pressure. To avoid facing his limitations, he has physically clamped down, causing limited range of motion on every level of his life. He is over-controlling his world instead of looking inward. He is caught in a *hyper-reaction condition*, with an underlying belief system that conflates his ability to handle stress with his underlying emotional stoicness.

A thirty-year-old writer is a classic over-corrector. She either powers through stress mercilessly, placing impossible demands on herself, or heaps herself in self-criticism when she can't rise to the impossible goals she's set. She generally feels disconnected from her body but is starting to experience some pain in her shoulders and lower back—limiting her range of motion—and feels weakened from her constant chase to keep up. Because she vacillates between these two extremes, she is experiencing a *hyper/hypo-reaction condition*. She needs to feel the balance of contraction and release.

Create Your Own Workout

Creating a BodyLogos workout goes far beyond choosing the exercises. In addition to choosing the muscle groups and exercises appropriate for meeting your physical goals, you are deciding on the mental outlook and emotional viewpoint you want to create. Will you accentuate your energy's active force for a dynamic, action-oriented outlook or accentuate the counter-active force for a more introspective, self-reflective outcome? Will your active meditation focus on a specific psyche-muscular component or the greater energy orbit direction to which it's attached? Your artistry creates the experience and shapes your resulting life.

What you learn about yourself will ebb and flow exercise by exercise, day by day, week by week, and month by month. We are all unique in our survival patterns and the speed in which they transform.

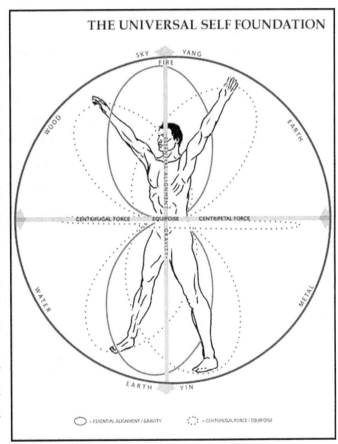

To address hyper or hypo conditions, you manage your energy to create alignment and balance.

- 75 percent counter-action to 25 percent action brings balance to hyper-reaction conditions. This places greater focus on feeling aligned and connected.

- 75 percent action to 25 percent counter-action brings balance to hypo-reaction conditions. This places greater focus on acknowledging alignment and connection.
- 50 percent counter-action to 50 percent action brings balance to hyper/hypo-reaction conditions.

Correcting Physical Complaints

When our pattern's strongest manifestation is in our bodies, we must listen to its divine wisdom and give it what it needs. Your body, either through pain or numbness, rigidity or weakness, may be sending you a message loud and clear that your patterns of survival need to be transformed.

Pain

Pain is a hyper-reaction to resistance. For handling pain, release the muscular tension in your overall posture and evaluate your essential alignment's vertical reach. This disengages your attention from the muscular holding pattern creating the discomfort and offers you an expanded skeletal position, which in turn expands your mental viewpoint. Next, choose an energy pattern that places the counter-active force in the area of pain. Visualize an active force that equals the force of your pain's tension. Do this without physical movement or deliberately contracting the active muscles. Treat the pain as the resistance and meet it with an equal force of orbiting energy. This step will concentrate the releasing effects of a counter-action on the painful area. Allow the active psyche-muscular component to be empowered as the counter-active component is subdued. You will be soothing the traumatized counter-active muscle by surrendering its psyche-muscular—physical and emotional—grip.

For example, if you are experiencing lower back pain, choose a lower abdominal crunch energy pattern—coming home—so the counter-active force is in the lower back. As you energize or actualize the lower abdominal crunch, feel the energy in your lower abdominals lift to the level that it takes to make the pain in your lower back subside—no more, no less. The pain is your resistance. Meet it with an equal amount of force. Find that sweet spot where the pain releases—too much force, and your back will get involved or react adversely; too little, and it will have no effect. Contain your movements to a size where the lower back remains pain free. With time, the tension will release.

Continue running energy this way until the pain is managed and meditative insights are experienced that can maintain your postural transformation. Once the pain is handled, choose exercises that continue to place the counter-active energy in the traumatized muscle group. This develops long-lasting resolution in the area.

Numbness and Weakness

Numbness or achiness in a muscle is a hypo-reaction to resistance. To address a lack of sensation and muscle weakness, increase the force of your energy orbits. Reach vertically through your essential alignment and notice where impingements (tension) disrupts your vertical stretch. With improved energy flow in your essential alignment, you will instantly feel more connection. Choose an energy pattern that places the active force in the area of weakness. Excite the energy orbit's force with curiosity about the active muscle's psyche-muscular component. Recognize this physical weakness as a challenge to connect with this aspect of your emotional self. Recognize your present state as an honest measure of your strength in the area. Be assured that building from this honesty will awaken the psyche-muscular holding pattern that has kept the area unresponsive. Continue running energy in this way until the muscle is able to maintain its state of being awake. This fosters trust in your own ability to handle opposition.

~ feel into this ~

Meditation to Defuse Reactivity

When you find yourself reacting to a life circumstance or interpersonal relationship, or when you just feel resistance toward life in general, you are being triggered by a psyche-muscular holding pattern that already exists in the body. Use musculoskeletal opposition to restore a neutral and open connection with your sense of self and the world.

Take a moment to discern whether you are experiencing a hyper- or hypo-reaction and feel where the emotional reaction is expressing itself in your body: an energy center; a muscle, bone, or joint; or possibly your mind is jumping from worry to worry. Extend energetically from the dan tien energy center toward earth and sky until your essential alignment stretches beyond the energy body and your reaction quiets its combative voice. Once you are aligned and poised, introduce an energy pattern that addresses the reactive psyche-muscular location.

Suppose You Are Having a Hyper-Reaction and Are Using Creating Forward Energy Pattern

First, balance the counter-active and active energy forces without engaging either muscle group. Focus your internal energy movement through the isolated connection being triggered (chest and back energy orbit) until it encourages the active muscle group to wake up (chest) and take notice of its psyche-muscular connection and meaning (smile of truth).

Second, meditate on your counter-active muscle's component (back's protection)—75 percent—as you use the action's force (chest's smile of truth)—25 percent—to drain the over-stimulated reactive expression. Cycle energy until you experience a notable surrendering of the mind-body reaction. In other words, you may be suspicious of your lover's behavior, causing your heart center to collapse into your back triggering mid-back discomfort. As the energy force down through the back increases, you release upwardly through your smile of truth (chest), and it becomes clear that you resent needing to protect yourself in the domain of this core relationship; so you have resisted using the balancing force of protection (back). This is the hyper-reactive controlling reaction showing itself. At this point, you may defend your reaction, stirring up a core belief. In other words, I deserve to be taken care of. If this happens, restretch your essential alignment and continue to cycle energy through the isolated connection until the reactive energy of the holding pattern is successfully channeled back to the dan tien energy center. This reorganization of tension will bring about a shift of consciousness—in other words, protecting myself in a relationship means staying self-possessed so I can stay honest with the relationships evolution and trusting I will be taken care of if I stay aligned within myself. Then a physical transformation ensues—in other words, relaxed muscular strength and/or joint space and/or reduced pain and/or sudden sweats.

The final step is to extend your focus to the unified connection of your energy pattern. With the entire body in on the reorganization of your muscular rebalancing, the core muscle group(s) needed to support the triggered area will become evident. In other words, the blockage may have been in the chest, but the core area of collapse can stem from the upper abdominals (spirit self). The resurgence of energy flowing from your core to the newly unblocked area feels like a sigh of relief, and from your newly expanded viewpoint, you feel safe and distant from the circumstances that triggered you. You are being energetically drawn into gravity's universal alignment rather than staying in your muscle's habitual outgrown beliefs. Continue practicing this new energy pattern until the old reactive pattern has fully dissolved.

For a hypo-reaction, you would follow the same protocol but reverse the hyper or hypo percentage of force, while a hyper/hypo-reaction remains a fifty-fifty split. By actively addressing your condition's pattern, emotional hope that change is in motion accompanies each insight made along the way.

Cultivating Physical Strength Workouts

The following workouts will be in consideration of a physical goal or concern. These exercise choices are for you to become familiar with how to combine exercises for an intended goal and a teaching methodology for safe execution. These workouts are suggested approaches for the sake of learning; however, each condition will have subtle differences that require artistry and know-how from you. Use these examples to inform your own instincts and intuition.

Notes:

Super Sets (SS): This is used to combine two or more exercises into one set.

Repetitions (reps): This refers to the number of times you perform an exercise without stopping.

Dyna-Band (DB): This is a latex strip used for freestanding resistance training.

Emotional Expression

Action: Meditate on developing action's psyche-muscular component.
Counter-action: Meditate on releasing counter-action's psyche-muscular component in relation to the action's psyche-muscular component.

Lumber Jack

Client Description

Lumber Jack is a forty-nine-year-old carpenter who handles heavy lumber daily yet is somewhat oblivious to his body's nuances. His complaint is general aches, pains, and fatigue. He wants to improve flexibility; ease the tension in his neck and shoulders, which causes headaches; alleviate foot fatigue; and increase overall energy. Lumber Jack has never engaged in a structured exercise program due to concern that it would exhaust him more.

Bone and Joint Placement

Wrist Roll (p.57)—Precede Crucifixion Curl.
Supine Tube Lie (p.62)—Finish workout.

Muscular Awareness

Flat-Footed Calf Raise (p.331)—Precede Hyperextended Calf Raise SS.
Single-Leg Hamstring Stretch with Flexed Foot (p. 274)—Follow Dead Lift SS.
Dyna-Band Circle (p.234)—Precede Seated Chest Press SS.

Workout

Lower Abdominal Crunch, 30 reps (p.116)/ Upper Abdominal Crunch, 30 reps (p.126)/Oblique Crunch, 30 alternating reps (p.140)

Dead Lift, 2–3 sets and 10–15 reps (p.302)—SS with Hyperextended Calf Raise
Hyperextended Calf Raise, 2–3 sets and 10–15 reps (p.334)

Seated Chest Press, 2–3 sets and 10–15 reps (p. 238)—SS with Lat Pull Down
Lat Pull Down, 2–3 sets and 10–15 reps (p. 196)

Crucifixion Curl, 2–3 sets and 10–15 reps (p.160)—SS with Triceps Push Down
One-Arm Triceps Push-Down, 2–3 sets and 10–15 reps (p. 220)

Note: Super sets with a common goal teach movement principles. In Super Set 1, because the arms aren't involved in the exercise, focus on dropping the shoulders through relaxed arms and shoulder blades. In Super Set 2 and 3, focus on understanding and exploring muscle opposition.

Emotional Expression

Focus on the following psyche-muscular meditations:

Action: Abdominals: Embody spirit self.
Action: Buttock: Embody comfort.
Counter-action to calves: Shins: Release groundedness.
Action: Chest: Embody a smile of truth.
Action: Back: Embody protection.
Counter-action to biceps: Triceps: Release pushing undesirables away.
Counter-action to triceps: Biceps: Release pulling desirables inward.

Note: Create a strong foundation (abdominal and buttock) to give him comfort in his own abilities. Strengthen his willingness to explore unconscious postural concerns (chest and back) that he may have never before considered, both as an active focus and counter-active focus (biceps and triceps).

Fire Dancer

Client Description

Fire Dancer is a twenty-seven-year-old belly dancer and aerobics instructor. Her hip joints and neck are problematic, and she has trouble sleeping through the night. She wants pain-free full range of motion in her hips and neck to unblock her connection with her center for better balance and more stable energy.

Bone and Joint Placement

Supine Tube Lie (p.62)—Begin workout.
Prone Straight-Leg Lie (p.61)—Precede Standing Hamstring Curl with DB.

Muscular Awareness

Forward Body Rock (p.295)—Precede Sumo Squat SS.
Praying Hands (p.233)—Precede Chest Press.
Supine Frog (p.316)—Finish workout.

Workout

Lower Abdominal Crunch, 30 reps (p.116)/ Upper Abdominal Crunch with Crossed Legs, 50 reps (p.130)/ Oblique Crunch, 20 reps––right and left (p.140)

Sumo Squat, 3 sets and 15 reps (p.306)—SS with Lying Adduction
Lying Adduction, 3 sets and 15–30 reps (p.320)

Standing Hamstring Curl, 3 sets and 10–15 reps––right and left (p.280)
Lying Chest Press, 3 sets and 15 reps (p.236)
Kickback, 3 sets and 15 reps (p.216)

Parallel Squat, 3 sets and 15–25 reps. (p.260)––SS with Calf Raise
Calf Raise, 3 sets and 15–25 reps (p.338)

Note: An early super set combination focused on the same big muscles produces muscle failure, grounding her hyper energy. Single exercise sets follow to focus her mind on relaxed connected movement.

Emotional Expression

Focus on the following psyche-muscular meditations:

Counter-action to Abdominals: Low Back: Release fear.
Counter-action to Buttocks: Inferior Iliopsoas: Release control.
Action: Hamstrings: Embody movement back.
Action: Inner Thigh: Embody movement inward.
Counter-action to Chest: Back: Release protection.
Action: Triceps: Embody pushing undesirables away.
Counter-action to Quadriceps: Hamstrings: Release movement hack.
Action: Calves: Embody determination.

Note: Release the fear (lower back), control (iliopsoas), and protection (back) congested in her neck and hip areas. This will increase joint space for mobility while strengthening core muscles to restore a sense of center (abdominals). Balance her attention and alternate the focus between actions and counter-actions to teach energy control in and out of workouts. Her sleeping and waking hours become more energetically stable.

Earth Mother

Client Description

Earth Mother is a fifty-three-year-old motorcyclist with lower back pain and tight hip joints who suffers from neck and shoulder discomfort. She wants to be fit for long motorcycle outings and to strengthen arms and abdominal muscles. Weight loss is an ongoing concern and frustration.

Bone and Joint Placement

Dead Cow (p.50)—Precede Seated Row.

Muscular Awareness

Shoulder Blade Grab (p.193)—Precede or place between Seated Row sets.
Iliopsoas Seated Knee Lift (p.296)—Precede Seated Abduction SS.
Door Breaker (p.169)—Precede Standing Overhead Press SS.
Supine Ball Abdominal Stretch (p.113)—Finish workout.

Workout

Lower Abdominal Crunch, 20–50 reps (p.116)/Lower Abdominal Touchdown, 20–50 reps (p.118)/Extended Upper Abdominal Crunch, 20–50 reps (p.128)

Seated Row, 2–3 sets and 15 reps (p.198)

Seated Abduction, 2–3 sets and 15 reps (p.304)—SS with Lying Overhead Triceps Extension
Lying Overhead Triceps Extensions, 2–3 sets and 15 reps (p.214)

Parallel Squat Static, 2–3 sets and 30 reps (p.260)—SS with Standing Overhead Press
Standing Overhead Press, 2–3 sets and 15 reps (p.180)

Note: Use super sets that alternate between upper and lower body to increase cardio and calorie burning. Add weight-bearing cardio (for example, treadmill), which is more calorie burning than non-weight-bearing cardio (for example, bike), for thirty to forty-five minutes on alternate days between strength-training workouts.

Emotional Expression

Focus on the following psyche-muscular meditations:

Counter-action to abdominals: Low back: Release fear.
Counter-action to back: Chest: Release smile of truth.
Counter-action to buttocks: Inferior iliopsoas: Release control.
Action: Triceps: Embody pushing undesirables away.
Action: Quadriceps: Embody movement forward.
Action: Shoulder exercise: Embody values or morals.

Note: Releasing tension from hip (quadriceps and buttock) and shoulder (shoulder and triceps) muscles to restore bone placement will support her upper body to freely open her smile of truth (chest).

Help her recognize the fear (lower back) and control (iliopsoas) she's holding unnecessarily.

Actively asserting her triceps, quadriceps, and shoulder muscles develops confidence for moving ahead in her life without the extra baggage.

Iron Man

Client Description

Iron Man is a sixty-year-old swimmer and bodybuilder with knee problems and elbow discomfort.

He wants to rehab his knees and elbows, maintain his strength, and become more aerobically fit without losing muscle mass.

Bone and Joint Placement

Prayer Position (p.58)—Begin workout.

Muscular Awareness

Lying Leg Extension (p.251)—Precede Leg Press.
Prone Knee Bend with Tube (p.273)—Precede Seated Leg Curl.
Supine Elbow Bend with Flexed Wrist (p.151)—Precede Biceps Curl.

Workout

Lower Abdominal Crunch, 30 reps (p.116)/Lower Abdominal Touchdown, 30 reps (p.118)/Leg Extensions, 30 reps (p.120)/Lower Abdominal Six-Inch Raise, 30 reps (p.122)/Upper Abdominal Crunch with 90-Degree Leg Raise, 50–100 reps (p.132)

Leg Press, 3 sets and 10 reps (p.258)—SS with Weighted Hyperextended Calf Raise
Weighted Hyperextended Calf Raise, 3 sets and 10 reps (p.336)

Standing Anterior/Posterior/Side Lateral Shoulder Raises, 3 sets and 10–15 reps each (p.172-177)

Seated Leg Curl, 3 sets and 10–15 reps (p.276)—SS with Ball Squeeze
Ball Squeeze, 10 reps (p.282)

Seated Biceps Curl with Hammerhead Grip, 3 sets and 10 reps (p.154)
Seated Straight-Leg Raise, 3 sets and 10–15 reps—right and left (p.254)
Standing Chest Fly, 3 sets and 8–12 reps (p.242)

Note: Alternate between upper- and lower-body exercises to increase cardio fitness; perform single muscle sets to continue building muscle mass. Add non-weight-bearing cardio for joint ease fifteen to twenty minutes before or after a strength-training workout. Limit range of motion in leg and bicep curls as needed for pain-free joint mobility.

Emotional Expression

Focus on the following psyche-muscular meditations:

Counter-action of Abdominals: Lower back: Release fear.
Counter-action to Quadriceps: Hamstrings: Release movement back.
Counter-action to Calves: Shins: Release groundedness.
Counter-action: Shoulder: Release values or morals.
Counter-action to Hamstrings: Quadriceps: Release movement forward.
Counter-action to Biceps: Triceps: Release pushing undesirables away.
Counter-action to Chest: Back: Release protection.

Note: Release the need to attack resistance and explore the idea of uniting with resistance. Focus on the counter-action to align and support his weakened joints.

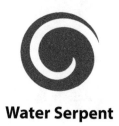

Water Serpent

Client Description

Water Serpent is a thirty-eight-year-old with a newborn. She used to run marathons and now has time for only the occasional group fitness class. Her lower back continues to tighten up since the birth of her child. She wants to alleviate pain in her lower and middle back, improve her posture, increase her energy level, and lose inches in her waistline. Her time limitations give her a feeling of defeat before even starting, causing her to become hyper-vigilant with her child's well-being.

Bone and Joint Placement

Prone Straight-Leg Lie (p.61)—Precede Hyperextension SS.
Prone Ball Lie (p.62)—Finish workout.

Muscular Awareness

Abdominal Breathing Exercise (p.113)—Precede abdominal exercises.
Kneeling Butt Tuck (p.297)—Follow Hyperextension SS.
Hollow Thigh Hug (p.193)—Follow One-Arm Row SS.

Workout

Seated Combo Crunch, 3 sets and 30 reps (p.134)—SS with Standing Straight-Leg Adduction
Standing Straight-Leg Adduction, 3 sets and 15 reps––right and left (p.322)

Hyperextension, 3 sets and 15 reps (p.300)—SS with Seated Overhead Press
Seated Overhead Press, 3 sets and 15 reps (p.178)

Leg Extension, 3 sets and 15 reps (p.256)—SS with One-Arm Rows
One-Arm Rows, 3 sets and 10–15 reps––right and left (p.200)

Seated Adduction, 3 sets and 10–15 reps (p.318)—SS with Seated Chest Fly
Seated Chest Fly, 3 sets and 10–15 reps (p.240)

Note: Bring attention immediately to alignment by making her aware of her central plumb line in the abdominal to inner-thigh progression. This step will neutralize her misguided hyper-reactivity.

Each super set alternates between lower and upper body to increase her calorie burning.

Emotional Expression

Focus on the following psyche-muscular meditation:

Action: Abdominals: Embody spirit self.
Action: Inner thigh: Embody movement inward.
Action: Buttock: Embody comfort.
Action: Triceps: Embody pushing undesirables away.
Action: Quadriceps: Embody movement forward.
Counter-action to back: Chest: Release smile of truth.
Action: Chest: Embody smile of truth.

Note: Focus her attention toward personal power (abdominals, inner thighs, and buttocks).

Clear away the emotional defeat that prevents her from moving forward freely (triceps and quadriceps). Transform the worry to protect her child into the quest to reassure her child (chest and back).

Stay connected to her smile of truth (chest) rather than the protection of it through mindful alignment in all exercises.

Meeting a Challenge

When challenging a psyche-muscular area in strength training, work with an outside resistance that challenges the strength you already have in the area. Feel the strength needed in relation to a resistance and meet it maintaining postural integrity. Don't demand the next level of strength before you are there. If you compromise postural integrity, you separate from your inward connection and wind up feigning an actual connection—and separate from the intended psyche-muscular area. Allow your strength to develop by actively being in it. Explore your strength's character as if being introduced to yourself anew with each exercise. Experience the strength and flexibility each isolated muscle group has in the moment by keeping your range of motion, speed, and intensity at a level that matches your subtle but constantly fluctuating abilities. An exercise that doesn't produce joint pain or emotional struggle while challenging the belly of your intended muscle is an example of meeting resistance successfully.

Recognize the ways you resist outside resistance. Experience the details of your avoidance by first paying attention to your physical posture, mental insights, emotional responses, and energy qualities. Train for personal ease. When that ease is disrupted, train for positive change by aligning skeletal placement, balancing muscular forces, and connecting energy centers to both your inside foundation and the outside resistance. Going through the motions of an exercise without taking the necessary steps to feel connected often creates the experience of empty or dutiful hard work rather than feeling energized and empowered. With heightened physical sensitivity and competent isolation skills, however, muscles develop greater acuity, and psyche-muscular insights become more and more cognizant. Use the "How to Isolate" sections throughout Part 3 to guide you in gaining isolated muscle sensitivity and skill.

Emotional Transmutation Chapter

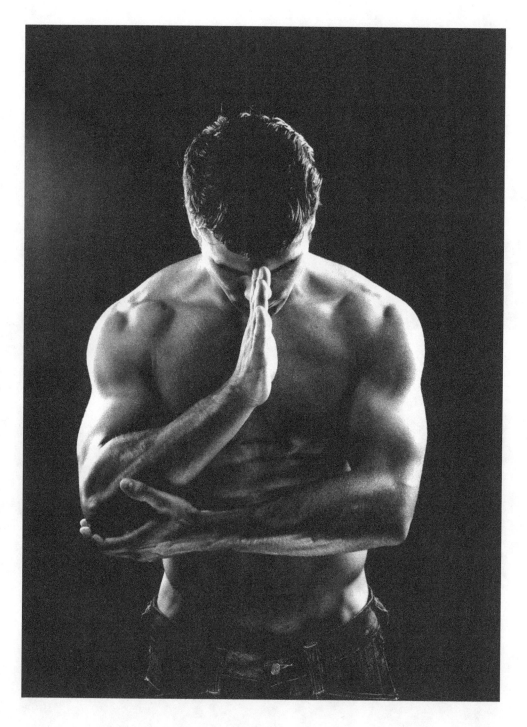

Explore physical-spiritual strength.
Move from the equipoise of your human trilogy.
Commit to standing in your original nature fearlessly.

Lesson 14
Train the Mind

Though there are beautiful things to be seen,
The Master remains unattached and calm.

If you let yourself be blown to and fro,
You lose touch with your roots.
If you let restlessness move you,
You lose touch with who you are.

—Lao Tzu, *Tao Te Ching*

Individual beauty matures as one's purpose unfolds.
Please others, and the Master is lost,
Please yourself, and the purpose is lost.

—Tammy Wise, BodyLogos

The Purpose of Spirit

BodyLogos follows Tao values. Mind and body are equal but not the same. Where the body's intelligence is in feeling and expressing emotion, the mind's intelligence is in collecting information and thinking. When you add the spirit's supreme intelligence, positive change is possible. Resolving inner conflict avails you to a meaningful purpose that makes you truly happy—content with your life's path. Ignoring inner conflict disengages you from meaningful connections with life; discontent plagues your life's path.

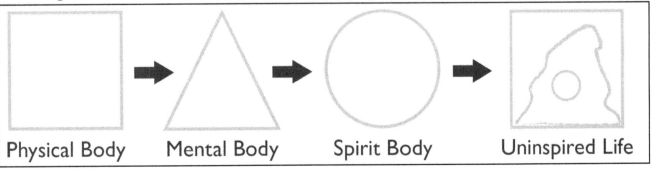

Think of your body, mind, and spirit as three islands. BodyLogos helps you to build a bridge between the three. Some of us have built whole towns and cities on one or two islands and almost nothing on a third. If you are conscious of physical patterns, you are well acquainted with your body; if you are conscious of your mental patterns, you are well acquainted with your mind; if you are conscious of a supreme intelligence, you are well acquainted with spirit. Becoming conscious of all three aspects of the self is the first step toward personal resolution. Releasing the tension that keeps your body, mind, and spirit separated is what allows you to permanently forgo a reactive pattern with ease. Wherever your greatest consciousness lies, BodyLogos offers a way in to build the infrastructure of your internal archipelago—the trilogy of you.

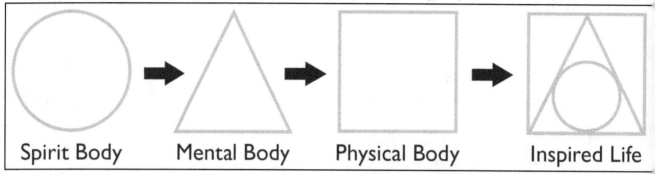

To build the bridges between body, mind, and spirit, start where you are most acquainted.
- If spirit guides you, the psyche-muscular blueprint will help you see how the body and mind mirror each other.
- If the body carries you, balance hyper or hypo muscular patterns to help you recognize how mind and spirit need unity to release tension.
- If the mind manages you, stretch your skeletal alignment into equipoise to help you feel how both spirit and body originate from the organized and well-established strength of life force.

Becoming Conscious

Stepping into unknown territory, like your first day of school or your first day at the gym, is always a reminder that you're vulnerable, ignorant, and imperfect. You may be a straight-A student at school, but at the gym you flounder, and it's scary (or vice versa). Often your biggest obstacle in expanding consciousness is handling the emotional fears of not being good enough. How often do you think, *I should have known that* or *I should be able to do this*? Why should you? From a Tao perspective, the fact that you are human means you are imperfect, and your life is the canopy that teaches you of the perfection of spirit. To step into the unknown, with the intent to improve yourself, is to step closer to the ideal of perfection. Be at ease knowing you are on a journey. Can you be okay with wanting more?

Whether it's psyche-muscular insights, muscular balance, or discovering equipoise that renders you conscious of internal misalignment and its origin, it is introducing you to an unfamiliar aspect of you. Because this is a physical practice, at first this can feel like it's specifically related to your workout. But like your mind and body mirroring each other, how you work out in the gym and how you work out in your life mirror each other. Acknowledge your reactive patterns as yours. They aren't the fault of gym challenges or life challenges—they are yours to own. The challenge is in facing the pattern physically, mentally, and spiritually. And this doesn't mean toughing out the trigger that elicited the pattern. It means facing the reaction you are having, getting curious about its outrage, and discovering an alternate relationship with the irritant. New consciousness will lead you back to your body anew. This newness can resemble Bambi trying to stand up for the first time. It's a little shaky at first.

The less practiced muscle groups of the body can feel humbled in their lack of know-how. Whether physically uncoordinated, uncomfortable, or limited in mobility, they can become emotionally unwilling to make an effort. Getting past defensive psyche-muscular reactions like "I don't know how" or "I feel uncomfortable" is the first layer of defense you might encounter. Any number of value judgments may follow as a second line of defense, such as, "I'm not good at this," "I'm not making a difference," or "I'm not strong enough." Before feeling the deeper and more insightful expressions that live in the muscle's belly, you will experience the layers of armor you have built against feeling deeply. All these fear voices are held as psyche-muscular holding patterns in the muscular system. Once given the permission to be experienced fully, your energy orbit's counter-action can disengage and release the held pattern.

For example, if you experience "I'm not good at this" while doing bicep curls, whose psyche-muscular nature is pulling desirables inward, you would focus instead on the bicep counter-action. Instead of focusing on not being good at this, meditate on the triceps counter-action (pushing undesirables away). "What do I need to let go of, to get better at this?" Maybe you need to decrease the weight. Maybe you need to sit down to stabilize. Maybe you need a trainer to keep you accountable to maintain your alignment. Before you know it, you are feeling, *I wasn't good at this, but I'm getting the hang of it now.* Or you might first experience a deeper emotional sadness, such as, "Am I not good at this because I wasn't allowed to play sports as a kid?" This experience is a stepping-stone toward feeling successful at your present effort or ability.

The permission to feel your fears as you release a muscle group's psyche-muscular hold allows the self-sabotaging pattern blocking your action to surrender and makes room for your current emotions to come forward to inform and inspire you. Repressing a defensive reaction keeps it intact. It keeps you from accessing the less assertive and subtle muscle groups in the body and discourages the deeper aspects of yourself to emerge. Atrophy is an unnecessary paralyzing disability for an otherwise-healthy mind and body.

Reactivity defends who you have been while stunting who you could become. The theory of yin and yang has shown that strength is found by allowing opposition; in fact, it is through opposition that you develop greater alignment and stability in your position. To gain strength in any practice or philosophy, you start as a beginner. If a defensive reaction exists, no matter how practiced you are in a discipline, it must be approached with a beginner's mind. A beginner need not ever feel defeated by weakness; by its very nature, it is triumphant to explore weakness. You are awakening an area that before now was undeveloped or even latent. Rather than avoiding the discomfort of being unable to do something, or unaware of doing something, can you appreciate your effort in becoming able and aware? Can you recognize that the reason you are experiencing weakness is because you are evolving past your previous level of strength? Muscle failure indicates you have undertaken a greater level of personal responsibility. Can you permit this feeling to be one of success? Can you go so far as to find the experience of weakness valuable and encouraging?

The psyche-muscular blueprint brings meaning to every strength and weakness, every hyper and hypo condition in your mind and body. Whatever you are being physically is what you are being emotionally. This added dimension of understanding can be cause for greater humiliation or appreciation. Regret helps enforce change, but to strive freely as your highest self is worth the price of a little humiliation. You are being made aware of a drain to your energy system. It is a drain you created in a time of great need, but it is a new time with changed needs. An unconscious or conscious avoidance of a personal imbalance robs you of vitality and strength. Once you are made aware of it, you can choose to accept it or change it. You are now in a position to train your mind by way of deliberate physical posturing. You are now in a position to change and stand in a revised viewpoint.

Correcting Psychological Complaints

Emotional Pain

When being self-critical or judgmental, recognize this is due to a reluctance to feel the uncomfortable emotions beneath the judgment. This is evidence that you have muscled your way through something that is so painful that you have buried it in your subconscious. Psyche-muscular conflict is locked inside your musculoskeletal system, blocking your energy flow.

To unravel the judgment, first allow yourself to feel your emotions as a valid viewpoint. Find the truth behind the judgment. "I am carrying more weight around my midsection than I'd like to be" is a valid and true statement. "And therefore I am disgusting and unattractive" is the judgment. Your first step is to allow this uncomfortable truth to exist without twisting it with judgment. It's vital that you allow your feelings and yourself to mourn when things aren't the way you want them to be. We must own the things we don't like about our present situation without justifying or damning them—it has to be okay that things aren't okay.

Check in with your body. Where are you feeling judgment's grip? You might very clearly feel it in a specific part of your body—for example, hunched shoulders or a collapsed chest. Other times, you may not feel it in your body at all because you just can't feel it, or you're in too much emotional pain and are over-stimulated. In this case, recognize what you like or dislike to work out and use the psyche-muscular blueprint to analyze its significance. Discern the energy pattern that's right for you to work intuitively. No matter what, when referencing the psyche-muscular blueprint, remember that you have the option to use the active or counter-active force to activate or release energy.

Recognize your judgments as a departure from spirit, since they are defensive against what is authentically being experienced. You appreciate that personal alignment includes all your emotions, pleasant and unpleasant, and knowing them intimately is crucial for a successful relationship with yourself and outside resistance.

From this vantage point, you become aware of how buried emotions fracture your life and how allowing emotions makes life whole. From here, you can discern whether you are having a hyper-reaction or a hypo-reaction to your emotional truth.

For example, the truth of an emotion may be, "The people who love me don't feel the need to protect me, and that makes me feel less valuable." A hyper-reaction would follow with, "So I need to protect myself from them. I can't depend on anyone else but myself in this world." A hypo-reaction would say, "So I guess I'm not really worth protecting." In both instances, I would need to work my back, which is connected to my sense of protection. But if it's a hyper-reaction, my meditative focus would be on my chest's release (smile of truth), not on my back's contraction. And if I had a hypo-reaction, my meditative focus would be on contracting my back (protection).

Now the workout itself is inspiring your performance and dissolving the judgments that hinder you by truthfully connecting with and balancing your emotions.

Spiritual Disconnection

When feeling disconnected from yourself, your sense of purpose, or your life, recognize it as a reluctance to be yourself. The expansion needed to be your highest self is compressed inside your physicality, leaving you trapped by the limitations of your mind and body.

Though unmotivated, use your will to bring this reluctance into a workout to explore it more deeply. Curiosity is your motivation until a clear intention is realized. Meditate on your feelings of reluctance through the psyche-muscular component being worked. As you perform the exercises, maintain a strong stance as a neutral witness. From this stance, it will feel like you are with the experience rather than being the experience. The distance between you and your reluctance allows you to recalibrate skeletal, muscular, emotional, and mental misalignments.

Witness your misalignments adjusting and recognize them as unconscious reactions to being yourself. This offers you greater awareness regarding the intentions you need to set to create positive change. As you continually explore your energy alignment, you are consciously changing your relationship with yourself, your practice, and your life. To be self-motivated is to pay attention to what inspires you as well as where conflict around being inspired exists. Acknowledging and experiencing discontent unveils your habitual reactions to living your life, reactions that can be transformed into inspired actions you would prefer. Actions that align personal choices with personal needs inspire a self from the Self. Intention and purpose are revealed and manifest the life you were born to live.

~ feel into this ~

Meditation to Establish Intention

When you want to connect to a situation, an individual, or life in general with a specific or more refined outlook, you are creating a new psyche-muscular pattern. Use musculoskeletal opposition and clear intention to empower both your inward and outward alignment with that outlook.

Take a moment to feel into your intended outlook. What is being expressed in mind and body other than the refined perspective you want? Where does this obstacle exist in your body? What is it saying? Discern whether you are experiencing a hyper- or hypo-reaction. Extend energetically from the dan tien energy center toward earth and sky until your essential alignment stretches beyond the energy body and you feel neutral. Once aligned, introduce an energy pattern that addresses the obstructed psyche-muscular area.

Suppose you are having a hypo-reaction and are using determined power energy pattern.

First, balance the counter-active and active energy forces without engaging either muscle group. Focus your internal energy movement through the isolated connection of the obstacle until the counter-active muscle group surrenders.

Second, meditate on your refined outlook in relation to the active muscle's psyche-muscular component. Contemplate the intermingling of your intended outlook and your active muscle's component—75 percent—as you use the counter-action's releasing force—25 percent—to drain the obstacle. Let the internal movement enliven the refined outlook so its intention burrows into the obstacle as if asserting itself into being. You will gradually experience a transmutation, an insight that explains the obstacle; in other words, the intention to feel relaxed when with your family is accompanied by a collapse in your upper back and an emotional crash, directing your meditation toward protection (back). Interrelating your intention to feel free and your emotional habit to collapse your back from its judgments leads you to realize, "To sincerely protect myself, I have to stop valuing their judgments and value my own." And an emotional transmutation ensues; in other words, your fresh intention overpowers and unveils the persistent belief from the past, "My family doesn't value who I am," and replaces it with, "I value who I am."

Finally, extend your focus to the unified connection of your energy pattern. As your entire body becomes energetically reorganized, you recognize your ability to intend an outlook into being and recognize what energy pattern is needed to secure that intention moving forward. Celebrate your willingness to change—to stop blaming others for the way you feel—and retreat from the defensive posture of your past beliefs. Recognize the ways this longstanding belief gets triggered in your life and become inspired to strengthen that psyche-muscular area in your posture. Design your workouts to specifically strengthen postures and perspectives that support this change. Be curious about the trial and error of change and enjoy creating yourself anew every day. Continue to use the active force to strengthen the refined outlook as the counter-action gives the old pattern an exit. Continue until you fully experience the refinement you intend to create.

By actively addressing obstacles, new beliefs that create positive change will rapidly unfold.

If you are unable to choose how you want to connect with life after doing the meditation to establish intention, and instead feel something unwanted is being done to you, you are still in the trauma of a reaction. Take time to explore the previous meditation to defuse reactivity exercise (p.353) and then return to the former exercise.

Cultivating Psychological Strength Workouts

The following workouts will be in consideration of an emotional condition or need. These exercise choices are for you to become familiar with how to combine exercises for an intended goal and how to best empower the will. These workouts are suggested approaches for the sake of learning. However, each individual will have subtle differences that require artistry from you. Use these examples to inform your own instincts and intuition.

Notes:

Super Sets (SS): This is used to combine two or more exercises into one set.

Repetitions (reps): This refers to the number of times you perform an exercise without stopping.

Dyna-Band (DB): This is a latex strip used for freestanding resistance

Emotional Expression

Action: Meditate on developing action's psyche-muscular component.
Counter-action: Meditate on releasing counter-action's psyche-muscular component in relation to the action's psyche-muscular component.

Strong as an Oak

Client Description

Strong as an Oak is a sixty-two-year-old CEO with a grown child of forty-two years and a newborn of nine months. Once a college football star with great athletic ability, he now finds himself fifty pounds overweight, out of shape, and struggling with a heart condition. He has built a business empire, taken financial responsibility for two families, rides a Harley-Davidson motorcycle, and is the oldest son in a demanding family. He needs emotional support to face his physical condition, motivation to do something about it, and confidence that being a beginner again will reintroduce him to his strength by way of his weaknesses.

Bone and Joint Placement

Prone Ball Lie (p.62)—Precede Standing Lateral Raise SS.
Supine Tube Lie (p.62)—Finish workout.

Muscular Awareness

Abdominal Breathing Exercise (p.113)—Begin workout.
Shoulder Blade Grab (p.170)—Precede Lat Pull Down SS.

Workout

Lower Abdominal Crunch, 20 reps (p.116)/Lower Abdominal Touchdown, 20 reps (p.118)/Upper Abdominal Crunch, 40 reps (p.126)

Seated Abduction, 2–3 sets and 15 reps (p.304)—SS with Standing Lateral Raise
Standing Lateral Raise, 2–3 sets and 15 reps (p.172)

Leg Press, 2–3 sets and 15 reps (p.258)—SS with Weighted Hyperextended Calf Raise
Weighted Hyperextended Calf Raise, 2–3 sets and 15 reps (p.336)

Lat Pull Down, 2–3 sets and 15 reps (p.196)—SS with Seated Chest Press
Seated Chest Press, 2–3 sets and 15 reps (p.238)

Note: Orient his breath with his center using basic abdominal exercises. Super Set 1 alternates upper and lower body exercises to invigorate workout and burn calories. Super Set 2 focuses on understanding muscle opposition and how to release tension. Seated exercises consider his heart condition and performance success.

Emotional Expression

Focus on the following psyche-muscular contemplations:

Action: Abdominals: Spirit self
Action: Buttocks: Comfort
Action: Shoulders: Values or morals
Action: Quadriceps: Movement forward
Action: Calves: Determination
Action: Back: Protection
Action: Chest: Smile of truth

Note: Open with motivation; help him feel comfortable and valuable within himself. Movement forward and weighing his protective behavior against his smile of truth pose greater challenge. Allow personal insights to be private but continue to inspire his commitment to well-being with your commitment to the mind-body connection.

Flame Resistant, Not Flameproof

Client Description

Flame Resistant is a fifty-year-old assistant in a high-power financial firm. Her job is to know her boss better than he knows himself. If her sensitivity to his needs is off, his sensitivity toward her is off. Her life is predominantly her job, or shall I say her boss. She eats on the run, has little time for socializing, and has stopped working out. She's grown nervous, insecure, antisocial, defensive, and exhausted. She wants her life back, a loving relationship, and some much-deserved fun.

Bone and Joint Placement

Prone Straight-Leg Lie (p.61)—Precede Dead Lift.
Supine Tube Lie (p.62)—Finish workout.

Muscular Awareness

Supine Elbow Lift with Pressed Fingertips (p.211)—Precede Triceps Extension.
Overhead Shoulder Blade Touch Down (p.211)—Follow Triceps Extension SS.

Workout

Lower Abdominal Crunch, 30 reps (p.116)/Lower Abdominal Leg Extensions, 30 reps (p.120)/Extended Upper Abdominal Crunch, 50 reps (p.128)

Dead Lift, 2–3 sets and 15 reps (p.302)—SS with Seated Adduction
Seated Adduction, 2–3 sets and 15–25 reps (p.318)

Hydrant Hamstring Curls, 2–3 sets and 10–15 reps each leg (p.278)—SS with Lying Overhead Triceps Extension
Lying Overhead Triceps Extension, 2–3 sets and 10–15 reps (p.214)

Parallel Squat, 2–3 sets and 15 reps (p.260)—SS with Seated Biceps Curl with Outward Rotation
Seated Biceps Curl with Outward Rotation, 2–3 sets and 15 reps (p.158)

Note: Super Set 1 focuses on aligning the buttock and inner-thigh strength to give a sense of personal power and readiness to commit to her personal life. Super Sets 2 and 3 alternate between upper and lower body, focusing on cardio and weight loss as well as encouragement of movement in life

Emotional Expression

Focus on the following psyche-muscular contemplations:

Action: Abdominals: Spirit self
Action: Buttocks: Comfort
Action: Inner thighs: Movement inward
Action: Hamstrings: Movement back
Action: Triceps: Pushing undesirables away
Action: Quadriceps: Movement forward
Action: Biceps: Pulling desirables inward

Note: Super Set 1 focuses on being comfortable moving inward toward herself. Super Set 2 focuses on recognizing when to say no to undesirable life conditions. Super Set 3 looks ahead at the life she would like to create.

Misplaced Earthling

Client Description

Misplaced earthling is an eighteen-year-old high school senior who feels like she doesn't belong anywhere. She's a competitive gymnast who struggles with an eating disorder, flip-flops from happy to horrid, and has a need for acceptance that leads her into dangerous relationships. She exists in a perpetual state of uncertainty and is resolute in covering it up. She wants to feel more grounded and connected with her goals.

Bone and Joint Placement

Dead Cow (p.59)—Precede abdominals.
Door Breaker (p.169)—Precede Standing Posterior Raise.

Muscular Awareness

Forward Body Rock (p.295)—Precede Sumo Squat.
Praying Hands (p.233)—Precede Seated Chest Fly.
Seated Heel Kiss (p.315)—Precede Calf Raises Turned Out.

Workout

Lower Abdominal Crunch, 30 reps (p.116)/Lower Abdominal Six-Inch Raise, 50 reps (p.122) /Upper Abdominal Crunch, 30 reps (p.126)/Oblique Crunch, 3 sets and 20 reps (p.140)

Sumo Squat, 3 sets and 15-20 reps (p.306)—SS with Standing Straight-leg Adduction
Standing Straight-Leg Adduction, 3 sets and 10–15 reps––right and left (p.322)

Seated Chest Fly, 3 sets and 15 reps (p.240)—SS with Standing Overhead Triceps Extension
Standing Overhead Triceps Extension, 3 sets and 15 reps (p.218)

Standing Posterior Lateral Raise (p.176)/Standing Anterior Lateral Raise, 3 sets and 15 reps each each (p.174)
Calf Raises Turned Out, 3 sets and 15 reps (p.340)

Note: Pyramiding abdominal intensity helps her relax into her body's weight. Super Set 1 aligns the buttock power with her central plumb line, offering a sense of empowerment. Super Set 2 lifts her body up while pushing resistance away. The shoulders can then move her outward as the turned-out calf work keeps her connected inward.

Emotional Expression

Focus attention on the following energy forces:

Action: Abdominals: Spirit self
Action: Buttock: Comfort
Action: Inner thighs: Inward movement
Action: Chest: Smile of truth
Counter-action to triceps: Biceps: Pulling desirables inward
Action: Shoulders: Values or morals
Action: Calves: Determination

Note: Inspiring comfort in feeling her feelings is essential to recognize what inspires her heart. Ask what she wants to make room for (triceps)? What makes her feel valuable (shoulders)? Encourage her to feel her answers in the movement rather than talk about them.

Iron-Clad Grip

Client Description

Iron-Clad Grip can carry a pipeline on each shoulder. He has got the spirit of a bull; he plows his body through things without thinking or testing them first. As a result, he is regarded as accident prone. He is forty-six years old and riddled with joint pain, headaches, and lower-back weakness. He is never without pain medication. He has always been a manual workman, not a gym rat. He wants to feel well enough to work without pain or pain medication.

Bone and Joint Placement

Wrist Roll (p.57)—Precede Seated Row.
Prayer Position (p.58)—Precede Chest Press.

Muscular Awareness

Abdominal Breathing Exercise (p.113)—Precede Abdominals.
Hollow Thigh Hug (p.193)—Follow Seated Row.
Supine Elbow Bend with Flexed Wrist (p.151)—Precede Seated Biceps Curl.
Supine Elbow Lift with Pressed Fingertips (p.211)—Precede Triceps Push Down.
Lying Leg Extension (p.251)—Precede Seated Leg Extension.

Workout

Lower Abdominal Crunch, 2 sets and 30 reps (p.116)/Upper Abdominal Crunch, 30 reps (p.126)
Seated Row, 2 sets and 15 reps (p.198)
Lying Chest Press, 2 sets and 15 reps (p.236)
Seated Biceps Curl with Hammerhead Grip, 2 sets and 15 reps (p.154)
One-Arm Triceps Push Down, 2 sets and 15 reps (p.229)
Leg Extension, 2 sets and 10–15 reps (p.256)
Seated Leg Curl, 2 sets and 10–15 reps (p.276)

Note: Teaching awareness is primary in this workout. The Wrist Roll will take the control out of his hands so he can refocus on isolating larger muscle groups. Rest enough between sets to avoid overloading the joints and demand proper alignment.

Emotional Expression

Focus on the following psyche-muscular contemplations:

Counter-action of abdominals: Lower back: Fear
Action: Back: Protection
Action: Chest: Smile of truth
Action: Biceps: Pulling desirables inward
Action: Triceps: Pushing undesirables away
Action: Quadriceps: Movement forward
Action: Hamstrings: Movement backward

Note: Recognizing and releasing the fear in his lower back will connect him to his spirit self and slow down his approach to all exercises. Focus on isolating muscle groups and exploring their emotional holding patterns. Introduce an internal world rather than allowing his sole concern to be his effect, or lack thereof, on the outside world.

Wallowing Water Works

Client Description

As a twenty-nine-year-old single Jewish woman, Wallowing Water Works is under great pressure to marry. She's up for partner at her law firm and is in a constant battle between her firm and her faith.

She feels unattractive, desperate, and hopeless about the predicament of her personal life—and uninspired, lazy, and resentful about her work. Wallowing Water Works wants to lose twenty-five pounds, improve her posture, and strengthen her resolve.

Bone and Joint Placement

Prone Straight-Leg Lie (p.61)—Precede Hyperextension.
Supine Tube Lie (p.62)—Finish workout.

Muscular Awareness

Abdominal Breathing Exercise (p.113)—Precede abdominal exercises.
Praying Hands (p.233)—Precede Seated Chest Fly SS.

Workout

Seated Combo Crunch, 2–3 sets and 25 reps (p.134)/Oblique Crunch with Lower Torso Twist, 2–3 sets and 25 reps––right and left (p.138)

Hyperextension, 2–3 sets and 15 reps (p.300)—SS with Seated One-Arm Row
One-Arm Row, 2–3 sets and 15 reps––right and left (p.200)

Parallel Squat, 2–3 sets and 20 reps (p.260)—SS with Seated Chest Fly and Standing Biceps Curl
Seated Chest Fly, 2–3 sets and 15 reps (p.240)
Standing Biceps Curl, 2–3 sets and 15 reps (p.156)

Ball Squeeze, 2–3 sets and 15 reps (p.282)—SS with Lying Adduction and Kickbacks
Lying Adduction, 2–3 sets and 25 reps (p.320)
Kickbacks, 2–3 sets and 15 reps (p.216)

Note: Coordinating upper and lower abdominals balances the two foundational aspects stabilizing her spirit self. Super sets alternating from upper to lower body add a cardio element and continue the dual focus for personal and work alignment

Emotional Expression

Focus on the following psyche-muscular contemplations:

Action: Abdominals: Spirit self
Counter-action of Buttock: Iliopsoas: Control
Action: Back: Protection
Action: Quadriceps: Movement forward
Action: Chest: Smile of truth
Action: Biceps: Pulling desirables inward
Action: Hamstrings: Movement backward
Action: Inner thighs: Movement inward
Action: Triceps: Push undesirables away

Note: Direct her contemplation toward what she genuinely wants for herself. In regard to her comfort (buttock exercise), direct her focus on who or what is controlling her wants.

Evolve Your Intention

Your intention is central to your personal transmutation. Your mind-body collaboration is central for environmental transformation. Set your intention, maintain your mind-body connection, and listen to hear the soft voice of spirit throughout your workouts. Bring the aligned, balanced energy you practice in your workout into your world. The reference points for relaxed strength in relationship to an outside resistance in the gym are the same reference points needed to align with and balance other relationships in the world at large. Continue to explore in your practice and apply in your life. Stay curious, and you will be the cultivator of your life's evolution.

Living Change Chapter

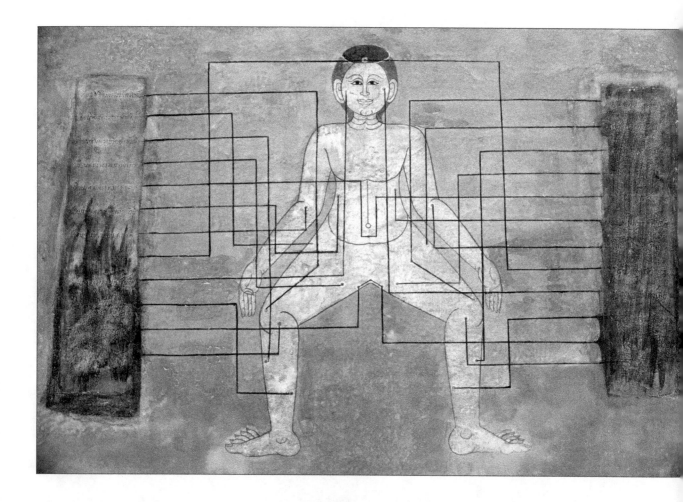

Personal responsibility
Is a choice and a privilege.
The BodyLogos gift
Is an inside look at your inherent beauty,
Beauty that depends on your esteem to be recognized
And comprehended in the world.

Lesson 15
Aligned Living

A good artist lets her intuition
Lead her wherever it wants.
A good scientist has freed himself of concepts
And keeps his mind open to what is.

They are ready to use all situations
And don't waste time.
This is called following the light.

—Lao Tzu, *Tao Te Ching*

Be with the present experience of all that you do.

—Tammy Wise, BodyLogos

When You Align with Spirit, Spirit Aligns with You

BodyLogos's analytic capabilities mirror your response to life back to you. BodyLogos practice offers energy alignment and balance that cuts through the unnerving aspects of your story that have been passed over in the name of survival and transforms the holding patterns that resulted into the liberating experience of personal equipoise. Consciously letting go of the beliefs and judgments that your survival impulses so carefully constructed to feel safe, but are no longer necessary, is the underlying goal of a BodyLogos practice.

Although musculoskeletal opposition offers a foundation for personal balance, personal balance and survival choices cannot coexist. To fully attain the personal balance musculoskeletal opposition yields, survival choices first need to be recognized and reconciled. Acknowledging the time, space, and vitality survival choices have robbed from you gives you the courage to let go of the hardship of survival and embrace your right to thrive. This courage, however, asks you to step back into the original struggle and fully feel what created the survival reaction or belief and make a new choice.

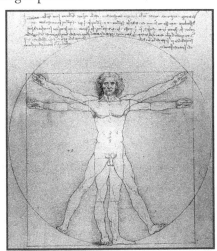

Coming into contact with blocked energy alters your life by transforming the block into awareness. Once we can accept the ways we have been considerate and inconsiderate to ourselves and to others, we can relax with ourselves. We can accept all the world offers as an opportunity for greater connection within ourselves and offer the world greater connection in return.

As you become energetically reorganized, you can disengage from triggers and become a neutral witness to new postures and perspectives. Disengaging from a trigger disengages the muscle carrying the trigger. More often than not, the triggered muscle group is tired of holding on and needs support. The key to creating long-lasting change in your posture lies in balancing the entire energy pattern supporting that disengagement and infusing it with your intention. Then strengthen the secondary muscle groups that may carry the unfamiliar weight of surrendering the trigger. Choose exercises for your workouts that develop these specific muscle groups and nurture the energy shift. As you design your workout meditations, work on developing the specific qualities and beliefs needed to support what you deliberately intend.

The specific relief you are experiencing exposes the neglect you underwent in your past and continue to experience from the past through real-time resistances. As you disentangle yourself from triggers, recognize the personal acceptance that has welled up in you. Aligning with the universe directs your will to change the beliefs that keep triggers intact. Mental and physical freedom is being firmly adopted to accept, without question, being you. In this adoption, you have broken the cycle of neglect in your story. A new chapter with a new story is allowed to unfold because your new real-time beliefs are creating new outcomes. The universe is always responding to the beliefs you carry. To stand in your strength, believe you are strong; to be comfortable being you, believe you are valuable; to be inspired by living, believe you are inspired.

Surviving to Thriving

Your central nervous system cannot distinguish between what is real or imagined. So to quiet mental stress and physical tension, first realize you experience all images as if they were real. If you focus on the image of a past event, you will reexperience the stress and tension of that event again now, even though it's not currently happening. If you focus on negative ideas, real or imagined, you will experience negativity. If you focus on creating equipoise, whether it is precise yet or not, you will experience a quiet mind and relaxed body. The validity of your various experiences can be distinguished, however, if you allow the intuition of spirit to guide you. Feelings are always accompanied by a deep level of knowing—a sense of truth—that is often bypassed. When your mind and body attain equipoise and you develop it into balanced action, you will experience an all-knowing grace. Your spirit self and universal spirit align, and authentic action flows between you and your world. Cultivating discernment between what is imagined and what is real leads to this authentic flow.

Authenticity, validity, and genuineness all require equipoise. Most of us have experienced equipoise in moments of contentment, when a healthy sense of self is attained unconsciously. Newfound consciousness is needed to bring equipoise into an area of discontent. The decision to develop consciousness will change your life, for the development of your future will develop from what you truly are rather than from what you are afraid you might be. And even more notably, you may be surprised by how easy it is to genuinely value yourself.

So what gets in the way of self-acceptance?

All the functions of the mind and spirit are housed in your physical being. It is the mind's technician and the spirit's instrument. You depend on the body as your ambassador to the world. *But when your body's survival instincts fail due to impacted outgrown holding patterns, your mental and emotional states easily sense danger and get derailed.* For your physical body to evolve beyond surviving past threats, it needs the mind's intelligence and the spirit's knowledge. If you were to interpret feeling unsuccessful as a mark of your present limitations, rather than a mark of rejection, you would use the feeling to stretch beyond the limitations without struggle. This nonreactive interpretation of a limitation directs your ever-evolving intention. Do you need to strengthen an area or transfer a challenge to an appropriate place? If you can't pull a window down from your triceps muscles, for example, you could strengthen your triceps or transfer the challenge to your stronger back muscles or call a repairman to fix the window. There is no reason to interpret yourself as unsuccessful.

You are learning truths about yourself and your surroundings. To maintain equilibrium in the face of resistance, you are asked to integrate the strength of all aspects of the body with its isolated muscle groups, the mind with its isolated data points, and the spirit with its unifying wisdom. Unsuccessful feelings simply reveal a new area to explore and expand. And as a result, you find an opening where you can bring about a more meaningful life experience. Becoming successful isn't due to the absence of limits; it's earned through the realization of limits. In the gym, muscle failure is success; in life, realizing limited equilibrium is success.

So how do we develop equilibrium?

It is aligning with who we are rather than who we think we're supposed to be or should be. Where did this fictional should-be archetype come from anyway? Why do we buy into it? It's inauthentic and unreal. We're not copies of one another. We're unique individuals with unique expressions that, when nurtured, bring meaning to that individual's life and cohesiveness to the world. Crisis happens when we don't look inward and start integrating the parts of who we are accurately and sincerely.

Time Is of the Essence

According to Tao concepts, as you mature, your increasing spiritual awareness will inevitably encounter your degenerating physical body. If spiritual and physical energies cross paths in an unbalanced or unsuccessful manner, you experience "crisis," a downward spiral, in which the degeneration of your physical energy is predominantly felt. Alternatively, if you have developed spiritual awareness—you are living life consciously and in accordance with your authentic self—you will experience the abundance of energy held within the spirit body.

The same dynamic happens whether you are at the age of midlife crisis or quarter life crisis, or are facing an arbitrary crisis. Spiritual awareness carries a higher energy vibration than the physical body, so developing it is crucial to your quality of life. Your spirit relies on your mind and body to nurture its existence and bring it forth into the world. Postponing this emergence at any age means letting time slip away.

Visualize your progressive spiritual awareness as following an ascending line that begins opposite the degeneration of the physical body. Then add to this picture a fixed central dividing line, a line that represents wholeness. If the two lines representing the spiritual and physical bodies cross paths above this central line, harmony and growth will follow. If, however, you ignore or avoid your spirit self, your spiritual awareness will be suppressed. Your opposing physical and spiritual energies will cross paths below their central division. When this occurs, the degeneration of the body is self-evident and drags both "lines" downward into a state of sickness, lethargy, and/or depression.

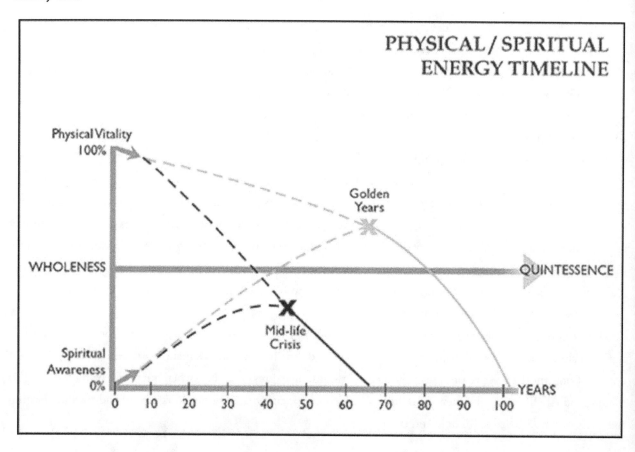

What is more, if these three lines merge, becoming one, you will have attained what the ancient sages referred to as the grace of quintessence—a physical body guided entirely by the spirit, experiencing and acting wholly out of love. Jesus Christ is a popular example of the transmutation of quintessence. It is recorded through history that about two thousand Tao sages have attained quintessence.

Moving through maturity repositions your inner and outer alignment constantly. The energetic balance between mind and body, and the connection between inner and outer spirit, is what constitutes good health. Good health is more than "not being sick." It reflects happiness—the ability to authentically express yourself. Logos—logic—tells you that by design your body is a blueprint of who you've been; your body is also what propels you toward who you're becoming. Being present in your body places you in a convergence point whereby you experience what is essential to create the life you want. "Spiritual fitness" creates a spirited life, a life with meaning, presence, and action.

Relieving Crisis and Conflict

Constant pain in an area tells you that an energy blockage exists. To actively participate in restoring the area, acknowledge that both your "psyche" and "muscular" systems are in this blockage together, and both need attention. An active meditation workout considers the psychological triggers the pain elicits while it gently brings circulation, suppleness, and strength to the affected area. If workouts are too aggressive for your condition, non-action is the remedy. Non-action, however, asks you to stop exercising the area, not to stop engaging energetically with the area. To practice non-action,

- analyze your psyche-muscular condition;
- align your bones and stretch into essential alignment;
- incorporate an energy pattern;
- place the counter-action in the area of hyper-reactivity or the action in the area of hypo-reactivity; and
- maintain equipoise.

Apply this plan to your everyday posture. Pain relief, physical and/or emotional, will be your guide to recognizing when your energy is running properly and will determine which energy pattern best restores the condition. When using the BodyLogos method, start in stillness. You are holding a space for your present condition to express the nature of its blockage and change its stance. Continue to align and run energy for as long as the pain persists. Insights will come, and peaceful moments will build. Active stillness unlocks your body's inherent intelligence. When more support is needed to remedy physical or emotional trauma, use BodyLogos in conjunction with medical attention or other healing modalities.

The following case studies describe what is under the surface of mind-body conflicts. These examples apply BodyLogos techniques for running energy so you learn how to transform physical pain and emotional chaos. Rather than focusing on specific exercises, these examples explore how to run energy for specific conditions. These solutions for correcting alignment and managing energy, with or without strength-training exercises, also reveal what you can expect mind-body change to feel like. This is a general how-to for a conscious relationship with your pain and a caring deliverance from its grip.

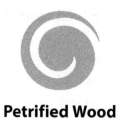

Petrified Wood

Client Description

Petrified Wood is a retired fifty-nine-year-old professor who developed her hobby as a dog trainer and handler into a second career. Her breed in show was standard and toy poodles. With the toy poodles, her challenge was flexibility—the constant need to bend over and reward the dog. Competing with the standard poodles required strength training for hauling crates and gear. As Petrified Wood advanced into agility competitions, her fitness needs intensified. Cardio, coordination, and balance were now mandatory. Petrified Wood was enthusiastic about competing as an agility handler, and she was a disciplined hard worker in her training. It was a stretch athletically, but she was managing. This was the timing of her unfortunate diagnosis of frozen shoulder.

Challenge

The cause of frozen shoulder is uncertain, but the symptoms are limited range of motion, rigidity, and pain. Inflammation occurred in her shoulder to such an extent that simple daily activities were difficult; hence, the demands of agility competitions were agonizing for Petrified Wood. She refused to take a break from competitive life, so we moved carefully into a more rehabilitative training rhythm. Heat preceded exercise, and ice followed in addition to icing one other time during the day and heating before bed. Though her personality was to give to others, she now needed to give to herself—to learn to receive.

Psyche-Muscular Holding Pattern

Shoulders (values) frame one's stance, be it their psychological or physical posture. Frozen shoulders indicate that there are locked-up feelings in regard to one's value or values. It is no wonder that 70 percent of people inflicted with frozen shoulder are around the age of midlife, a crisis time when one's value and values are traditionally questioned. This situation requires tenderness in mind and body, so gentle probing can occur. A daily regimen of moderate stretching and lightweight rehabilitation exercises for the shoulder's range of motion was recommended. Keeping all movements connected to the dan tien energy center was essential to recognize the subtle mind-body nuances that were aggravating the freeze. Coming home energy orbit supports shoulder (value), bicep (pulling desirable inward), and abdominal (spirit self) exercises. Because of their shared energy orbit, Petrified Wood had an unexpected opportunity to learn the ways her shoulders carried burdens that have separated her from her spirit self (abdominals) and have misled her to pulling delusions rather than desirables inward (biceps).

Musculoskeletal Remedy

By extending neutral alignment into essential alignment, Petrified Wood was able to bypass the pain of her shoulders' holding pattern in everyday activity. In her exercise regimen, essential alignment kept her connected to her dan tien energy center and the unknown root of her chronic condition. As she related to the pain of her limitations using the coming home energy pattern, she began to experience herself in the reality of the present moment rather than the want-to-be stance of her determination. Valuing her internal center over her limited external range of motion repositioned her viewpoint to value her needs and desires over the judgments and expectations of her prior self. This was a radical change from a lifetime of letting the needs of her supervisors and students as well as competition judges and dogs supersede her own.

Spiritual Fitness

Recognizing the ways she abandoned herself for the love and acceptance of others unraveled a slew of emotions, emotions locked in her heart center and narrowing her shoulders—punishing her sense of value. Punishing emotions she previously mistook as her hard-driving determination to succeed were revised. She now recognized her abandonment of self as her determination to hide behind the needs of others. As her heart opened inwardly, her shoulders opened outwardly. Being kind to others no longer meant sacrificing herself.

Flourished by Fire

Client Description

Flourished by Fire, a concert pianist with arthritis in both hands, broke her wrist one year ago. She learned that she had the beginnings of osteoporosis. She was advised to start strength training to increase bone density and improve her diagnoses, yet she couldn't hold anything in her hands, since doing so would exacerbate the curled-in nature of her wrist or hand condition.

Challenge

An inward softening of Flourished by Fire's bones was accompanying an outward stiffening in mobility. Weakness was uncomfortably evident in her day-to-day activities, while tension intruded on her piano-playing demands. The physical curling inward had followed her long-standing emotional curling inward—a conscious protective mechanism that protected her through her upbringing. But it unconsciously continued though she was no longer in an abusive situation. She wanted to reverse this degenerative pattern.

Psyche-Muscular Holding Pattern

Problems that affect superficial areas, such as the hands and feet, are indicators that life challenges are being superficially handled. Superficial responses to life challenges are characteristic in traumatized children. Flourished by Fire's soft bones indicated that essential alignment was unable to reach outwardly due to postural limitations. And her stiff hands indicated that the aggression of outside resistances was greater than her ability to manage. An abusive childhood established a pattern of withdrawal into her energy body, using it as a protective cave. From this vantage point, Flourished by Fire could feel a sense of safety dodging the onslaught of outside aggression. That cave turned into a protective shelter that forbids her freedom of movement today.

Musculoskeletal Remedy

Flourished by Fire employed the skeletal alignment and energy extension of essential alignment. This newfound central plumb line gave her a renewed outlook on life. In addition to experiencing an energy boost, she gained a reference point to step out of her habitual reaction to hide and experienced emotional connection. The constant outward stretch of essential alignment, challenged by the force of gravity, proved to be bone building, and she simultaneously released the compressed tension she was experiencing. Once essential alignment was mastered, Flourished by Fire began practicing coming home, universal connection, and creating forward energy patterns in her everyday posture. The counter-active energy force of these two patterns could flow outwardly through the backs of her hands and wrists.

As Flourished by Fire maintained musculoskeletal opposition through everyday activities, she began transforming the holding patterns that curled her inward. When she continued to use these energy patterns through her rehab exercises, her mind and body came out of the protective cave. Slowly, her hands began to relax more and react less. Once ready for strength training, Flourished by Fire used wrist weights to keep her hands and wrists relaxed for the outward unleashing of tension through each exercise's counter-action. She started strength training in the muscle groups from the above-mentioned energy patterns, working buttocks, calves, inner thighs, chest, and quadriceps. In time, she was able to introduce all muscle groups.

Spiritual Fitness

By connecting her dan tien with gravity, Flourished by Fire experienced her spirit self aligning with universal spirit, giving her a sense of belonging in her own life. Her present thoughts and feelings as well as triumphs and limitations became a self-realizing tapestry that replaced the unresolved past experiences. "You'll never amount to anything" was replaced with the realization that "I am a recognized and successful musician and woman." She transformed her sense of self by using the restorative properties of running energy. And through active meditation, she gained greater and greater trust in connecting outwardly by relating to the insights experienced inwardly.

Family Terrain

Client Description

Family Terrain is one of two daughters overseeing an aging mother facing open-heart surgery. It was decided that Mom would permanently move in with Family Terrain's more local, older sister after the hospitalized rehabilitation. Family Terrain had six weeks to select the most treasured valuables from her mom's home and downsize her living quarters from an entire house to a single room. Family Terrain's sister, frustrated by Family Terrain's inconvenient geographical distance from family situations, left Family Terrain alone in the task and objected to every idea Family Terrain had. What could have been a uniting time for the siblings was instead divisive. Family Terrain was alone and lonely.

Challenge

The decisions Family Terrain made would frame the rest of her mom's life, so a certain degree of fret accompanied all her choices. She was unnerved and guilt ridden by the state of her mother's house and wounded by a lack of appreciation coming from her sister and brother-in-law, no matter how much she worked to stabilize the family's crisis. For four months Family Terrain traveled six hours and worked her entire weekend to support the family crisis. At the end of her mom's transition, Family Terrain felt like a slave to, rather than a member of, her family. She returned to her regular life, feeling sad, taken for granted, and angry. She had a constant pain in her neck.

Psyche-Muscular Holding Pattern

The pain in Family Terrain's neck was a bone pain in thoracic vertebrae one and two. It had no range-of-movement limitation but rather a pain when touched and when she carried anything heavy. The location of her pain pointed to a stagnation of energy in the upper back and shoulder muscles, which characterizes a psyche-muscular reaction Family Terrain knew too well—protecting (back) her value (shoulders). After all, these same people had raised her in the same disparaging manner she was facing now. Being surrounded by the same disregard amid every effort to be loved and valued brought Family Terrain face-to-face with a long-standing childhood holding pattern. This was an opportunity for Family Terrain to recognize her overprotective posture and surrender the habit to guard her heart and defend her value.

Musculoskeletal Remedy

Family Terrain's essential alignment needed to stretch beyond her energy body to detach from this long-standing holding pattern. Once essential alignment was connected to earth and sky, Family Terrain's reaction to protect and defend herself could be transformed into loving and appreciating herself without the habitual fear of being wronged. To support the traumatized area in Family Terrain's neck and upper back, she temporarily abstained from strength training and practiced creating forward energy pattern in her everyday posture. Energy cycled up through her chest, opening her heart and down through the back without any muscular contraction. She released the pain in her neck and upper back downwardly through the counter-action by lifting the chest upwardly through the action.

Releasing physical and emotional pain with a counter-force that lifted Family Terrain's chest and heart supported her need to right herself and shifted her posture into a restorative placement. This rebalancing of Family Terrain's posture relieved the neck and upper back's reactivity and brought awareness to the holding pattern's trigger. In other words, *I need to protect myself when I'm not seen*. Once the pain subsided, Family Terrain introduced chest exercises using a counter-active meditation—to release hyper-reactive tendencies and free her smile of truth. *I need to love myself when I am not seen*. When totally pain free, she was able to reintroduce back exercises and train for balance between back and chest strength.

Spiritual Fitness

Temporarily abstaining from strength training and instead adjusting her day-to-day posture, Family Terrain began to recognize the treatment from her loved ones, both in the past and present, as a reflection of them rather than a judgment of her. The chest meditations developed in her a greater capacity to love because she stopped trying to be loved. When reintroducing back exercises into her workout, she found her approach had shifted. She remembered being aggressive toward outside resistance when doing back exercises; now she felt tenderness toward developing her heart's expansion.

Tammy Wise

Nerves of Steel

Client Description

Nerves of Steel was attending university abroad in the USA and met a fellow who was also living away from his homeland. They fell in love. University life was ending for Nerves of Steel, and she needed a job that would sponsor her to work in the USA and be permitted to stay stateside. Graduation came and went, as did job placements that would launch her into an academic career path. At the last minute, the school from which she'd graduated offered a short-term position. With this position, she had one year to understand the potential of her international love relationship and her career's future in the USA. She felt bewildered by the pressures of love and vocation, and uncertain about where to call home. Would Nerves of Steel and her man be separated due to citizenship or career paths?

Challenge

Exhaustion, tightness below her shoulder blades, and rigidity in her hip flexors (iliopsoas) kept Nerves of Steel in a state of physical and emotional irritation. She wanted more certainty about her future, both personally and professionally, so she could move into the next chapter of her life. She was tired of living in dorms and being short of cash. Unable to take nonacademic jobs due to visa restrictions—and uncomfortable making any promises to her man that could prove impossible to keep—Nerves of Steel feigned a free-flowing attitude. But underneath this calm-mannered exterior was tremendous trepidation and insecurity.

Psyche-Muscular Holding Pattern

Tightness around the shoulder blades indicated the need to protect her heart from collapse. An over-pinching of the shoulder blades forced her chest up (smile of truth) and heart center forward, and it elevated her upper abdominals (sense of self). This forced elevation matched the enforced need to be quickly recognized as exceptional in her vocation. An overactive effort was being imposed, be it conscious or unconscious, to feel hope and happiness; rather than hope and happiness being the effortless result of Nerves of Steel's energetic alignment. This overactive effort exhausted her energy, leaving her in a state of physical and emotional depletion. Add her hip-flexor rigidity (control) to the mix, and the controlled focus of being in graduate school quickly turned to out-of-control frenzy. Focus was replaced by the fret of losing all she'd worked for professionally and personally.

Musculoskeletal Remedy

Nerves of Steel needed to find more space in her skeletal alignment and more reliance in her muscular stability. She was using her core-alignment muscles (abdominals, back, chest) as her core-stability muscles (abdominals, inner thighs, buttocks), placing her muscular foundation above her center of gravity. This is like building a house on cinder blocks aboveground. A powerful storm will eventually overpower it. Nerves of Steel needed to trust and depend on her core-stability muscles in her everyday posture and workouts so her core-alignment muscles would be free to manage her alignment's intention.

With this adjustment, her essential alignment was able to stretch outside of her energy body. She learned to use less effort and more release. In this way, energy orbits could become more effective in restoring her energy and setting up the environment for active meditations. Once essential alignment connected to earth and sky consistently, she added the universal connection energy pattern to her everyday posture and workout. This brought greater strength and awareness to her buttock and inner-thigh muscles, connecting her to the security of her center through the united power of her core stability muscles. With buttocks and inner thighs strengthened, she was then able to incrementally surrender the controlling grip of her iliopsoas muscles. This psyche-muscular restructuring balanced her need to control (iliopsoas) and replaced it with inner comfort (inner thighs and buttocks).

Spiritual Fitness

Nerves of Steel felt more confident as her essential alignment extended beyond her energy body. What she needed for her spirit self became more and more evident and important. As she awakened her buttocks and inner thighs into action, she started making decisions about her future, both in regard to and not in regard to her fellow. She was now connected to her needs rather than the needs of him or her career. In workouts, she needed less weight to be challenged—a sign that she was feeling—and her hip flexors' discomfort became a measurement of how reactive she was being from one moment to the next. She felt an emanating truth permeating her movements and her life choices.

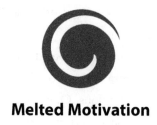

Melted Motivation

Client Description

The dread starts with a pinch in the lower back, sometimes right side and sometimes left side; then it progresses into a searing pain that radiates down the back of Melted Motivation's legs. He compares it to a toothache that, in addition to pain, carries a fragility that feels like he could break with each impending step. Any wrong move could lead to him being left behind socially or professionally in a crippled state. This recurring event renders Melted Motivation helpless, making him wary of the life pressures that are the precursors to these events.

Challenge

This feeling of helplessness deeply affected gregarious Melted Motivation's sense of self. Motivation to take on greater challenges at work, confidence in personal relationships, and exploring new experiences had been replaced with isolation, solo ventures, and a deep need to control his environment. His posture expressed a man getting punched in the gut. Melted Motivation wanted his zest for life back.

Psyche-Muscular Holding Pattern

The inward compression at Melted Motivation's abdominal center (spirit self) indicated a constant concern about losing himself. The pain in his lower back (fear) and collapse of his upper back (protection) indicated that he was also concerned about living up to the pressures of the outside world. These concerns steered Melted Motivation's energy inward, away from the outward reach of essential alignment, challenging his ability to see beyond his present perceptions. This situation paralyzed him in a sense of loss, and he feared anything that made demands on him and protected what little esteem was still intact.

Musculoskeletal Remedy

Establishing neutral alignment was the foremost concern. Melted Motivation's vertical and horizontal posture needed complete restructuring. Shifting his body's center of gravity forward, out of the lower back, he stretched his central plumb line out from his abdominals and unfurled the gut-punched appearance. Rather than him feeling trapped by his lower back (fear), his newfound skeletal position unleashed energy from his dan tien energy center (sense of self). By applying the creating forward energy pattern in stillness, Melted Motivation directed its counter-action down the posterior body. Releasing tension through the heel stirrups, his shoulder blades dropped, and lower-back dimples opened. Without deliberately contracting active muscles, the upward direction of energy through his anterior body connected the dan tien energy center to his heart center.

Once he could maintain neutral alignment and the energy pattern restored muscular balance, Melted Motivation stretched beyond the energy body into essential alignment. Immediate relief from fear and uncertainty followed, while the long-standing holding pattern in his lower back continued to gradually ease by working with creating forward energy pattern. When he was ready to work out, Melted Motivation used the creating forward energy pattern exercises to build a stronger connection between his spirit self (abdominals) and heart center (chest). His lower back was now able to surrender its habitual pain-filled grip, and his energy-filled abdominal support stepped up. As this happened, he was freed to reclaim his zest for life and soon returned to a full workout.

Spiritual Fitness

Melted Motivation's reactivity to stress was the root of his crippling back pain and low self-esteem. The experiences that created his hypo-reactive posture were long gone, but daily triggers kept them engaged. As his back (protection), lower back (fear), and hamstrings (movement backward) relaxed, his chest (smile of truth) and quadriceps (movement forward) awakened. He restored his connection with life by taking greater personal responsibility. Through his active meditations, insights influenced Melted Motivation's mind-body experience daily, reinforcing his connection with life and people. Melted Motivation was soon exploring new things both inwardly and outwardly.

The Will to Align

Lao Tzu said, "Give attention to the smallest things to simplify the complicated." We have a cultural tendency to slough off the small things in pursuit of grandeur. In our constant agitation to beat the clock, we subscribe to the narrative that there simply isn't time for the small things—that they are a luxury. But your life is the sum of your smallest choices: how you stand on your feet, where your shoulder blades rest. These subtleties generate the tension in your body, place you in poor posture, and ultimately place you in a life you don't want, because how we choose to act in the smallest things is how we train ourselves to react in the biggest moments.

We use up all our energy fighting the resistance from jobs we hate, lives that don't fit, and labels that stunt our growth. We drown underneath mental fog, anxiety, and exhaustion until it morphs into crippling pain—and zaps all our energy for anything else. This, at its core, is misalignment. By denying yourself permission to attend to the smallest details of your posture—to listen to your body's wisdom and treat it with compassion—you reinforce the message that pain is acceptable. You unconsciously become more familiar with tension than you are with ease or strength. Most importantly, you submit to the confining belief that you are defined by what happens to you, thus surrendering your agency and identity.

Your life doesn't have to be defined by your pain. Your blocks, your pains and tensions, your insecurities and faults aren't inherent to who you are—and it's possible to remove them. We've adopted them because of our life story, but they don't define us. They can be released and reforged in positive pathways.

The will to align is the courage to stand up for yourself and live boldly. It is the confidence to make choices and craft a life simply because it contributes to a soundness of body, mind, and spirit—and not because it adheres to an external pressure to do or be anything else. It is the will to invest in your highest good and self even—and especially—in the minutiae. It means building on what is meaningful, not what is guaranteed. The will to align abandons the need to build strength and instead excavates it from our core selves and adapts it to meet life's challenges.

Committing to the BodyLogos lifestyle and stepping outside your tension leaves you vulnerable to the possibility that you might be wrong. They allow the possibility that your patterns might need correcting. My gift to you through BodyLogos is a system that takes the shame out of correction. It replaces judgment with compassion and neglect with curiosity. It allows you to master improvement in the subtleties with ease so you can align with your highest good. Then when life does its absolute worst, it may cause pain, but it cannot cripple your soul for good.

You were born to be a creator. You are constantly creating your life in each small moment, every tiny decision. BodyLogos is the conscious practice of that creativity in our bodies and lives. When you summon the will to align, you shed your anonymity and claim your life as your own masterwork.

Venture Forth

As you embark on the BodyLogos practice, use all you have learned in these pages to influence your posture, workout, and life. What you do in one of these life applications affects what you do in all applications. You are venturing into a holistic strength-training practice built on the sensitivity of subtle energy rather than the competitiveness of brute force. You are being asked to approach the experience of strength from the inner origins of your deepest vulnerability and desires. To stand in your strength is to have the courage to stand in your frailty. This courage is based in curiosity, not fearlessness. It is the search for the actual experience of "standing in strength" as opposed to chasing that experience.

We are born out of a dark, wet, and insulated place. We can experience this vivid description as dreary, familiar, or liberating. Deliberate change in our consciousness is a rebirth that asks us to come into contact with a raw environment that can feel disorienting and vulnerable, but it is at this juncture that we choose our experience. And the choice directs the quality and evolution of our lives.

What do you need to choose to create the life you want?

>Physical alignment sustains your creative life force for a long life.
>Mental alignment restores your creative life force for a happy life.
>Mind-body alignment coordinates your creative life force
>For a meaningful life.

—Tammy Wise, BodyLogos

Index

A

Abdominal Breathing Exercise	113
Alignment Stabilizers [graphic]	42

B

Ball Squeeze	282
Body Planes [graphic]	36
Breathing Exercise [video]	14

C

Calf Raise	338
Calf Raise Turned Out	340
Centripetal of Centrifugal Force Exercise [video]	71
Chin-Up	202
Coming Home Energy Pattern [graphic]	107
Coming Home––Seated Lap Lay and Active Meditation [video]	108
Connection Point Exercise [video]	99
Creating Forward Energy Pattern [graphic]	227
Creating Forward––T-Shirt Strip and Active Meditation [video]	228
Crucifixion Curl	160

D

Dead Cow	59
Dead Lift	302
Determined Power Energy Pattern [graphic]	187
Determined Power––Standing Ponder and Active Meditation [video]	188
Door Breaker	169
Dyna-Band Circle Stretch	234

E

Experience Active Meditation [guided]	102
Experience Alignment Stabilizers [video]	44
Experience Equipoise Exercise [video]	67
Experience Essential Alignment [video]	49

Experience Neutral Alignment [video]	39
Experience the Bone [video]	46
Extended Upper Abdominal Crunch	128

F

Five Forms of Expression [description]	12
Flat-Footed Calf Raise	331
Forward Body Rock	295

H

Hollow Thigh Hug Stretch	193
Hydrant Hamstring Curl	278
Hyperextended Calf Raise	334
Hyperextended Oblique Crunch	142
Hyperextension	300

I

Iliopsoas Seated Knee lift	296
Isolated Muscle Opposition [graphic]	94

K

Kickback	216
Kneeling Butt Tuck Stretch	297

L

Lat Pull Down	196
Leg Extension	256
Leg Press	258
Lower Abdominal Crunch	116
Lower Abdominal Leg Extension	120
Lower Abdominal Six-Inch Raise	122
Lower Abdominal Touchdown	118
Lying Adduction	320
Lying Chest Press	236
Lying Leg Extension	251
Lying Overhead Triceps Extension	214

M

Meditation to Defuse Reactivity [guided]	353
Meditation to Establish Intention [guided]	373

N

Neutral Alignment [graphic]	38
Neutral Witness [video]	19

O

Oblique Crunch	140
Oblique Crunch with Lower Torso Twist	138
One-Arm Row	200
One-Arm Triceps Push Down	220
Overhead Shoulder Blade Touch Down Stretch	211

P

Parallel Squat	260
Physical/Spiritual Energy Timeline [graphic]	392
Prayer Position	58
Praying Hands	233
Prone Ball Lie	62
Prone Knee Bend with Tube	273
Prone Straight-Leg Lie	61
Psyche-Muscular Blueprint [graphic]	10

S

Seated Abduction	304
Seated Adduction	318
Seated Biceps Curl with Hammerhead Grip	154
Seated Biceps Curl with Outward Rotation	158
Seated Chest Fly	240
Seated Chest Press	238
Seated Combo Crunch	134
Seated Heel Kiss	315
Seated Leg Curl	276
Seated Overhead Press	178
Seated Row	198
Seated Straight-Leg Raise	254
Shoulder Blade Grab	193
Shoulder Blade Hug	170
Single-Leg Hamstring Stretch with Flexed Foot	274
Stair Heel Drop Stretch	332
Standing Anterior Lateral Raise	174
Standing Biceps Curl	156
Standing Chest Fly	242

Standing Foothold Stretch	252
Standing Hamstring Curl	280
Standing Overhead Press	180
Standing Overhead Triceps Extension	218
Standing Posterior Lateral Raise	176
Standing Side Lateral Raise	172
Standing Straight-Leg Adduction	322
Sumo Squat	306
Supine Ball Abdominal Stretch	113
Supine Buttock Release Stretch	296
Supine Elbow Bend with Flexed Wrist	151
Supine Elbow Lift with Pressed Fingertips	211
Supine Frog Stretch	316
Supine Lie	61
Supine Tube Lie	62
Suspending Judgment Energy Pattern [graphic]	267
Suspending Judgment––Standing Prayer and Active Meditation [video]	268
Swan Dive with Flexed Wrist	152

T

Tao Eagle Active Meditation [video]	6
Trilogy of the Self [guided]	21

U

Universal Connection Energy Pattern [graphic]	289
Universal Connection––Standing Corkscrew and Active Meditation [video]	290
Upper Abdominal Crunch	126
Upper Abdominal Crunch with 90-Degree Leg Raise	132
Upper Abdominal Crunch with Crossed Legs	130

W

Weighted Hyperextended Calf Raise	336
Wrist Roll	57